Pulmonary Circulation in Health and Disease

ETTORE MAJORANA INTERNATIONAL SCIENCE SERIES

Series Editor:
Antonino Zichichi
European Physical Society
Geneva, Switzerland

(LIFE SCIENCES)

Volume 1   BLADDER TUMORS AND OTHER TOPICS IN UROLOGICAL
ONCOLOGY
Edited by M. Pavone-Macaluso, P. H. Smith, and F. Edsmyr

Volume 2   ADVANCES IN RADIATION PROTECTION AND DOSIMETRY
IN MEDICINE
Edited by Ralph H. Thomas and Victor Perez-Mendez

Volume 3   PULMONARY CIRCULATION IN HEALTH AND DISEASE
Edited by G. Cumming and G. Bonsignore

Pulmonary Circulation in Health and Disease

Edited by

G. Cumming

The Midhurst Medical Research Institute
Midhurst, Sussex, United Kingdom

and

G. Bonsignore

University of Palermo
Palermo, Italy

Springer Science+Business Media, LLC

Library of Congress Cataloging in Publication Data

Main entry under title:

Pulmonary circulation in health and disease.

(Ettore Majorana international science series: Life sciences; v. 3)
"Proceedings of a symposium on the pulmonary circulation held July 16—21, 1979,
at the Ettore Majorana Center for Scientific Culture, Erice, Sicily, Italy."
Includes index.
1. Pulmonary circulation—Congresses. 2. Lungs—Diseases—Congresses. I. Cumming, Gordon. II. Bonsignore, G. III. Series. [DNLM: 1. Pulmonary circulation—Congresses. 2. Lung diseases—Physiopathology—Congresses. W1 ET712M v. 3 / WF600 P9823 1979]

QP107.P85	612'.2	80-20154

ISBN 978-1-4757-1723-5   ISBN 978-1-4757-1721-1 (eBook)
DOI 10.1007/978-1-4757-1721-1

Proceedings of the Symposium on the Pulmonary Circulation, held at the Ettore Majorana Center for Scientific Culture, Erice, Sicily, Italy, July 16—21, 1979.

FOREWORD

        This volume documents the proceedings of a symposium on "The
Pulmonary Circulation" held at the Ettore Majorana Center for
Scientific Culture, in Erice, Sicily, between 16th July and 21st
July 1979. This was attended by about 200 participants drawn from
Europe as a whole, but the majority were from Southern Europe.

        The discussion was recorded either in English or Italian and
the tapes were reduced to a verbatim typescript by the Ente
Nazionale Interpeti Congresso. The verbatim typescript has been
edited using a few guiding principles as follows:

1.   Titles and honorifics have been eliminated unless the
        statement is addressed to a specific person.

2.   The style of the speakers in the discussion has been
        preserved as far as possible and not reduced to a strictly
        grammatical format.

3.   Where references to illustrations (e.g., on the blackboard)
        are made, the comments have been left unaltered and many
        are understandable. Removing them detracted from the
        sense.

4.   The air of informality in the proceedings has been
        preserved so far as possible.

5.   The responsibility for the discussion rests solely with
        the editors, and no contributor has had the opportunity of
        correcting what he said.

6.   No manuscript was received from one participant, but the
        discussion of his presentation has been included since it
        contains some points of substance.

                                    G. Cumming and G. Bonsignore

CONTENTS

CONTENTS

FUNCTIONAL MORPHOLOGY OF THE PULMONARY CIRCULATION

Keith Horsfield

Midhurst Medical Research Institute
Midhurst
West Sussex

GENERAL ARRANGEMENT

The main bronchus enters the lung hilum, and by a series of
dichotomous divisions, gives rise to about 25,000 terminal bronchioles,
each of which supplies an acinus. At each division the diameters
of the bronchi decrease, but at a rate which is less than the
increase in numbers, so that the summed cross-sectional area at
any given level increases down the tree (Fig 1). Within the acinus
dichotomous division continues down to and including the first
generation of alveolar ducts, but thereafter branching is more
profuse and irregular. Reduction of diameter at each division is,
however, less (Fig 2) so that there is a very rapid increase in
summed cross-sectional area with respect to distance down the acinus.

The pulmonary artery branches in similar fashion to the
bronchial tree (Fig 3) and follows it closely, although near the
hilum the two branching patterns differ slightly. Within the acinus
the pulmonary artery is applied to the respiratory bronchioles
along their non-alveolated sides, and finally gives rise to branches
which course over the alveoli arising from alveolar ducts. As in the
bronchial tree, branches decrease in diameter at each dichotomy,
and this decrease continues all the way along the acinus to the
alveolar capillaries (Fig 4) while the summed cross-sectional area
increases. Although the two trees are similar, the arteries branch
more profusely, especially peripherally, where they give off
branches to supply alveoli on respiratory bronchioles and immediately
adjacent alveoli of neighbouring acini (Fig 5).

The pulmonary veins arise from capillaries at duct junctions, on
respiratory bronchioles, on the pleura, and in septae, those starting

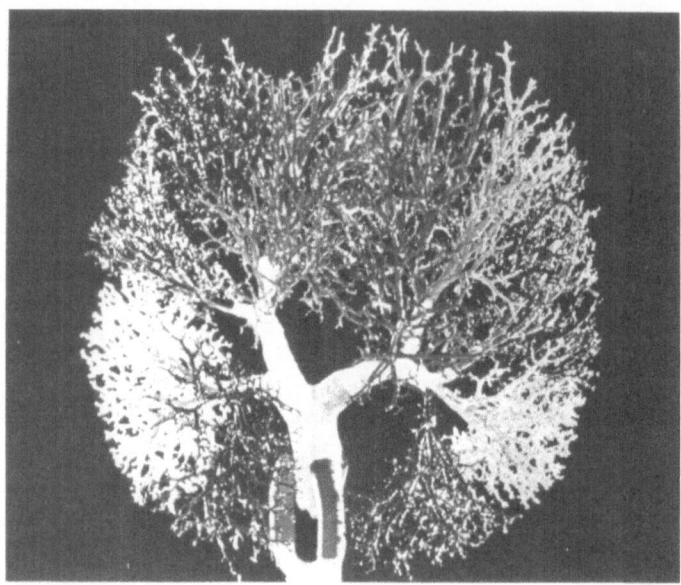

Fig. 1   Cast of the human bronchial tree showing dichotomous
          branching, and decrease in diameter peripherally with
          rapidly increasing numbers of branches.

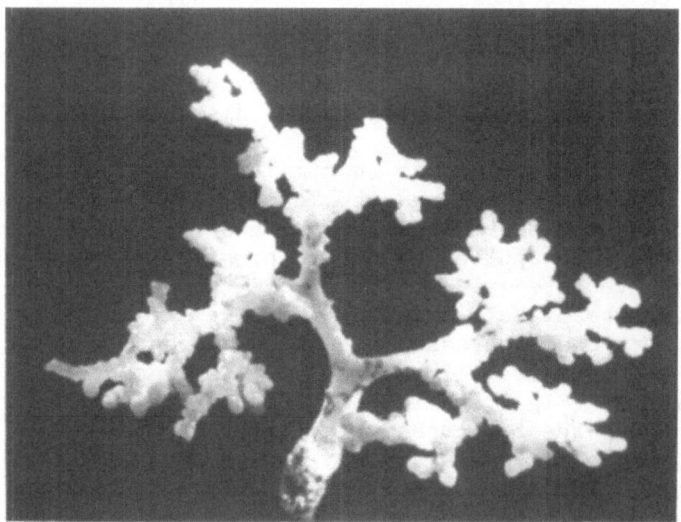

Fig. 2   Cast of the airways of an acinus, showing terminal
          bronchiole (no alveoli), respiratory bronchioles (few
          alveoli), and alveolar ducts surrounded by alveoli.

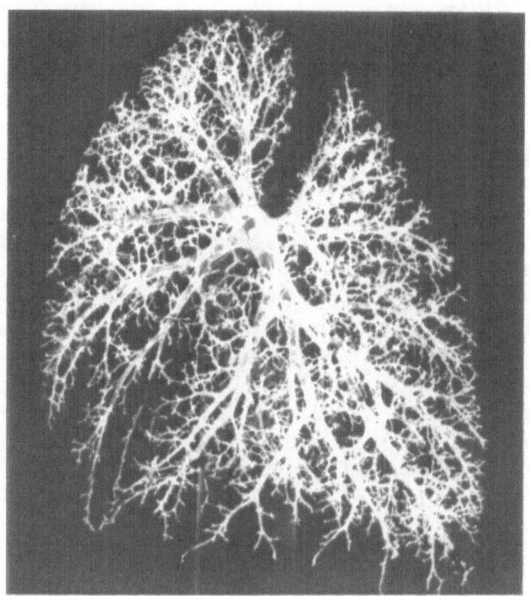

Fig. 3.   Cast of the human pulmonary arterial tree (lateral view),
           showing features similar to the bronchial tree in Figure
           1. (From Cumming and Semple, 1973, Disorders of the
           Respiratory System, Blackwell Scientific Publications,
           London).

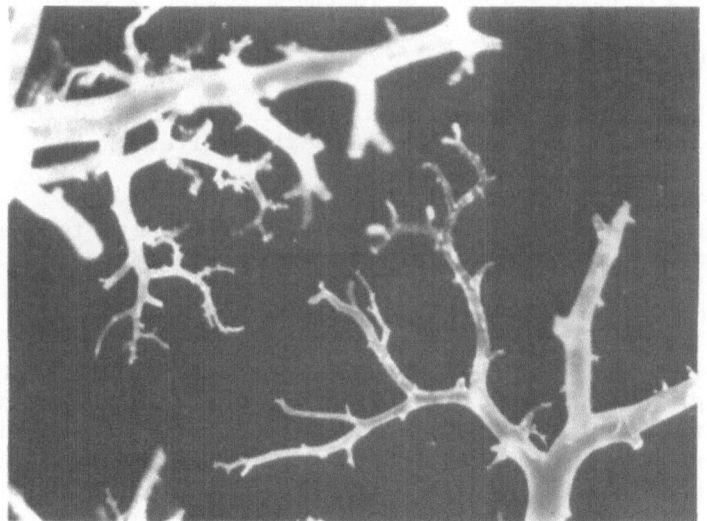

Fig. 4.   Cast of the pulmonary arteries supplying an acinus.

within the acinus coursing centrifugally to the periphery of the
lobule. There they join veins running between the lobules, situated
away from the airways (Fig. 6). Veins, arteries, and the airways
only come together as they approach the hilum. The general
arrangement of the pulmonary vessels is shown in Fig. 7.

Functional Consequences

It has been shown that blood may become oxygenated in small
arteries, oxygen diffusing across the vessel wall direct from the
contiguous airways and alveoli. This direct access which gas in the
airways has to small arteries makes possible a very rapid and
localised vascular response to changes in gas composition. Thus a
low PO_2 and raised PCO_2 in the airways due to regional
hypoventilation can produce localised vasoconstriction and a
balancing up of the local Va/Q ratio. Conversely the possibility
exists that chemical or humoral substances, carried in the pulmonary
arterial blood or produced in the vessel wall, can reach the
adjoining bronchus directly and cause localised bronchoconstriction.

THE ARTERIES

Both bronchi and arteries run within the lung in a connective
tissue sheath, arising at the hilum as an invagination of the pleura
and ending at the bronchioles (Fig. 8). Distally both arteries and
bronchi are attached directly to the lung substance. A potential
space exists between the artery and its sheath, in much the same way
as the potential pleural space lies between the two layers of the
pleura. Valved lymphatics also run in the sheath.

Mechanical Consequences

Lymphatics in the periarterial sheath are exposed to arterial
pulsation which, in conjunction with the valves, helps to propel
lymph towards the hilum.

Because the lung is elastic, and when in situ in the closed
chest is partly expanded, retractile forces are set up by the lung
tissues which act in all directions. With respect to the arteries,
however, they can be considered as acting radially and
longitudinally. Distally, the arteries attached to the lung tissues
are subject to a longitudinal pull which is transmitted along the
arterial tree to structures in the mediastinum. The tissues
surrounding the perivascular sheath exert a radial traction on it,
and this force is normally transmitted across the potential
perivascular space to the bronchi and arteries, tending to hold them
open and increase their diameters. In the presence of pulmonary
oedema, fluid accumulates in the perivascular space thereby

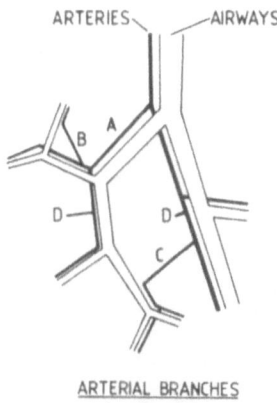

Fig. 5. Diagram of the branching of the pulmonary arteries showing how they differ from their parallel airways (After Reid, 1968).

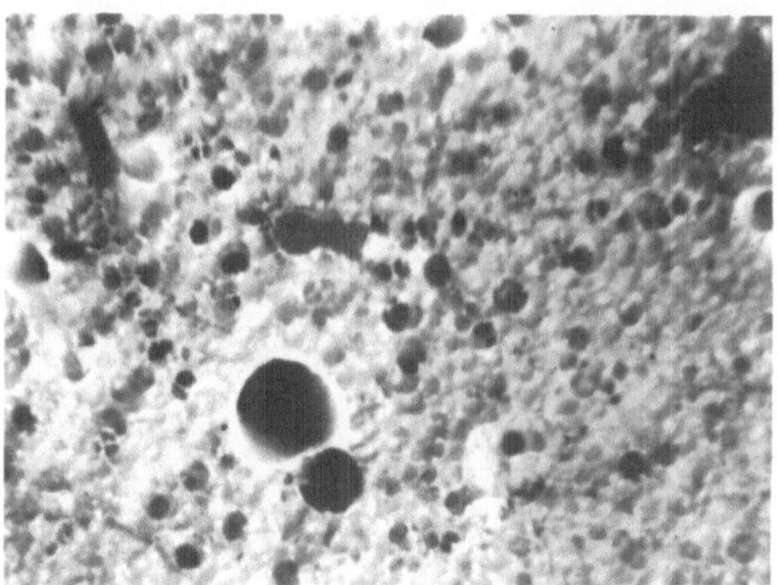

Fig. 6 Frozen section of lung showing bronchus with accompanying artery in left lower quadrant, and separate vein, left of centre (From N. C. Staub).

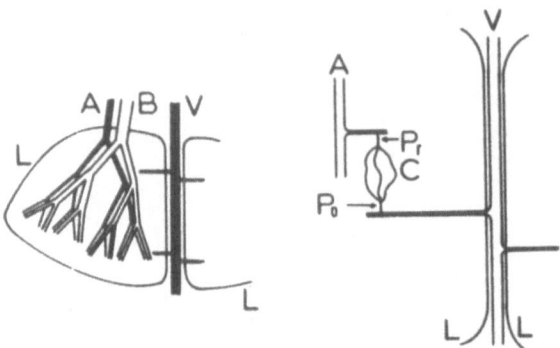

Fig. 7   Diagram of the general arrangement of the pulmonary
          vessels: A - artery; B - bronchus; C - capillaries; L -
          lobule; Po - post-capillary vessel; Pr - Precapillary
          vessel, V - vein.

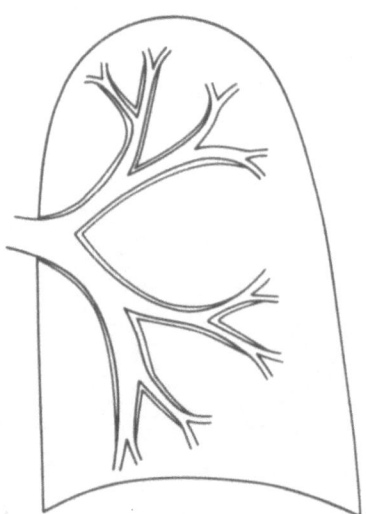

Fig. 8   Diagram of the peri-vascular and peribronchial space.
          (From British Journal of Disease of the Chest, 68, 145,
          1974).

partially isolating the artery from the radial traction (Fig. 9). The diameter of the artery will thus decrease, with a consequent rise in vascular resistance at that site. Because the arterial tree is elastic and filled with fluid under pressure, it physically supports the lung to maintain its shape.

MORPHOMETRY OF THE ARTERIES

In order to express the morphometry of the arterial tree quantitatively it is necessary to have some method of classifying or grouping together branches of a similar kind. Asymmetrical trees can usefully be classified by the method of ordering described by Strahler (Horsfield and Cumming, 1976). In this technique peripheral branches are order 1, two order 1 branches meet to form an order 2 branch, two order 2 branches meet to form an order 3 branch, and so on up the tree. Where branches of different order meet, the next branch continues with the same order as the higher ordered meeting branch. Finally, contiguous branches of the same order are taken together to represent just one branch of the order (Fig. 10). In vascular trees order 1 branches can be difficult to define, as can be seen from Fig. 11 which shows various modes of origin of the capillary nets. When, for practical purposes, arteries of 10 to 15 um diameter are defined as order 1 branches, the human pulmonary arterial tree is found to have 17 orders (Horsfield, 1978). The number of branches in successive orders up the tree decreases logarithmically, and the mean diameter and mean length increase logarithmically, as shown in Fig. 12. These data can be used to calculate haemodynamic variables, given suitable equations.

Functional Consequences

The design of the pulmonary arterial tree is appropriate for a distribution system. Proximally, the wider and longer higher-ordered vessels have a low resistance, as can be shown at cardiac catheterisation by the fall in pressure along them. This permits distribution of the blood at low energy cost. Distally, the short and narrow vessels capable of increasing their resistance by vasoconstriction, are ideally placed for local regulation of flow. It can be shown that if the fall in pressure is equal in each order of the tree, then entropy production is minimised (Horsfield, 1977). This concept of entropy is based on a statistical approach, that the energy in the system has the most probable distribution. No data are available to test the hypothesis that the pulmonary arterial tree is designed in this way, except that most of the fall in pressure is known to be peripheral. This observation is compatible with an equal pressure drop in each order, as shown in Fig. 13.

It is interesting to note that the pulmonary arterial pressure is similar in a wide variety of mammals, from the mouse to the elephant, although the reasons for this are not clearly understood.

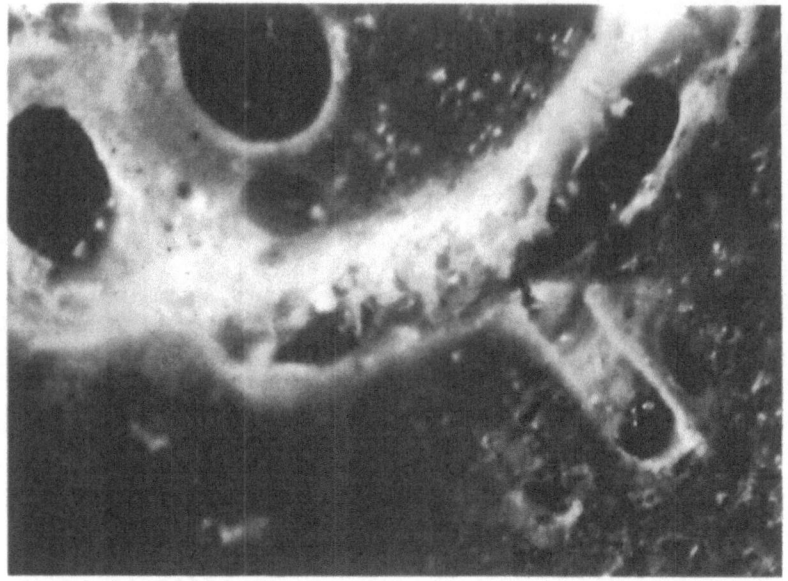

Fig. 9   Frozen section of the lung showing fluid in the
            peribronchial and perivascular space (From N.C. Staub.)

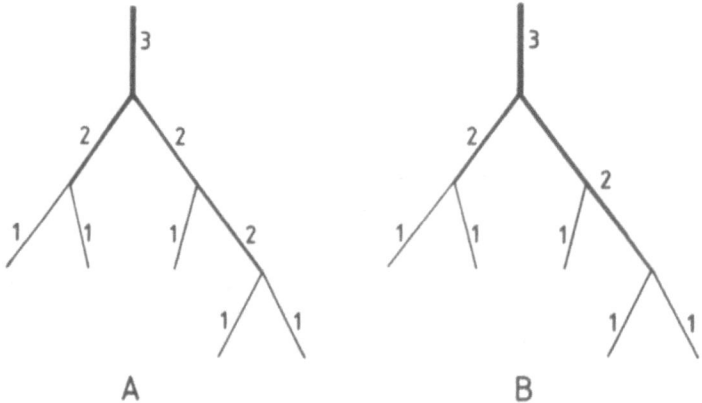

Fig.10   Strahler ordering and asymmetrical tree. A, stage one; B,
            stage two in which contiguous branches of the same order
            become one branch.

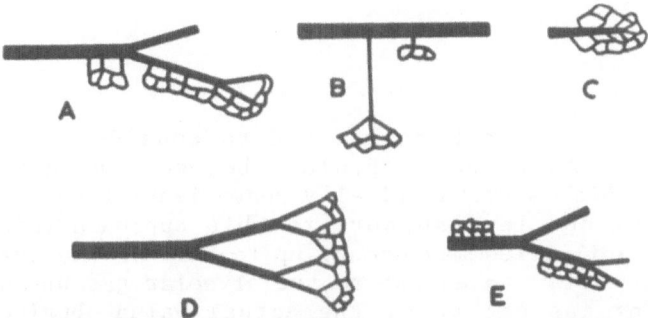

Fig. 11   Diagram of some of the different ways in which capillaries
           originate from small arteries. (From Horsfield,
           Morphometry of the small pulmonary arteries in man.
           Circulation Research, 42, 593, 1978, by permission of the
           American Heart Association, Inc.)

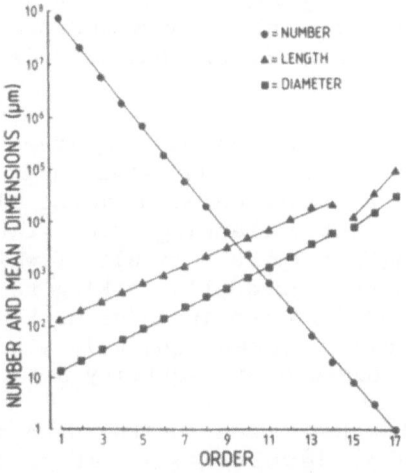

Fig. 12   Plot of data from the human pulmonary arterial tree,
           showing number of branches in each order, and mean length
           and mean diameter of branches in each order. Ordinate –
           number of branches, and mean diameter and length in
           micrometres, on the same logarithmic scale. Abscissa
           Strahler orders.

Certainly the level of this pressure must be of considerable physiological importance.

THE CAPILLARIES

Although there has been a vogue to consider the alveolar capillary network as a sheet of blood between two flat surfaces, partly because this is mathematically convenient, inspection of the capillaries does not lend support to this approach (Fig. 14). In plan view the capillaries may occupy up to half of the surface area of an alveolar wall, and expose to the alveolar gas up to 80 m^2 of surface area for gas exchange. The actual value obtained for the surface area depends on the magnification employed, the higher the magnification the higher the surface area. This phenomenon has been demonstrated by the study of fractals.

Functional Consequences

The remarkably large area available for gas exchange in the lungs, equal to that of a tennis court, is sufficient to meet the body's requirements for oxygen uptake even during severe exercise. This large functional reserve is well illustrated by disease processes such as emphysema which can destroy 75 per cent or more of the lung without killing the patient. The surface area of the red cells in the capillaries is about 80 m^2, and given that the red cell membrane and the alveolar capillary membrane offer approximately equal impedances to the diffusion oxygen, this is the most efficient arrangement.

When pulmonary capillaries are observed through a window implanted in the chest wall, at any given moment most capillaries are seen not to have any red cells flowing through them. The pattern of flow is constantly changing, flow starting in some loops and stopping in others, partly as a result of white cells impacting at branching points and then gradually working their way through. On exercise pulmonary blood flow can increase markedly with only small changes in pulmonary artery pressure, mainly because of capillary recruitment, and partly because of capillary dilation.

Very little work has been done on the three dimensional aspects of blood flow at lobular level. Wagner et al (1967) showed that blood flow to the distal part of a lobule is less than that to the proximal part. Such an arrangement might represent an adaptation to the gradient of oxygen concentration down the lobule resulting from incomplete diffusive mixing, thereby maintaining a normal Va/Q ratio (Fig. 15). Ewan et al (1978) also obtained some evidence to support this hypothesis.

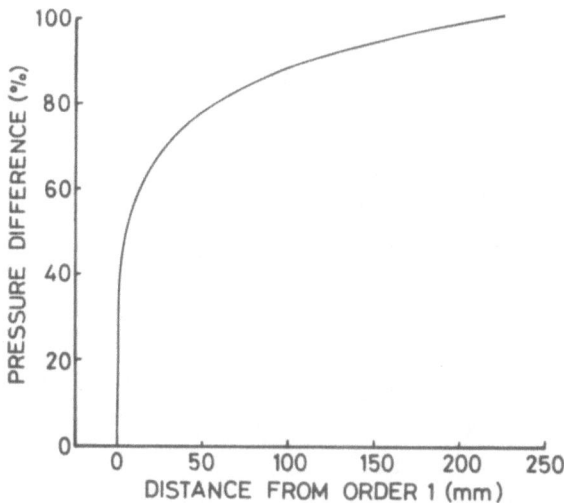

Fig.13   Plot of blood pressure in the pulmonary arteries versus
           length from the start of order 1 vessels. Ordinate
           pressure as a percentage of the pressure difference from
           order 1 to order 17. Abscissa - distance from the origin
           or order 1 vessels.

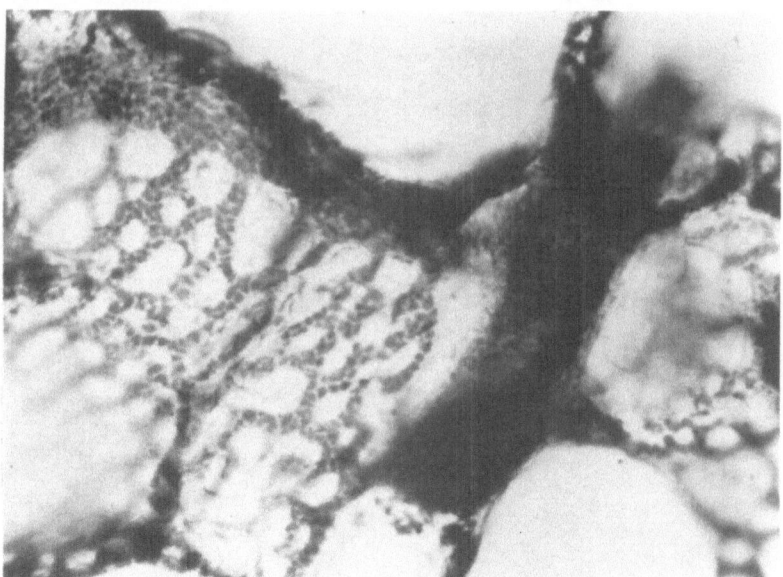

Fig. 14   Pulmonary capillary networks and their origins from small
           arteries. Individual red cells can be seen in the
           capillaries. (From N. C. Staub).

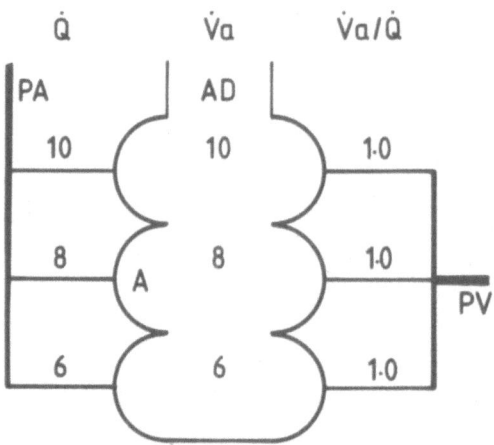

Fig.15   Diagram of stratified perfusion of an acinus matching
          stratified fresh gas ventilation. Q – blood flow to a
          segment, in arbitrary units; Va – fresh gas ventilation to
          a segment, in arbitrary units; Va/Q –
          ventilation/perfusion ratio to a segment, maintained at
          unity, A – alveolus, AD – alveolar duct system, PA –
          pulmonary artery, PV – pulmonary vein.

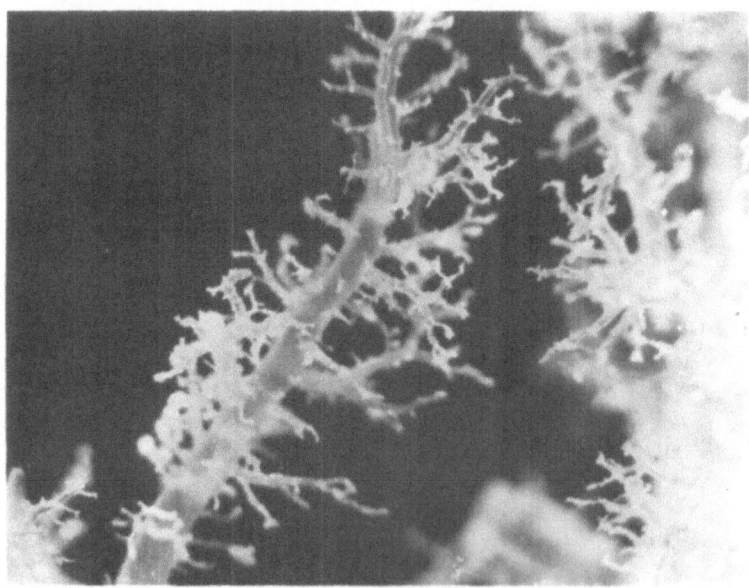

Fig.16   Cast of an interlobular vein, being joined at right angles
          by veins draining the lobules.

THE VEINS

The general arrangement of the venous drainage has already been described. Short and long venules run to the periphery of the lobules and join at right angles the considerably larger veins running between the lobules (Fig. 16). Further up the tree veins join at more acute angles, in the manner of the conventional branching of arteries and bronchi. It can be seen from casts of arteries and veins (Figure 17) that the venous system has a larger volume than the arterial, and at any given level has a larger cross-sectional area. Unlike arteries, veins do not have a perivascular space, so that veins within the lung are connected directly to the lung substance and are held open by the elastic forces. Veins situated beween the hilum of the lung and the left atrium are not so attached, and can change volume relatively easily by becoming flattened.

Functional Consequences

Most of the available driving pressure in the pulmonary circulation has been dissipated by the time the blood reaches the end of the capillaries. Therefore there is only a small pressure available to drive the blood along the venous side

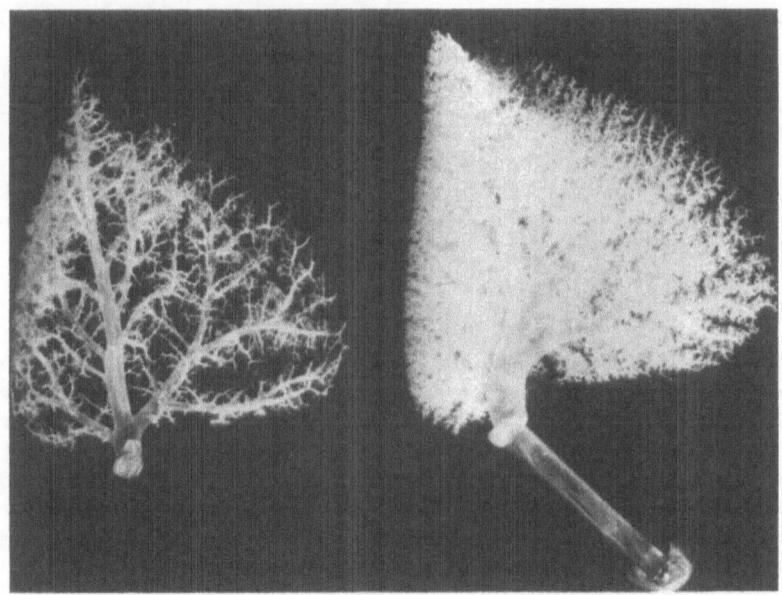

Fig.17   Arterial and venous casts of the right lower lobes of two dog lungs. Veins on the left, arteries on the right.

of the system. The large cross-sectional area of the veins makes for
a low resistance system which can function with the low driving
pressure available. Under experimental circumstances the
extrapulmonary veins can be observed changing in volume, taking up
temporary differences between the outputs of the right and left
ventricles (see the chapter by Lee on this topic). In order for the
intrapulmonary veins to have a reservoir function it would be
necessary for them to be able to actively contract against the
radial elastic forces. There is little evidence available on this
point at present.

COLLATERAL CIRCULATION

        The lung has a double vascular supply, the bronchial and the
pulmonary, and the interconnections between their various parts are
widespread, complex, difficult to investigate, and subject to
interspecies differences. Interconnections have been described
between the following structures:
1)   Parallel branches of the bronchial artery.
2)   Pulmonary artery and bronchial artery.
3)   Capililary networks of the pulmonary and bronchial systems
     meeting at the level of the terminal bronchioles.
4)   Venules draining the pulmonary capillaries and the bronchial
     plexus.
5)   Bronchial venous plexus, and pulmonary and bronchial veins.

        Connections between the pulmonary and bronchial arteries have
been demonstrated in man and guinea pigs. In congenital heart
disease with reduced pulmonary blood flow, for example severe
pulmonary stenosis, these communications are well developed.
Muscular "Sperr" arteries have been described by von Hayek (1960)
arising from these connecting veins on the pleura. Other authorities
doubt their existance.

Functional Consequences

        A careful distinction must be made between the demonstration of
an anatomical connection and the presence of a route through which
blood actually flows. For example, the pulmonary and bronchial
arterial connections may not normally take any flow, but in the
presence of pulmonary stenosis they open to form a major source of
the pulmonary blood supply. The enormous potential for variations
in the route of the blood flow presented by the above anastomoses is
obvious. Arteries, capillaries and veins from both systems
respectively are connected, and direct arterio-venous anastomoses
may exist too. Thus almost any part of the lung may potentially be
supplied by blood from either artery, and be drained by either set
of veins. Under these circumstances collateral supply of tissues

distal to blocked arteries and shunting of blood help maintain a
normal Va/Q ratio are among the possible responses to pathological
changes in the lungs and vessels.

REFERENCES

EWAN,P.W., Jones,H.A., Nosil,J., Obdrzalek,J. and Hughes,J.M.B.,
     1978, Uneven perfusion and ventilation within lung regions
     studied with nitrogen-13, Respir. Physiol., 34: 45.
HAYEK,H.von., 1960,"The Human Lung", Hafner, New York.
HORSFIELD,K., 1978. Morphometry of the small pulmonary arteries in
     man, Circ. Res., 42: 593.
HORSFIELD.K., 1977. Morphology of branching trees related to
     entrophy. Respir. Physiol., 29: 179.
HORSFIELD,K. and Cumming,G., 1976, Morphology of the bronchial tree
     in the dog, Respir. Physiol., 26: 173 .
REID,L., 1968, Structural and functional reappraisal of the
     pulmonary arterial system, in "The Scientific Basis of Medicine"
     Annual Reviews, Athlone Press, London.
WAGNER,P., McRae,J. and Read,J., 1967, Stratified distribution of
     blood flow in secondary lobules of the rat lung, J.Appl.
     Physiol., 22: 1115.

Discussion

HEATH: The first thing I would like to ask is this: are these data related only to sea-level man? because it seems to me that what we are talking about here is very closely related indeed to the level of alveolar oxygen tension. I am quite sure, if you had a look at the normal pulmonary circulation of the millions of people throughout the world who live above an altitude of about three thousand meters you would find that all these data would not be applicable. Arias-Stella has shown that there is a pronounced muscularisation of the distal peripheral portion of the pulmonary arterial tree and I think that whilst all these numbers are interesting, you want one system of data for sea level and another for anything above three thousand meters. I'd be interested to know what you think about that.

HORSFIELD: I entirely agree, and I do not have data for altitude. Indeed at one time we expected to get them, but we have not yet done so.

DENISON: I am sure that Professor Heath would agree that although 25 million people live above three thousand meters, they only represent one twentieth of the world's population. It's only fair to point out that what follows from Horsfield's description still applies to 19 out of 20 lungs.

HEATH: I take that point about the normal, but I think what we must bear in mind all this week is that we are going to be talking about conditions in which the oxygen tension in the alveolar spaces is diminished. I know we are not going to spend a week talking about the Sherpas or the Quechuas of Peru, but we are going to be talking about many many people throughout the world that have diminished alveolar tension. People who have things like chronic lung disease, and I think that you ought to keep that in mind. The actual data reported would not be applicable to anybody in which the alveolar oxygen tension diminishes.

CUMMING: It's always a great pleasure to engage in controversy with Donald Heath, especially when it's in public. So I am going to begin by disagreeing strongly with what he just said, in one respect. He suggested that Strahlers method of describing anatomy might be different in lungs from altitude. No so. The system refers to gross anatomy, and Donald knows and will agree with me that as far as the gross anatomy is concerned, the number of branches and how they arise is almost certain to be the same. Where we'll agree is how the vessels structure itself changes with altitude.

HEATH: You say, Gordon, that it may be the same. Now, it may be, but it may not be. And let's be frank about it. Nobody has looked.

CUMMING: I accept that absolutely.

HORVATH: How much is the fine structure, ultrastructure, in the lung, genetically determined?

HORSFIELD: Well, I don't know, I am not an expert at that level.

CORRIN: I think you suggested that increased interstitial fluid produced pulmonary hypertension. Is there any concrete evidence that it does?

HORSFIELD: I don't think so.

CUMMING: It occurred to me during the presentation that if the vessel is in contact with parenchyma through a molecular layer of liquid, as it normally is, then the adhesive forces between the vessel wall and the parenchyma are transmitted through fluid. If that monomolecular layer becomes two molecules thick, it is identical. If it becomes one thousand molecules thick, I think it is still identical, because the cohesive forces of the liquid are not dependent upon the length of the liquid through which the force is transmitted. I suppose that what may happen is that the vessel may be more readily deformed, because the liquid is more readily deformed than the lung parenchyma. But I take Brian Corrin's point:
  I wonder whether there is a rational argument for saying that this would produce pulmonary hypertension.

CORRIN: The reason I asked is that at capillary level I have observed phenomena whereby the lumen is completely blocked. But when we observed this we were measuring ventricular thickness and there was no evidence of pulmonary hypertension in the way of right ventricular hypertrophy. So we presumed that this phenomenon was a focal affair able to be accompanied by a vast vascular reserve of the lung.

BARER: Experimentally we produce pulmonary oedema without pulmonary hypertension. They very often concur, but you can often bring down the pressure with dilator substances while retaining the oedema.

BRONCHIAL CIRCULATION: ANATOMICAL VIEWPOINT

Antonio Blasi

Professor of Respiratory Diseases
Naples University
Ospedale "V. Monaldi"
Camaldoli
Naples 80131, Italy

Problems associated with the bronchial circulation are currently of great theoretical and practical interest. Our present knowledge in this field is derived both from anatomical investigations (blood vessel injection of surgical and autopsy material) and from radiological investigations such as general or selective arteriography.

1. BRONCHIAL ARTERIES AND BRONCHIAL CIRCULATION IN NORMAL CONDITIONS

1a. In the first four weeks of embryonal life the IVth aortic arch provides the peribronchial plexus, which supplies the trachea and bronchi, and the common pulmonary plexus, which supplies the lungs. About the 7th to 8th week the definitive bronchial arteries can be seen, which remain in communication with the pulmonary circulation via numerous anastomoses.

In the adult the bronchial arteries arise by one or two trunks from the aorta and there may also be many supplementary or accessory branches, derived from: the subclavian artery, the upper posterior intercostal arteries, the right internal mammary artery, the diaphragmatic arteries, or the abdominal aorta.

1b. Distribution is alongside the peripheral bronchi (with anastomotic communication between the left and right sides at the roots of the two principal bronchi) and along the lobar bronchi.

Arterial branches can be identified as far as 3rd, 4th or 5th order bronchi and then they ramify in a peribronchial network which extends to the lobule periphery.

Throughout their course the bronchial arteries give off the vasa vasorum of the pulmonary arteries.

1c. <u>Venous Return</u> is by the bronchial veins which form two distinct systems. The superficial bronchial veins drain the principal and lobar bronchi and empty into the azygos vein on the right, the hemiazygos and mediastinic veins on the left. The deep bronchial veins drain the segmental and distal bronchi and empty into the pulmonary veins.

In a normal adult flow through the bronchial artery system is less than 20% of left ventricular output.

2. RELATIONS AND CONNECTIONS BETWEEN THE BRONCHIAL AND PULMONARY CIRCULATIONS

Most arterial broncho-pulmonary anastomoses occur at perilobar and intralobar levels; they may be:-

        side-to-side (H anastomoses)
        end-to-end (Y anastomoses)
        end-to-side.

3. BRONCHIAL ARTERIES AND BRONCHIAL CIRCULATION IN SOME PATHOLOGICAL CONDITIONS

The bronchial circulation undergoes brisk local development with new vessel formation in certain disease conditions, such as:-

- in some prolonged, non-specific pneumonic or broncho-pneumonic infections;

- in relation to cavities (tuberculous, abscess) or cysts (due to malformations or parasites);

- in relation to bronchiectasis or peribronchiectatic infection;

- in relation to neoplastic tissue (solitary tumours, primary infiltrating carcinoma of the lung) with new vessel formation around and within the lesion;

- in atelectatic areas of the lung, where marked unfolding of the newly formed bronchial vessels occurs, with numerous anastomoses between the bronchial and pulmonary circulations.

The increase in the bronchial circulation under the above-mentioned pathological conditions is often responsible for repeated, sometimes serious episodes of haemoptysis. This may necessitate selective bronchial arteriography both for a precise diagnosis and so that adequate treatment may be carried out by embolization of the bronchial artery involved.

Discussion

MORPURGO: I would like to ask the speakers how they practically proceed to embolise the bronchial arteries.

BLASI: Naturally we first carry out selective arteriography of the bronchial artery. Once we have seen the bronchial circulation we inject, under microscopic control, a very small amount - a few cc's - of contrast medium associated with Spongostan. This is a gelatine substance which has been very finely ground into particles and this is injected under fluoroscopic control. We use this because it is a reversible substance. It is not a very good emboliser but given the readiness with which the bronchial circulation is damaged this substance allows us not to run too many risks when we carry out embolisation. Some authors have recently been using irreversible embolising agents for tumor embolisation procedures; these in practise close the artery at the origin and allow complete occlusion of the pathological part of the circuit. This is very very dangerous in the case of bronchial arteries. We must tread very carefully here. After embolisation, we wait a few seconds and then after that we inject the contrast medium without an embolising agent to see whether embolisation has taken place or not.

RIEDEL: I would like to add another important indication for measuring the bronchial collateral circulation and the flow, and this is the differential diagnosis of primary against thromboembolic pulmonary hypertension. We have never found collateral bronchial circulation in primary pulmonary hypertension.

BLASI: We have no experience in this field, however, this is important and I thank you for your comment.

SCHIAVINO: I would like to ask if, as well as the embolisation you describe, you have carried out embolisation with an autologous withdrawal of blood. In other words, an embolus of the patient himself.

BLASI: We have never used this because we turned to bronchial embolisation after a certain amount of experience in the embolisation of renal tumours. Here we used the patient's own blood in nephrogenous hypertension and renal tumours with scant results. Since we have good results with Spongostan we didn't think it worthwhile to use the patient's own blood. Also because this method of embolising affords us a fairly long period before recanalisation.

SCHIAVINO: One last thing. There is a very interesting aspect of bronchial circulation in the presence of bronchial embolism. This is a fairly controversial point, it's not very clear what happens and I would like to ask whether you have any experience of this. Some say that the circulation is in fact a support in the course of bronchial embolus in some way and that as such it would seem possible to distinguish between pulmonary emboli which give just emboli and pulmonary emboli which give rise to haemorrhage and infarction. If the embolus is massive, there is no haemorrhage or infarction; if it is not massive, if it is a micro-embolus in other words, there is a haemorrhage and infarction, because the bronchial circulation behaves in a different way. There is a complete substitution and the pressure does not cause haemorrhage. There is a partial substitution in the small embolus and the extreme pressure creates extravasation, with haemorrhage and hence infarction. And from this we have a different way of considering pulmonary embolus and therefore a different succession of events: embolus - haemorrhage infarction. I would like to ask your opinion of this.

BLASI: What my colleague has said is most interesting and in fact the fundamentals are those he has described. In relationship to a request by the bronchial circulation in some emboli, those which are fairly distal, this is true. Because if they are proximal branches, since on sub-segmental and distal branches anaestomoses are opened through those pulmonary bronchial arteries which have been outlined some time ago and which we mentioned here today. The problem becomes important when we consider the future recanalisation of embolised or thrombosed pulmonary branches - embolised because some are autologous thrombosis of pulmonary branches in a pathological region. For example: a sub-segmentary pulmonary artery adjacent to a pulmonary abcess or near a focus of post-tubercular fibrosis. In these case the bronchial artery completely disappears. We have seen and studied these anatomically in the case of an autologous thrombosis; for example, in that region where there is a slowing down of the circulation and alteration of the parenchyma this produces autologous thrombosis of the pulmonary artery. In these cases recanalisation is very frequently observed. The permeation of the pulmonary artery throughout by bronchial vessels with anatomic pictures that are indeed very elegant because they are very small bronchial arterial branches which spiral, as it were, around the thrombosed vessels and which go into and recanalise with many of the aspects that I showed you in my last slides. This is an important and interesting aspect which is linked up with what my colleague asked.

HORVATH: The important collateral role of the broncho-pulmonary flow is well known in the progressive stages of silicosis; what is your opinion and experience as regards the classification of the stages of silicosis (since this does not indicate therapy)? I think that it does not cause embolisation of the circulation.

BLASI: We do not have a great deal of silicosis in Naples, however, I agree that probably embolisation does not occur.

LOCKART: We have been told that a lot of lung conditions will cause an abnormal bronchial or intercostal or mediastinal circulation to develop. I wonder, does anyone know what causes this growth of abnormal vessels. I can recall a paper in which it was suggested that following ligation of a main PA, administration of cortisone could hamper the development of collateral lung circulation.

CUMMING: Responding to the comment of Alan Lockart. It might interest the audience to know that Thurlbeck has recently shown a circulating substance which can recognise the absence of a piece of lung tissue. In other words, he has taken a developing rat, removed one lung, and the other lung grew to exactly the same volume that the two lungs together would have been. They took out one lung, and filled the remaining space with wax: the other lung developed to the size it alone would have been. So something permitted one lung to recognise the absence of another. Then he took out one lung and cross-circulated from the excised lung to a normal rat, which then developed lungs twice as big as they would normally have been. Now, if there is a circulating substance recognising lung absence, perhaps we should be looking for the cirulating substance which can cause hypertrophy of the bronchial circulation. Perhaps we should look for a molecule, a small molecule.

BLASI: What Cumming says is right from the pathophysiological point of view. As a pathologist - and I recall that I am a clinical pathologist and not a clinical physiopathologist, the important point here is this request and this originates in the need for nourishment. If there is newly formed tissue or an episode of tissue repair, along side this granulomatous cellular movement there is a need for nourishment and therefore the bronchial collateral circulation is set up. This always goes back to the concept that the bronchial circulation can produce new tissue. In my opinion the bronchial circulation does not have this ability. And the explanation was given to us by tuberculosis, old tuberculosis, which taught us a great deal and which helped us to explain the activity of pericavitary tissue which almost always wipes out the pulmonary circulation except in those cases of aneurysms of Rasmussens of the cavity, which was first seen by an Englishman. The pulmonary circulation is wiped out and the bronchial circulation takes over. And in the pericavitary granulomatous tissue we have the presence of bronchial circulation. This observation comes from anatomic studies which preceded the arteriographic data coming much later.

TRICOMI: I am a radiologist. I would like to put a question to fellow radiologists. For more than ten years now we know from Nordenstrom, who has been one of the greatest workers in the field of broncho-arteriography who has affirmed and indeed, struck a note of alarm, asserting the well nigh complete uselessness of bronchial arteriography or diagnostic purposes. It is not possible to make differentiations using broncho-arteriography between inflammatory and neoplastic processes.

But as Blasi has said, we know everything from pathological anatomy. Suffice it just to think of De La Rue's work and that of some of our fellow Italians, that whereever there is cessation of blood flow from the pulmonary artery, where there is an arrest of the functional artery at the level of the cavity, in destructive processes, in new formation, in bronchiectasis, we have hypertrophy, a thinning out of the bronchial system. Therefore I wonder what are the clinical indications for bronchial arteriography?

BLASI: We generally carry this out in cases of haemoptysis. We started to do this as a therapy to stop haemopysis of a severe nature. (We have had fairly good results.) We also have a revascularisation of the pathological circulation and therefore new autologous episodes. However, generally these are the only cases where we have employed this.

HEATH: One of the most interesting histological features of bronchial arteries is the very large amount of longitudinal muscle they have in their walls and this is often related to the fact that bronchial arteries are subjected to a constant stress of longitudinal stretch. But Horsfield has shown us this morning very beautifully that pulmonary arteries also lie in very close association with the bronchial tree and are subjected to the same stimulus of longitudinal stress throughout the life of the subject. This being so, why is it that pulmonary arteries don't have a longitudinal muscle in their walls, even to the same extent when there is a severe degree of pulmonary hypertension? What is the physiological stimulus for the characteristic microscopic structure of the bronchial artery.

BLASI: Thank you. Bronchial arteries are essentially muscular structures, strengthened by longitudinal muscle fibres and this in some pathological process becomes hyperplastic.

CORRIN: With regard to the growth stimulating factor, I think it is unlikely to be a circulating factor, because as we have seen the overgrowth of the bronchial circulation is limited to diseased tissue, whereas if it were a circulating factor we would have it in the other lung too. I'd like to ask if there is any data pertaining to diffuse lung disease. We had a wealth of data on a variety of local lung diseases, tumours, malformations, inflammations. What about diffuse scarring of the lung? Is that too supplied by the bronchial arteries? I am looking for a broad generalisation covering all lung diseases.

BLASI: As to diffuse fibrosis there has not been a great deal of
investigation carried out. There has been a great deal of study,
however, into circumscribed, massive fibrosis. Massive
circumscribed fibrosis differs from the diffuse type which might
have a different aspect but I have not found this either in the
literature or from my own personal experience.
malformations, inflammations. What about diffuse scarring of the
lung? Is that too supplied by the bronchial arteries? I am looking
for a broad generalisation covering all lung diseases.

BLASI: As to diffuse fibrosis there has not been a great deal of
investigation carried out. Thhere has been a great deal of study,
however, into circumscribed, massive fibrosis. Massive
circumscribed fibrosis differs from the diffuse type which might
have a different aspect but I have not found this either in the
literature or from my own personal experience.

BACKGROUND OF PHYSIOLOGY IN THE PULMONARY CIRCULATION

G. Bonsignore

Institute of Respiratory Physiopathology

University of Palermo - 90146 Via Trabucco 180

This paper has to be considered as an introduction to the physiology of pulmonary circulation: it can only introduce to some aspects of this topic which will be dealt with in more detail in the following presentations and actually are widely discussed in the literature.

Pulmonary circulation is a system working at low pressures (mean pressure in the aorta is about six times higher than in the pulmonary artery); arterial pressure in it is required to lift the blood to the top of the lung. At capillary level, in the upright human lung, pressures are very different varying from a low value at the top (1 cmH_2O) to an higher one (at least 20 cmH_2O) at the bottom.

Pressure-flow relationships of pulmonary circulation are influenced by alveolar pressure: this assumption has been firstly claimed by Banister and Torrance (1960) who demonstrated that a reduction of flow is a consequence of higher tracheal pressures, when the pulmonary arterial pressure remains unchanged, because the intraalveolar pressure exceeds the intracapillary pressure. This behaviour of the capillary bed is confirmed in the "Starling resistor's" model (Permutt et al., 1962) represented by a flexible rubber tube inside a glass chamber: when chamber pressure is greater than the pressure at the outlet of the tube, the tube collapses and the surrounding

pressure at this point limits flow, so that the driving
pressure is determined by the difference between upstream
pressure and chamber pressure.

Distribution of the flow is influenced also by the
hydrostatic pressure differences within the blood vessels,
which are particularly evident in the upright position,
between the top and the bottom of the lung: in this
latter position blood flow decreases almost linearly
from bottom to top, whereas in the supine position its
distribution from apex to base becomes almost uniform
and a pressure gradient becomes evident between dependent
and upper lung zones.

It is easy to find the effects of alveolar, arterial
and venous pressures on the distribution of blood flow
on the "three-zone model" (West et al., 1964), as is evidenced by the radioactive xenon method. This model includes: "zone 1" at the top of the lung, where the capillaries are collapsed as effect of alveolar pressure;
"zone 2" where the capillaries are open because pulmonary arterial pressure exceeds alveolar pressure, whereas
venous pressure is lower than alveolar one, so that
blood flow is determined by the difference between arterial and alveolar pressures; "zone 3", where capillaries
are more widely open, blood flow is influenced by the
arterial-venous pressure difference because, as an effect
of hydrostatic pressure increase at both vascular extre-
mities, venous pressure eventually exceeds the alveolar
one.

It must be pointed out now that the calibre of the
capillaries is influenced by some physical factors along
the lung, which are related to a) the dynamics of pressure in the pulmonary interstitial fluid, and b) the
distribution of vascular pressures through the capillary network. Concerning the former factor, the analysis
of fluid transport between the interstitial space and
the alveoli has shown that the interstitial fluid pressure in the normal lung cannot be more positive than
the fluid pressure in the alveoli; pressures generated
by the surface tension of the fluid in the alveoli tend
to expand the perivascular spaces and the capillary side
of the epithelial membrane (Guyton et al., 1976), in-

fluencing in such a way the calibre of capillaries, particularly at the level of the so-called "corner vessels" and in the upper zones.

The intervention of the second factor is consistent with the fall of the pulmonary vascular resistance when the pulmonary arterial or venous pressures increase; one mechanism, termed "recruitment", is represented by the opening of vessels unperfused at lower pressures; the second mechanism, termed "distension", is represented by the widening of individual capillaries previously open. Many experiments have been carried out about the role of the above-mentioned mechanisms in regulating the total blood content of alveolar septum: some of them demonstrated that "recruitment" is the main determinant of septal filling (Permutt et al., 1969), depending more on changes of pulmonary arterial pressure than on those of pulmonary venous pressure; some others (West, 1979) have suggested that "recruitment" occurs mainly as pulmonary artery pressure raises from low levels whereas "distension" is the predominant one intervening at relatively high vascular pressures.

Another important mechanical factor which influences the calibre of pulmonary vessels is represented by lung volume. In order to understand the intervention of this factor, we must distinguish the capillaries included in the alveolar septum and the extra-alveolar vessels which are arteries and veins larger than about 30 μm diameter. When a subject takes a deep inspiration, lung volume increases and the alveolar walls are stretched, whereas the perivascular pressure is reduced equalling pleural pressure: this makes the vascular bed of alveolar vessels "compressed" and that of extra-alveolar vessels "expanded"; the opposite, obviously, takes place during expiration. These findings, which were experimentally studied in excised lung by Macklin (1946) and Howell et al. (1961), were demonstrated in humans by Hughes et al. (1968), by means of radioactive xenon method; these latter demonstrated that at total lung capacity blood flow increases down the upright lung, whereas at functional residual capacity a region appears of reduced blood flow at the bottom of the lung which

is believed to be caused by the high resistance of the
extra-alveolar vessels, and finally at residual volume
the apical blood flow slightly exceeds basal flow. As a
result of these findings, taking into account particularly the effects of increased interstitial pressure in
the dependent zone, Hughes et al. (1968) suggested to
modify the above-mentioned "three-zone model" of the distribution of blood flow into a "four-zone model" where
the "zone 4" at the base is characterized by a reduction
in blood flow due to an increase in vascular resistance
of the extra-alveolar vessels.

Strictly connected with the capillary circulation
is that of the interstitial space: the background of
Knowledgde on this topic is represented by the measurement and calculation of forces acting on the two sides
of the pulmonary capillary membrane that cause fluid
and solute molecules to move through the capillary pores
(Guyton et al., 1970). It has been stated that the normal negative fluid pressure in the interstitial spaces
plays an important role in determining the reciprocal
topographic relationship between the alveolar epithelial cells and the pulmonary capillaries; this relationship is completely altered when the interstitial fluid
pressure rises above atmospheric pressure, making easy
to fluids to collect in the interstitial space, to compress mechanically blood vessels and to invade the alveolar space. In addition, in the field of the relationship between interstitium, capillary circulation and
alveolar space it has been demonstrated that: a) the
alveolar pressure influences the capillary one, so that
as the first increases, it reduces or offsets the fil-
trating effect of the increasead capillary pressure;
b) filtration induced by an increase in capillary hydrostatic pressure is limited by the reduction in the extra-
vascular colloid osmotic pressure determined by a small
transvascular shift of fluid, so that this last mechanism acts as an efficient and rapidly adjusting coun-
ter-force (Waaler and Aarseth, 1976).

The pulmonary capillary blood flow is pulsatile,
as it has been demonstrated by Lee and Dubois (1955)
in man, through the intermittency of the nitrous oxide

absorbtion, in time with the heart beat, during body-
plethysmography; the influences determined by the instantaneous pressure events which take place simultaneously at the arteriolar and venular ends of the capillary
system, on the pulsatile nature of lung capillary blood
flow, have been fully demonstrated by Lee (1971).

Many experiments have been carried out concerning
the effects of changing gas tensions on the local blood
flow in the lung, after the well-known observations of
Euler and Liljestrand (1946) who described, in cats ventilated with low oxygen or high carbon dioxide mixtures,
a rise in pulmonary artery pressure thought to be due to a
vasoconstriction. It has been demonstrated that there
is a relationship between the degree of unilateral hypoxia determined either in awake man or in anesthetized
dog and the reduction of blood flow in the same lung;
this relationship is expressed by some stimulus / response curves of pulmonary vessels to hypoxia (Barer, 1976).
The use of a control system theory to analyze the gain
of local pulmonary hypoxic vasoconstriction at different
levels of local PAO_2 and $\dot{V}a/\dot{Q}$ (experiments carried out
in the coati mundi), has demonstrated that the ability
of the local pulmonary circulation to stabilize PAO_2
and $\dot{V}a/\dot{Q}$ is greater in the physiological range, but relatively poor outside these limits (Grant et al., 1976).

The investigations carried out in this topic, mainly concern:
a) the site of action of pulmonary hypoxia;
b) the effects of hypoxia, of hypercapnia and of changes
   in blood pH on pulmonary vascular bed;
c) the mechanisms of pulmonary vasoconstrictor response
   to hypoxia, with emphasis on the hypotesis of intervention of a mediator, or of a direct effect, or of
   neuroepithelial bodies.

Attention has been paid to the following problems:
- the role of higher "sensitiviness" to hypoxia of "alveolar vessels" when compared with larger vessels
  (Bergofsky, 1969);
- the effect of alveolar oxygen tension on precapillary
  vessels and that of oxygen content of blood on the
  magnitude of vasoconstrictor response to ventilation

hypoxia (Hauge, 1969);
- the effect of sistemic hypoxia on distensibility of
  large pulmonary arteries mediated by a chemoreflex
  (Szidon et al., 1977);
- the effect of alveolar hypoxia on pulmonary venocon-
  striction (Bland et al., 1977).

When the pulmonary vascular responses to hypoxia
have been compared with the responses to infused histamine (Dawson et al., 1975), on the basis of the assumption that histamine released from mast cells is a mediator of the hypoxic vasoconstriction (Hauge et al., 1968;
Haas et al., 1972), it has been found that hypoxia decreases mainly arterial volume (indicating an arterial
site of action for hypoxic vasoconstriction), whereas
histamine decreases venous volume (indicating that it
increases venous resistance).

More recently (Tucker et al., 1977), histamine has
been demonstrated as acting as a pulmonary vasoconstrictor under normoxic conditions, and as a vasodilator
under hypoxic conditions, being thus a modulator, rather than a mediator, of hypoxic pulmonary vasoconstriction.

Investigations concerning the effects of hypercapnia on the pulmonary blood flow (Barer et al., 1970)
have demonstrated that as PCO_2 increases (to maximum 55
torr) flow falls sharply: the slope of regression line
indicates that a rise in PCO_2 of 20 torr would cause a
19.4% fall in blood flow; as PCO_2 increases further,
flow flattens, or can rise. Hypercapnia induces a con-
stricting effect at the level of larger vessels, thus
raising pulmonary vascular resistance (Bergofsky, 1969)
whereas it is not yet located the site of vasodilatation. Further experimental studies carried out by Barer
and Shaw (1971), have confirmed that the overall effects of CO_2 on the pulmonary vasculature depend on a
balance between a vasoconstrictor action probably due
to carbonic acid and vasodilation caused by some other
property of the molecule, and have suggested that in
the life the dilator mechanism may be important when
pH changes caused by CO_2 are minimized by renal compensation.

Attempts to identify the agents mediating the pulmonary vasoconstrictor responses to hypoxia and hypercapnic acidosis, have used pharmacologic antagonism, such as alpha and beta-adrenergic receptor blockade (Barer and McCurrie, 1969), or hystamine H_1 and H_2 receptor blockade (Tucker et al., 1976); more recently, Porcelli et al. (1977) have demonstrated that the three pulmonary vasoconstrictor agents, i.e. hypoxia, hypercapnic acidosis and histamine, have specific alpha-adrenergic activity and elicit most of their vasoconstrictive activity through the alpha-adrenergic system of the pulmonary circulation. Pharmacological beta-blockade or beta-stimulation alter considerably the vasoconstrictive response of alpha-adrenergic drugs, suggesting that the quantitative vasoactive effect of an adrenergic agonist is a result of the balance between alpha-constrictor and beta-dilator activity (Triner et al., 1971).

Several investigations on the constrictive effect induced by hypoxia on the isolated pulmonary artery (Lloyd, 1970), have highlighted the role of anaerobic glycolysis as source of energy to maintain the vascular smooth muscle contraction during oxygen lack (Souhrada et al., 1977), the potentiating effect of RBC's on hypoxic vasoconstriction possibly related to the depletion of circulating glucose by RBC metabolism (McMurtry et al., 1977).

Some others investigations have demonstrated the marked pressor activity determined in the pulmonary vascular bed by $PGF_2\alpha$ which was 10 times more active than serotonine in increasing resistance to flow (Kadowitz et al., 1975), inducing constriction at the level of intrapulmonary veins and upstream vessels presumed to be small arteries (Kadowitz et al., 1977); the effects of temperature changes (Nilsen and Hauge, 1968) and of anesthesia (Sykes et al., 1973) on the vasoconstrictor response to alveolar hypoxia; the role of angiotension II as an agent which is believed to permit the release or action of some other vasoconstrictor rather than causing directly the vasoconstriction (Berkov, 1974).

The above-mentioned mechanism are only a few among the very numerous illustrated to explain the vasoconstrictor pulmonary response. Conversely in spite of the large amount of investigations, at the present, what appears not questionable is that the pulmonary hypertension resulting from hypoxia is due to the contraction of pulmonary vascular smooth muscle, whereas it is not yet clear what is the cause of this hypoxic contraction (Bohr, 1977).

In conclusion, it appears clear that though the role of mechanical factors involved in the regulation of pulmonary circulation is well established, that of neuro-humoral factors is still a matter of debate which is mainly concerned with metabolic functions in the lung and release of vasoactive mediators.

REFERENCES

Banister J., Torrance R.W., 1960, The effect of the tracheal pressure upon flow/pressure relations in the vascular bed of isolated lungs.
Q.J. exp. Physiol., 45:352.

Barer G.R., 1976, The physiology of the pulmonary circulation and metods of study, Pharmac. Ther. B., vol. 2, 247.

Barer G.R., Howard P., Shaw J., 1970, Stimulus-response curves for the pulmonary vascular bed to hypoxia and hypercapnia, J. Physiol. (Lond.), 211:139.

Barer G.R., McCurrie J.R., 1969, Pulmonary vasomotor responses in the cat: the effects and interrelationship of drugs, hypoxia and hypercapnia, Q.J. exp. Physiol., 54:156.

Barer G.R., Shaw J.W., 1971, Pulmonary vasodilator and vasoconstrictor actions of carbon dioxide, J. Physiol. (Lond.), 213:633.

Bergofsky E.H., 1969, Ions and membrane permeability in the regulation of the pulmonary circulation, in: "The pulmonary circulation and interstitial space", A.P. Fishman and H. Hecht eds., pp. 269-285.

Berkov S., 1974, Hypoxic pulmonary vasoconstriction in the rat: the necessary role of angiotensin II, Circulation Res., 35:256.

Bohr D.F., 1977, The pulmonary hypoxic response: state
    of the field, Chest, 71 suppl.:244.
Dawson C.A., Forrester T.E., Hamilton C.H., 1975, Effects
    of hypoxia and histamine infusion on lung blood vo-
    lume, J. appl. Physiol., 38:811.
Euler U.S. Von, Liljestrand I.A., 1946, Observations on
    the pulmonary arterial pressure in the cat, Acta
    Physiol. scand., 12:301.
Grant B.J., Jones H.A., Davies E.E., Hughes J.M., 1976,
    Local regulation of pulmonary blood flow and venti-
    lation-perfusion ratios in the coati mundi, J. appl.
    Physiol., 40:216.
Guyton A., Taylor A., Drake R., 1976, Dynamics of sub-
    atmospheric pressure in the pulmonary interstitial
    fluid, in: "Lung liquids" Ciba Foundation Symposium
    38, Elsevier/Excerpta Med., Amsterdam.
Guyton A., Taylor A., Granger H., 1970, Analysis of types
    of pressure in the pulmonary spaces: interstitial
    fluid pressure, solid tissue pressure and total
    tissue pressure, in: "Central Hemodynamics and Gas
    Exchange", C. Giuntini ed., Minerva Med., Torino.
Haas F., Bergofsky E.H., 1972, Role of mastcell in the
    pulmcnary pressor response to hypoxia, J. Clin.
    Invest., 51:3154.
Hauge A., 1969, Hypoxia and pulmonary vascular resistan-
    ce. The relative effects of pulmonary arterial and
    alveolar PO_2, Acta physiol. scand., 76:121.
Hauge A., 1969, The pulmonary vasoconstrictor response
    to acute hypoxia, in: "Pulmonary circulation",
    J. Widimsky, S. Daum, H. Herzog eds., S. Karger,
    Basel.
Hauge A., Melmon K.L., 1968, Role of histamine in hypo-
    xic pulmonary hypertension in the rat. II. Deple-
    tion of histamine serotonin and catecholamines,
    Circulation Res., 22:385.
Howell J.B., Permutt S., Proctor D., Riley R., 1961,
    Effect of inflation of the lung on different parts
    of pulmonary vascular bed, J. appl. Physiol., 16:71.
Hughes J.M., 1977, Pulmonary circulation and fluid balan-
    ce, in: "Respiratory physiology II", vol. 14,
    J.G. Widdicombe ed., University Park Press, Balti-
    more.

Hughes J.M., Glazier J.B., Maloney J.E., West J.B., 1968,
     Effect of extra-alveolar vessels on distribution of
     blood flow in the dog lung, J. appl. Physiol.,
     25:701.
Kadowitz P.J., Joiner P.D., Hyman A.L., 1975, Physiologi-
     cal and pharmacological roles of prostaglandins,
     Ann. Rev. Pharmacol., 15:285.
Kadowitz P.J., Spannhake E.W., Knight D.S., Hyman A.L.,
     1977, Vasoactive hormones in the pulmonary vascular
     bed, Chest, 71 suppl.: 257.
Lee G. de J., 1971, Regulation of the pulmonary circula-
     tion, Br. Heart J., 33 Suppl.: 15.
Lee G. de J., Dubois A.B., 1955, Pulmonary capillary
     blood flow in man, J. clin. Invest., 34:1380.
Lloyd T.C., 1970, Responses to hypoxia of pulmonary ar-
     terial strips in nonaqueous bath, J. appl. Physiol.,
     28:566.
Macklin C.C., 1946, Evidence of increase in the capacity
     of the pulmonary arteries and veins of dogs, cats
     and rabbits during inflation of the freshly excised
     lung, Rev. Can. Biol., 5:199.
McMurtry I.F., Hookway B.W., Roos S., 1977, Red blood
     cells play a crucial role in maintaining vascular
     reactivity to hypoxia in isolated rat lungs, Chest,
     71 Suppl.: 253.
Nilsen K.H., Hauge A., 1968, Effects of temperature
     changes on the pressor response to acute alveolar
     hypoxia in isolated rat lungs, Acta physiol. scand.,
     73:111.
Permutt S., Bromberger-Barnea B., Bane H.N., 1962, Alveo-
     lar pressure, pulmonary venous pressure and the va-
     scular waterfall. Med. Thorac., 19:239.
Permutt S., Caldini P., Maseri A., Palmer W.H., Sasamori
     T., Zierler K., 1969, Recruitment versus distensibi-
     lity in the pulmonary vascular bed, in: "The pulmo-
     nary circulation and interstitial space", A.P.
     Fishman and H. Hecht eds., pp. 375-387. University
     of Chicago Press, Chicago.
Porcelli R.J., Viau A., Demeny M., Naftchi N.E., Bergof-
     sky E.H., 1977, Relation between hypoxic pulmonary
     vasoconstriction, its humoral mediators and alpha-
     beta adrenergic receptors, Chest, 71 suppl.: 249.

Sykes M.K., Davies D.M., Chakrabarti M.K., Loh L., 1973,
    The effects of halothane, trichloroethylene and
    ether on the hypoxic pressor response and pulmona-
    ry vascular resistance in the isolated perfused cat
    lung, Br. J. Anaesth., 45:655.
Szidon J.P., Flint J.F., 1977, Significance of sympathe-
    tic innervation of pulmonary vessels in response to
    acute hypoxia, J. appl. Physiol.: Respirat. Environ.
    Exercise Physiol., 43:65.
Triner L., Nahas G.G., Vulliemoz Y., 1971, Cyclic AMP
    and smooth muscle function, Ann. N.Y. Acad. Sci.,
    185:458.
Tucker A., Hoffman E.A., Kenneth E.W., 1977, Histamine
    receptor antagonism does not inhibit hypoxic pulmo-
    nary vasoconstriction in dogs, Chest, 71 Suppl.:261.
Tucker A., Weir E.K., Reeves J.T., Grover R.F., 1976,
    Failure of histamine antagonists to prevent hypoxic
    pulmonary vasoconstriction in dogs, J. appl. Phy-
    siol., 40:496.
Waaler B.A., Aarseth P., 1976, Interstitial fluid and
    transcapillary fluid balance in the lung, in:
    "Lung liquids" Ciba Foundation Symposium 38,
    Elsevier/Excerpta Med., Amsterdam.
West J.B., 1979, "Respiratory Physiology - the essen-
    tial", Williams and Wilkins Co., Baltimore.
West J.B., Dollery C.T., Naimark A., 1964, Distribution
    of blood flow in isolated lung; relation to vascu-
    lar and alveolar pressures. J. appl. Physiol.,
    19:713.

Discussion

A.N.OTHER   As regards what Bonsignore said regarding the possible
mechanisms of pulmonary arterial hypertension, I would like to point
out that the studies and assessments carried out on various
experimental animals are one thing and the results obtained on man
are quite another. I would recall that in human pathology there
exists a whole series of situations which show the pathogenetic
importance either of hypoxia or of hypercapnia - taken as an element
by itself, or else through acidosis. For example, intoxications
lead to metabolic acidosis, which is an extremely serious condition
for the patient. We have observed in these cases of metabolic
acidosis the presence of pulmonary arterial hypertension. In
additon there are pure hypercapnic syndromes usually due to an error
of the anaesthetist. During surgery they ventilate the patient by
hand with a balloon; they give the patient oxygen and therefore
maintain a normal arterial PO_2 but they ventilate the patient badly
and he becomes progressively hypercapnic developing pulmonary
arterial hypertension. Also in many cases we see the situation in
man of hyponemia in the hypercapnic patient where we have pulmonary
hypertension. All this shows that the mechanisms can be very
different but that probably they all go back to one single matrix.
At this point I would recall the excellent research work of Enson, a
pupil of Cournand. This was work carried out some time ago on a
dog. Enson was able to obtain with a heart-lung machine alveolar
hypoxia with normal capnia and normal partial pressure of oxygen in
arterial blood. This situation of hypoxia which is just alveolar,
with normal capnia and normal PO_2 gave rise to the appearance of
pulmonary arterial hypertension. Secondly, alveolar hypercapnia
with normal alveolar pressure of oxygen produced pulmonary arterial
hypertension. Thirdly, creation of acidosis by infusion of acid
substances, maintaining PO_2 and PCO_2 normal both at the alveolar and
arterial level caused pulmonary arterial hypertension. Fourthly the
opposite, the creation of alkalosis with normal PO_2 and PCO_2
produced alveolar hypotension. And for this reason, Enson's view
was that pulmonary hypertension is due to a situation of local
hypoxia. This hypoxia can be manifest on the ventilatory side of
the vessel or within the vessel in the blood flowing through it.
This hypoxia is caused by a local lactic acidosis which is the
determining factor in this hypertension. To conclude I would like
to ask one more thing. In one of the slides you showed how the fall
of the alveolar PO_2 always leads to a fall of the cardiac output.
The progressive fall of alveolar PO_2 brings about a reduction of
cardiac output. Did you refer to the local flow rate? I thought we
were talking about systemic flow. A slight in PO_2 corresponded in
man to an increase in cardiac output.

BONSIGNORE: I am completely in agreement and I wanted to bring the analytical and experimental data before you because they allow for an analysis of the influence of the single factors. For example, the influence of the pH, of alveolar PO_2, of the PO_2 at the capillary level: are all factors which coincide with the data reported by Enson? In my opinion, the reaction in man is always unforeseeable and depends on the state of preservation of the capillary structure which allows for vaso-motor response and also depends on the unforeseeable development of mediators which sometimes can abolish or prevent vaso-constrictive response. Therefore, in man the situation is more complex than what we have seen in the experimental animal data.

ZARDINI: The first question is this: at the present time, given the status of hypoxia etc I would like to know the role of Enson's experiments. I ask this of everyone. His experiments of 1951 which showed how hypoxic blood on reaching the lung gives vaso-dilation while alveolar hypoxia gives vasoconstriction. This is a famous work published in 1951 and as far as I am concerned it marked a turning point in the understanding of hypoxia. My second question refers to the pulmonary circulation since I have been concerned with this in the past. As regards the different blood flows at the different degrees of lung expansion and here I am pleased to see that a work of mine from 1966 has been mentioned with a slightly different emphasis being put on the data. What I would like to put to the audience is this: probably at the maximum degree of lung expansion, blood flow and its distribution is greatly influenced by the fact that the lung passes into zone 2. This is the interpretation that we gave to this and which Bonsignore seconded. That is, the interpretation of the maximum degree of lung expansion. The familiar thorny problem was recruitment or distensibility of the vessels. This has in part been resolved. I recall a series of experiments which we carried out last year on an isolated dog lung. There were 2 types of experiments: perfusing with the lung entirely in zone 2 - in other words, with venous pressure being less than alveolar pressure. The other experiment was with the lung in zone 3, and both phenomena are shown in the pressure-volume curve. The problem is that the pressure cost when perfusing the lung in zone 2 is much greater than the pressure cost with the lung in zone 3. Therefore, we can say that both phenomena take place but that we have a pressure volume curve which is completely different. These results are the fruit of a series of experiments carried out separately; it is obvious that probably with a human lung in situ these two factors will be integrated.

BONSIGNORE: I suppose that as regards your first question about the importance of alveolar hypoxia and on the other hand a low PO_2 at the capillary level, I think that I can refer to Hauge who has carried out experiments on this and has shown that if alveolar pressure of oxygen is normal and the capillary arterial pressure (wedge pressure) is lowered, we do not have vasoconstriction while on the other hand, if alveolar pressure is low and capillary pressure is normal, we do have vasoconstriction. Therefore, the first pathogenetic step starts in the alveolus. The partial pressure of oxygen at the capillary level is what alters or modulates the severity of the response. As far as West's results are concerned, regarding the filling of the lung and resistance, I confirm what you have said. With the lung in zone 2, the pressure cost is much higher than with the lung in zone 3. This corresponds to the U curve that I showed you earlier.

LOCKART: Do I have time to make a short comment and then ask a question? I'd like to come back very briefly to the problem of a mediator responsible for vasoconstriction in the lung vessels. I believe that if you accept the hypothesis that a mediator is involved, several criteria have to be fulfilled. The first one is to prove that a mediator increases in concentration with hypoxia. Second criterion: that vasoconstriction should be reproduced by application of an increased concentration of the mediator, usually by infusing it in blood. One is making a guess about the concentration which is actually operative in interstitial lung tissue, and tries to produce this concentration by a concentration in blood. The third criterion should be that vasoconstriction has to be blocked by administration of an antagonist agent. A fourth criterion has been also advocated, which is the proof that such a mediator is released, by the demonstration that its concentration is increased either in the effluent venous blood or in the lymph or in pleural exudate in isolated lung experiments. I do not believe that the last criterion is important because the mediator may be diluted by the huge blood flow in the lung circulation. The three first criteria are of paramount importance and I do not know one of the postulated mediators that meets them all in all circumstances. However, I do believe that a mediator is involved, and that vasoconstriction is due to such release because the direct effect of either hypoxia or acidosis on any smooth muscle that I know of, including smooth muscle of the pulmonary artery, is a relaxing effect. So there must be something other than this direct effect. Now, if I may come to the question I'd like to ask, do you believe that demonstration of vasoconstriction in isolated lung experiments rules out the release of a mediator by terminal nerve endings which accompany pulmonary vessels very distally?

BONSIGNORE: Its very difficult to give an answer because as far as appears from the literature the question is still very much open. There is much discussion about the validity of the models used for isolated lung experiments not perfused with blood. There is discussion about the mediators that appear in isolated lung which does have a blood perfusion. There is discussion about the reaction of vessels which are isolated from lung tissue because we have seen that when there is no lung tissue the reaction of these vessels is completely different or non-existant. Therefore, it is thought that a metabolic intervention is necessary and that this develops at the level of the lung tissue. All this research is under discussion and this all leads to the conclusion which I have set out here on a slide and that is, that vasoconstriction is the result of a muscle contraction of the smooth muscle. Or at least that is my opinion.

CUMMING: Thank you Giovanni. I think I will bring this mornings proceedings to a close at this point. It is quite clear that many items of controversy have been raised and I hope we shall have the opportunity during the remainder of the week to discuss these at length. If you will make a note of those things you wish to discuss we hope to provide the opportunity, for you to discuss them.

FUNCTIONAL ASPECTS OF THE PULMONARY COLLATERAL CIRCULATION

Alain Lockhart

Laboratoire d'explorations fonctionelles
Hôpital Antoine Béclère
Clamart, 92140, France

INTRODUCTION

The normal lung contains the pulmonary circulation which subserves the gas exchanging as well as the endocrine and metabolic functions of the lung and a systemic circulation, the pulmonary collateral circulation or bronchial circulation. Marked deviations from the normal anatomy of the pulmonary collateral circulation exist in certain acquired lung and liver diseases as well as in some congenital heart diseases. The aim of this presentation is twofold - to discuss the role of the normal pulmonary collateral circulation, and to review the functional modifications which take place in conditions which are accompanied by an abnormal development of the pulmonary collateral circulation.

FUNCTIONS OF THE PULMONARY COLLATERAL CIRCULATION

Anatomical survey

A comprehensive review of the anatomy of the pulmonary collateral circulation can be found in a recent monograph (1), and as certain of its features concern us here a short summary follows. The pulmonary collateral circulation originates from the aorta and from aortic branches (2) and supplies arterial blood to all lung structures proximal to the respiratory bronchioles. Bronchial blood is returned to the heart by bronchial veins and by pulmonary veins. The bronchial veins drain blood from the hilum of the lung and from large proximal bronchi and empty into the azygos, the hemiazygos, or one of the intercostal veins from whence blood is returned to the right atrium. Collateral blood from within the lung is returned to the left atrium through anastomoses at the level of the microcirculation between the bronchial and the pulmonary vascular networks. At the level of respiratory bronchioles, the bronchial arteries terminate in a capillary network which anastomoses with pulmonary capillaries. The blood from capillaries of the more distal bronchi (including some respiratory bronchioles) passes into venous radicles, called bronchopulmonary veins, which bypass the alveolar network and anastomose with pulmonary venules proper which drain oxygenated blood from the alveolar capillary network. The existence of precapillary anastomoses between bronchial and pulmonary arteries in the normal human lung is generally accepted. However, they are rare being clearly identified under the microscope in random sections of normal human lung tissue (3).

Normal pulmonary collateral blood flow.

Since part of the bronchial blood drains into pulmonary veins, the bronchial circulation contributes to the true venous admixture together with other sources of anatomic shunts, e.g. the Thebesian veins. In the normal lung breathing air at sea-level true venous admixture is the principal cause of the alveolar-arterial difference in O_2 partial pressure (4). Measured by indirect methods venous admixture is about 1-2% of cardiac output (5). It follows that pulmonary collateral blood flow is less than the above figure. With more direct techniques attempts have been made to measure pulmonary collateral blood flow in intact man. The elegant dye dilution method depicted in figure 1 has been validated in a physical model and was subsequently used in human studies. The rationale of the method is that left-ventricular output is larger than right-ventricular output, the difference being due to pulmonary collateral blood flow. In normal subjects left-ventricular output was 0.9 per cent above right-ventricular output, a barely measurable and non significant difference (6). By use of two different dilution techniques values of bronchopulmonary flow of about 3 per cent of cardiac output were found in the dog (7). However, experiments in 5 anaesthetized close-chested dogs involving injection of indocyanine green into the left ventricle and sampling from the left atrium yielded values for collateral pulmonary blood flow which were as high as 5.9 to 9.7 per cent of left-ventricular output (8). Since these surprisingly high values have not been confirmed by later work and are far in excess of the estimated physiological venous admixture, it is generally accepted that the normal pulmonary collateral blood flow is minute and places no haemodynamic burden on the left ventricle.

Nutritional function of the pulmonary collateral circulation

An obvious function of the pulmonary collateral circulation is nutritional. Early attempts to obliterate the bronchial arterial circulation in the dog by ligation of the bronchial arteries and of branches of the aorta going to the lung, and by stripping the bronchi free of loose aveolar tissue have been on the whole inconclusive or unsuccessful (9).

Conversely, occlusion of the bronchial arterial circulation of one lung in its entirety by injecting it with a plastic material caused varying degrees of ulceration of the main stem bronchus and of the lobar bronchi for a distance of a few millimetres from their origin. Distal to the hilar region mild submucosal congestion was present but the bronchi were viable. When occlusion of the bronchial arteries to the right apical lobe was carried out there was no evidence of infarction or ulceration of the hilar bronchi, a finding which was attributed to anastomosis with other sources of systemic blood supply such as the adjacent unoccluded bronchial arteries (9). These findings have been confirmed to some extent by the effects of transcatheter embolization of bronchial arteries in man for treatment of massive recurrent haemoptysis. In ten of 104 patients lactic dehydrogenase rose during 3 to 5 days following the procedure. Also observed in one subject was focal necrosis of a main stem bronchus which healed within a few weeks (10). There is also evidence that careful reconstitution of the bronchial arteries at the time of allotransplantation of one lung in the dog strikingly reduces the frequency of early disruption of the bronchial suture line and of bronchial ulceration which are associated with lethal post-operative pneumonia (11, 12). These animal experiments suggest that the high frequency of early bronchial complications in clinical lung transplantations may be reduced by reconstruction of the bronchial arterial system (11). Restoration of the bronchial arteries takes place within two to four weeks of lung transplantation (13, 14) and is complete in dogs killed from one to six months after lung autotransplantation (15). Unknown are the factors that govern the orderly restoration of bronchial arteries across the suture line. It is only known that cortisone seems to inhibit, and growth hormone to stimulate the growth of lung collateral vessels after ligature of one pulmonary artery in the rat (16).

Non-nutritional functions of the normal pulmonary collateral circulation.

It is not known whether any substances released in the body normally exert their action on the lung through the bronchial vascular system alone. For instance the bronchomotor

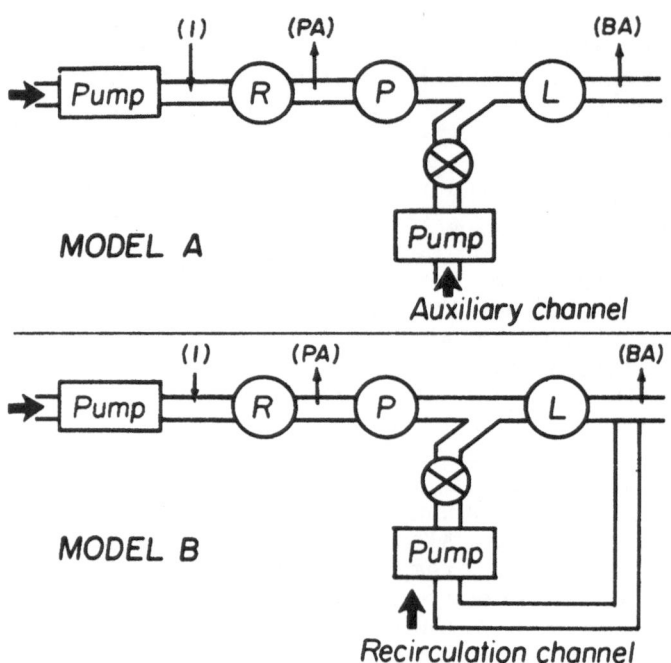

Figure 1.   Physical models used to validate a dye-dilution method for
            estimating the individual outputs of the ventricles when
            the output of the left exceeds that of the right. R,P
            and L are blood filled chambers representing,
            respectively, the vascular volumes of the right heart, the
            lungs and the left heart. Dye is injected in the venous
            circulation at point I and simultaneous dilution curves
            are inscribed from the pulmonary (PA) and systemic (BA)
            artery. In model A, the extra flow is delivered from an
            auxiliary channel whereas in model B it is derived from
            the aorta and recirculated into the pulmonary circulation.

            Reproduced from Fritts, H.W.Jr., et al. by permission of
            the American Heart Association Inc.

action of epinephrine and histamine on perfused lung is the same with bronchial arterial and pulmonary arterial injection (1).   Recent studies with veratrine have shown that the majority (67%) of pulmonary stretch receptors are accessible to drugs from both the pulmonary and bronchial circulation, whereas 28% and 5% of the endings are affected from only the pulmonary or bronchial circulations respectively. Thus, although a chemoreflex may be initiated as a chemical passes through the pulmonary circulation, the reflex may be potentiated as the drug reaches the receptor, albeit diluted, through the bronchial circulation (17). Histamine by any route of administration (airways, intravenously, subcutaneously) and bradykinin selectively cause the bronchial venules to leak thus causing interstitial pulmonary oedema while the permeability of the pulmonary vessels is unaffected (18). Unknown is how relevant is this observation to pathophysiology of clinical pulmonary oedema (18). Obviously much more work has to be done on the accessibility of different effector cells of the lung to naturally occurring substances or to exogenous chemicals before the physiological role of the pulmonary collateral circulation is completely understood.

Other physiologic or pathophysiologic functions of the pulmonary collateral circulation are poorly understood. It is generally accepted that inspired air is conditioned at body temperature when it reaches intrathoracic airways. However measurements of oesophageal temperature during exercise breathing ambient air have shown that the temperature in the oesophagus behind the trachea was several degrees lower than behind the heart or in the rectum. The difference was enhanced by inhalation of cold dry air (19). These findings prove intrathoracic airways play a role in conditioning the inspirate and makes credible the hypothesis that the lung collateral circulation contributes to the warming of inspired air (18). Indeed one may imagine that the extensive submucosal bronchial microcirculation subserves a counter-current heat exchange function whereby air is heated during inspiration and cooled during expiration.

PATHOPHYSIOLOGY OF THE PULMONARY COLLATERAL CIRCULATION IN LUNG DISEASES

Pulmonary collateral circulation as a cause of haemoptysis

Enlargement of the pulmonary collateral circulation in a variety of lung diseases associated with the development of inflammatory or neoplastic tissue, e.g., bronchiectasis, suppurative lung diseases, sequelae of pulmonary emboli,

tuberculous cavities, lung carcinoma, aspergilloma, has been
documented by many post-mortem studies (see references in 3,
20, 21) and more recently by bronchial arteriography (22-29).
By permitting selective transcatheter haemostatic techniques to
be carried out, bronchial arteriography has confirmed that
systemic arterial bleeding is the most common cause if not the
only one, of haemopysis in chronic lung diseases (27, 28).   In
a recent study immediate cessation of massive recurrent
haemopysis was obtained in 41 of 49 patients submitted to
selective embolization of the enlarged systemic arteries.
However, recurrence of haemoptysis within 2 to 7 months
occurred in 6 of the 41 patients because of recanalization of
the embolized artery or revascularization via small previously
insignificant arteries (28).

Pulmonary collaterals as a cause of left-to-right shunt

        In addition to being the principal cause of haemoptysis an
enlarged pulmonary collateral circulation represents a
left-to-right shunt originating from branches of the aortic
arch and opening into the pulmonary arterial tree.   Direct
evidence of a left to-right shunt in chronic lung diseases was
obtained some 25 years ago when it was shown that oxygen
saturation of blood sampled from distal sites in the pulmonary
artery in diseased zones of the lung was higher than true
mixed venous blood sampled above the pulmonary valve.
Moreover, in 2 of 11 patients blood samples from a pulmonary
vein of the diseased zone, obtained by catheterisation of a
patient with cor pulmonale had an oxygen saturation almost
identical to the corresponding artery (20).   Arterialisation of
pulmonary arterial blood sampled from distal branches of the
pulmonary artery in chronic destructive lung diseases e.g.
tuberculosis, bronchiectasis, polycystic lung disease has also
been confirmed (30, 31).   It has been proposed that the
collateral shunt causes a reversal of blood flow thus diverting
mixed venous blood away from the diseased territories and
minimising arterial oxygen unsaturation (32).

        To demonstrate pulmonary precapillary shunts in chronic
lung diseases different indicator dilution methods have been
found useful.   One method involves slug injection of a non
diffusible indicator proximal to the origin of the shunt and
recording of arterial dye curves before and during balloon
occlusion of the pulmonary artery of the diseased lung.
Appropriate sites of injection are the pulmonary artery
proximal to the occlusion or preferably the wedge position of
the unblocked lung (33).   Theoretically the downslope of the
control curve will be interrupted by the early recirculation of
the pulmonary collateral blood flow whereas the shape of the
dye curve will be normal during occlusion. Pulmonary arterial

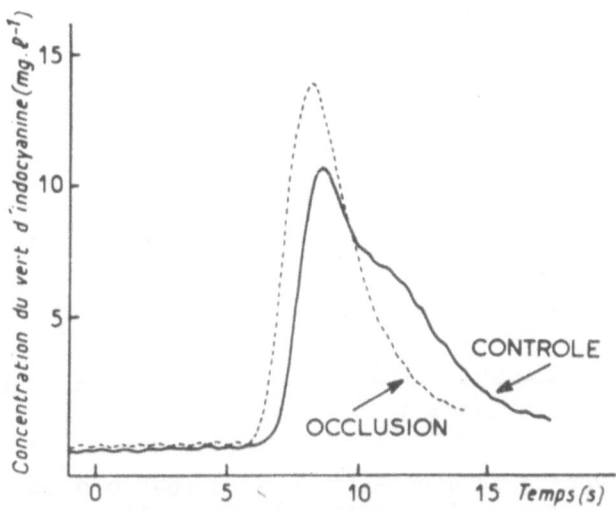

FIGURE 2   Unilateral bronchogenic carcinoma. Injection of dye
            in the pulmonary wedge position in the contralateral
            lung. Dilution curves inscribed from the brachial
            artery before (solid curve, control) and during
            balloon occlusion of the pulmonary artery of the
            diseased lung (interrupted curve occlusion.) Curves
            were redrawn in order to superimpose the moment of
            injection. Early recirculation during the control
            period suggested collateral blood flow in the
            carcinomatous lung.

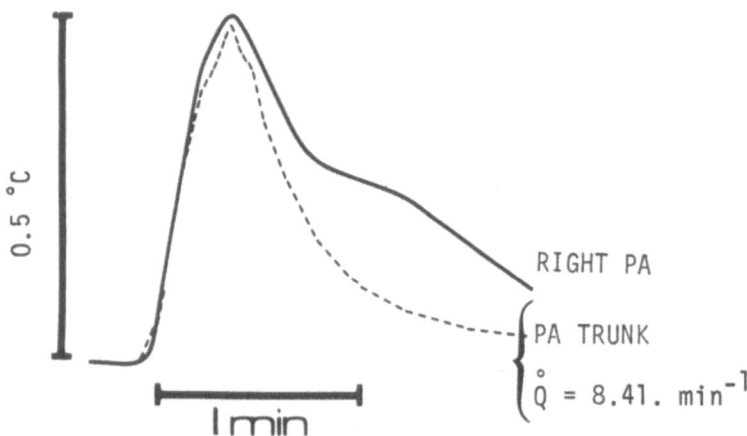

FIGURE 3   Severe bronchiectasis in a 22 year old man suffering
            from congenital agammaglobulinemia. Thermodilution
            curves inscribed from the pulmonary arterial trunk
            just above the valve (dotted curve) and from the
            distal part of the main right pulmonary artery
            (solid line). Injection of cold saline into the
            right atrium. Curves have been redrawn in order to
            superimpose baselines. Early recirculation
            suggestive of precapillary anastomoses between
            systemic and pulmonary arteries is clearly apparent
            on the right PA curve.

shunts less than about 20% of the pulmonary blood flow are unlikely to be detected (34). In fact this method failed to discern a left-to-right shunt in 2 cases of extensive unilateral lung disease (35). With pulmonary wedge injection a left to right shunt was found in only 4 of 40 cases of lung carcinomas (36) (figure 2). Another technique also makes use of balloon occlusion of the pulmonary artery of the diseased lung but the injection of dye is made into the blocked artery, i.e. dye is injected distal to the inflated balloon. The washout of the dye will be the more rapid the greater the flow of collateral blood into the blocked territory. Conversely in the absence of significant collateral blood flow the washout of dye will be markedly delayed. Varying degrees of pulmonary collateral blood flow were found with this technique in 5 of 6 cases of extensive unilateral lung disease (35). Still another technique makes use of venous indicator dilution curves recorded at different sites in the pulmonary artery (Figure 3). The early recirculation of indicator causes distortion of the downslope of curves recorded at the level of, or distal to the shunt whereas the contour of the curve recorded in the pulmonary arterial trunk is normal in the absence of reversal of blood flow. The above described methods do not represent the whole gamut of indicator dilution methods available for the detection of shunting of blood through an enlarged pulmonary collateral circulation. Neither do these methods lend themselves to precise measurement of the shunt. Nevertheless, they illustrate that measurement of cardiac output with indicator dilution may be in error in chronic lung diseases, because of inapparent recirculation (36). The same remark applies to the measurement of left ventricular output and of pulmonary collateral blood flow with the technique described in figure 1. A necessary assumption of the method is that the circulation times through the bronchial-pulmonary anastomoses are sufficiently long to prevent contamination of the downslope of the arterial indicator dilution curve with recirculated dye (6). Indeed the preceding discussion has shown that the assumption is not tenable.

Pulmonary collateral circulation and the Fick principle. Effective pulmonary collateral blood flow.

Notwithstanding the difficulty of sampling true mixed venous blood from the pulmonary artery when a large pulmonary left-to-right shunt is present, unwary use of the Fick principle with oxygen as an indicator to calculate cardiac output may also lead to erroneous results[6,37]. In the presence of pulmonary collateral pathways carrying inflowing arterial blood the Fick equation becomes:

$$M_{O2} = (\dot{Q}_R + \dot{Q}_B) \, Ca_{O2} - \dot{Q}_R \cdot Cv_{O2} - \dot{Q}_B \cdot Cb_{O2}$$

where M_{O_2} is oxygen uptake, $\dot{Q}_R$ and $\dot{Q}_B$ are pulmonary and pulmonary collateral blood flows respectively, Ca_{O_2}, Cv_{O_2} and Cb_{O_2} are concentrations of oxygen in the arterial, mixed venous and effluent collateral blood. By regrouping terms and dividing by the arterio-venous O_2 difference ($Ca_{O_2} - Cv_{O_2}$), the equation becomes:-

$$\dot{Q}_{Fick} = \dot{Q}_R + \dot{Q}_B \ (Ca_{O_2} - Cb_{O_2})/(Ca_{O_2} - Cv_{O_2})$$

where

$$\dot{Q}_{Fick} = M_{O_2}/(Ca_{O_2} - Cv_{O_2}).$$

This equation indicates that the calculated output represents right ventricular output plus an additional quantity which may or may not be equal to the collateral blood flow $\dot{Q}_B$. If $Cb_{O_2} = Ca_{O_2}$, $\dot{Q}$ Fick $= \dot{Q}_R$ and collateral blood flow is overlooked. Conversely if $Cb_{O_2} = Cv_{O_2}$, $\dot{Q}$ Fick $= \dot{Q}_R + \dot{Q}_B$ measures left ventricular output. If collateral effluent blood is more desaturated than mixed venous blood, $\dot{Q}$ Fick is larger than left ventricular output. Conversely, if the saturation of effluent collateral blood is less than Ca_{O_2} and greater than Cv_{O_2}, $\dot{Q}$ Fick is larger than $\dot{Q}_R$ and smaller than left ventricular output. Which of the above situations pertains in a given clinical situation is unknown because the actual value of Cb_{O_2} is not known.

During air-breathing the pulmonary collateral circulation has no gas-exchanging function in lung diseases because the partial pressure of oxygen in the alveoli and arterial blood are quite similar (38). Unequivocal demonstration of the absence of oxygen uptake has been obtained by use of bronchospirometry in patients in whom one lung was vascularised solely by systemic arterial blood. During ambient air-breathing there was no measurable oxygen uptake by the diseased lung (39). In order for the pulmonary collateral blood flow to participate in the gas-exchanging function of the lung two conditions are necessary. (i) arterial desaturation permitting loading of oxygen by the pulmonary collateral blood. (ii) presence of an alveolar-arterial O_2 gradient providing a pressure head for the diffusion of oxygen. The experimental approach used to demonstrate the potential for gas-exchange of the pulmonary collateral circulation and to measure "effective" pulmonary collateral blood flow in man (39) is as follows (Figure 4). The experimental procedure consists of interruption of pulmonary blood flow to the diseased lung with a balloon, bronchospirometry permitting administration of a low oxygen mixture (12% O_2 in nitrogen) to the normal lung and an enriched oxygen mixture (25% O_2 in nitrogen) to the diseased lung. This causes a fall of the arterial saturation to about

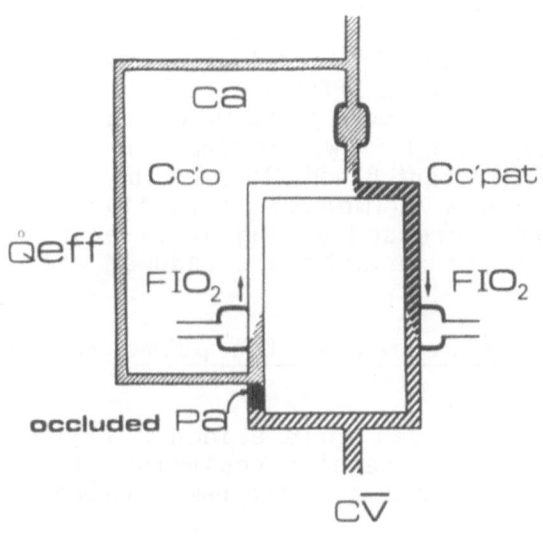

FIGURE 4   Estimation of "effective" collateral blood flow ($\dot{Q}$
eff) in unilateral lung diseases. The method
entails bronchospirometry and occlusion of the
pulmonary artery of the diseased lung.
Administration of an enriched (25%) oxygen mixture
to the occluded lung brings O_2 content in the
effluent blood $C_{c'o}$ close to the O_2 contralateral
lung whose pulmonary artery is patient lowers O_2
content of both effluent blood ($C_{c'pat}$) and of
collateral pathways. Also measured is the oxygen
uptake of the occluded lung. $\dot{Q}$ eff is calculated by
the usual Fick formula.

70% and a rise to about 135 mmHg of the partial pressure of oxygen in the diseased lung. By application of the Fick formula to the diseased lung "effective" pulmonary collateral flow was calculated. In 3 of 6 patients with temporary occlusion of one pulmonary artery and in 1 of 2 patients with permanent occlusion the oxygen uptake of the diseased lung was too low for calculation of blood flow by the Fick principle. In the remaining 4 patients effective collateral flows ranging from 0.19 to 0.95 $1.min^{-1}$ were found which represented 3 to 9% of total pulmonary blood flow. Whether these figures can be extrapolated to represent blood flows during air breathing is uncertain since both pulmonary blood flow and pulmonary arterial pressure increased during unilateral hypoxia and pulmonary collateral vessels are endowed with vasomotor activity.

Haemodynamic consequences of the pulmonary collateral left-to-right shunt

All-in-all the available evidence suggests that an expanded pulmonary collateral circulation in chronic lung disease does not constitute a haemodynamic burden for the left ventricle (38).

Distal anastomosis between systemic arteries and pulmonary arteries represent a potential cause of error in the measurement of pulmonary wedge pressure (40). For pulmonary wedge pressure to represent left atrial pressure there must be no blood flow in the blocked territory. If collateral channels open in the blocked territory, be it at the pre-capillary, capillary, or post-capillary level, pulmonary wedge pressure will be a function not only of left atrial pressure but also of the flow rate of collateral blood and of the pressure-flow relationships of the blocked portion of the pulmonary vascular bed. It is unlikely that this represents a significant cause of error in normal subjects in whom the good correlation of pulmonary wedge pressure in relation to left atrial (41) and left ventricular end-diastolic pressure (42) is well documented. Similarly pulmonary wedge pressure is well correlated with left atrial and left ventricular end-diastolic pressure in chronic bronchitis, a condition in which enlargement of the pulmonary collateral circulation is uncommon (43). I know of no such comparative studies in lung diseases associated with an enlarged pulmonary collateral circulation. I submit that in these conditions the measurement of pulmonary wedge pressure with a truly wedged open-end catheter is preferable to the measurement of pressure distal to an inflated balloon blocking a medium-size pulmonary artery, e.g. with a Swan-Ganz catheter; the smaller the blocked artery, the lesser the risk of distal opening of functional collateral channels.

PATHOPHYSIOLOGY OF THE PULMONARY COLLATERAL CIRCULATION IN MISCELLANEOUS CONDITIONS

Congenital heart disease

There is a spectrum of congenital heart diseases in which the lungs are perfused partially or solely by systemic arterial blood. In persistent truncus arteriosus a single vessel forms the outlet of both ventricles and gives rise not only to the systemic arteries but also to the pulmonary arteries. In tetralogy of Fallot stenosis of the right ventricular outflow is one of the four components of the malformation. When there is atresia of the pulmonary artery, pulmonary valve, or right ventricular infundibulum the condition may be called pseudo-truncus arteriosus. In Fallot's disease the lungs are perfused partially or entirely through enlarged systemic arteries and/or a patent ductus arteriosus. Similarly in some cases of tricuspid atresia the only route for blood to perfuse the lung is through enlarged systemic arteries. The above conditions share certain features which enable the systemic blood supply of the lung to take part or to take over the gas exchanging function of the lung. These common features are: (i) arterial oxygen unsaturation due to a coexisting right-to-left shunt; (ii) alveolar partial pressure of oxygen in the normal range or even slightly elevated due to hypoxic hyperventilation; (iii) increased alveolar-arterial O_2 gradient. Therefore, conditions for measurement with the Fick principle of pulmonary collateral blood flow ($\dot{Q}$ coll) breathing ambient air are met in theory (Figure 5). When the lungs are solely perfused by systemic arterial blood, $\dot{Q}$ coll = $M_{O_2}/(Cpv_{O_2}-Ca_{O_2})$ where Cpv_{O_2} is the O_2 content of mixed pulmonary venous blood. The latter can be taken as equal to the O_2 content of a pulmonary venous sample although it is not certain that blood sampled from one pulmonary vein is representative of mixed pulmonary venous blood. Alternatively the O_2 content of the end-capillary blood may be equated to the oxygen carrying capacity if the subject is given an enriched oxygen mixture to breathe. When the lungs are perfused by both pulmonary and systemic arterial blood, the calculation of pulmonary blood flow and of pulmonary collateral blood flow cannot be made with any degree of precision because there are too many unknowns in the mixing equation (Figure 6).

Liver Disease

Anatomical evidence of anomalous connections between the portal and pulmonary venous system in patients with cirrhosis of the liver has been shown by post-mortem vascular injection methods. In 2 of 6 satisfactory studies of cases of Laennec's

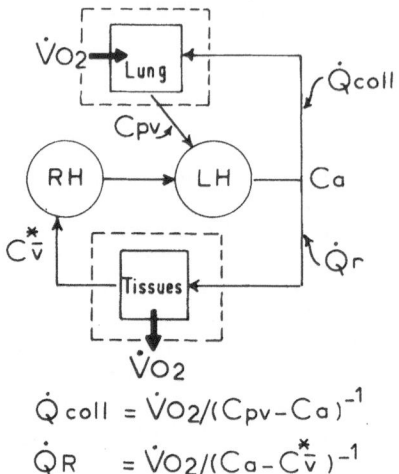

$$\dot{Q}\,coll = \dot{V}O_2/(C_{pv}-C_a)^{-1}$$

$$\dot{Q}_R \quad = \dot{V}O_2/(C_a-C\overset{*}{\bar{v}})^{-1}$$

FIGURE 5   Congenital atresia of the pulmonary artery; blood
             entering the lung (Qcoll) is entirely supplied by
             the aorta and is drained by the pulmonary veins into
             the left heart (LH). By straightforward application
             of Fick's formula to the upper box (interrupted
             lines):

$$\dot{Q}coll = V_{O2} \: / \: (Ca - C_{pv})$$

where the oxygen uptake (VO_2) and the concentration
of oxygen in arterial blood (Ca) are measurable
quantities. C_{pv} is the concentration of oxygen in
mixed pulmonary venous blood and cannot be actually
measured. It is usually assumed that it is equal to
O_2 concentration of blood sampled from an accessible
pulmonary vein. Alternatively it may be taken as
the oxygen carrying capacity of blood during
enriched oxygen breathing.

Similarly straightforward application of Fick's
formula to the tissues (lower box) yields right
ventricular output:

$$\dot{Q}_R = V_{O2} \: / \: (Ca - C^*_v)$$

in which the concentration of oxygen in mixed venous
blood (C^*_v) cannot be actually measured. It is
usually equated to the O_2 concentration of right
ventricular blood or derived by use of empirical
formulae from blood sampled from the superior and
inferior venae cavae.

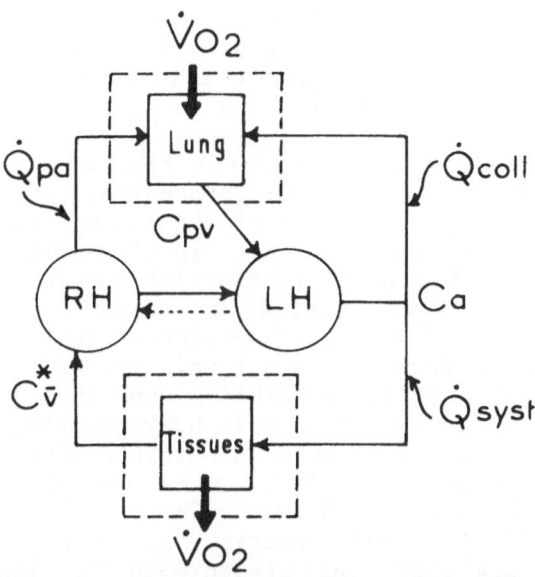

FIGURE 6   Congenital heart disease with both arterial ($\dot{Q}$coll)
and pulmonary ($\dot{Q}$pa) blood supply to the lungs.

Blood flow to the tissues ($\dot{Q}$syst) can be estimated
by Fick's formula applied to the lower box. The
concentration of oxygen in the mixed venous blood
can be measured if it is possible to catheterise the
pulmonary artery when there is no associated
left-to-right shunt (dotted arrow between left (LH)
and right heart (RH)). When the above requirements
are not mot mixed venous O_2 concentration has to be
assumed (see legend of Figure 5).

Fractionation of the blood supply to the lung in
collateral and pulmonary blood flow is not usually
possible. By application of Fick's formula to the
lung and rearrangement:

$$\dot{Q}syst = \dot{Q}pa \ \frac{C^*pv - C^*v}{Ca - Cv} + \dot{Q}coll \ \frac{Cpv - Ca}{Ca - Cv}$$

Even if the concentration of O_2 of the mixed
pulmonary venous blood and of the mixed venous blood
are assumed one is left with two unknowns, $\dot{Q}$pa and
$\dot{Q}$coll.

Bidirectional shunts create an utterly hopeless
situation in which use of the above mixing equations
is illusory.

cirrhosis, the injected material filled the pulmonary veins, left atrium and left ventricle (44). Subsequent investigators have attempted to find out whether these anastomoses carry blood in vivo, to provide a quantitative estimate of blood flowing through these channels, and to evaluate their role in the arterial hypoxaemia of cirrhosis of the liver. To investigate whether the anastomotic channels carry blood, arterial (Ca) and mixed venous (Cv) concentrations of ^{85}Kr were compared during constant infusion of the isotope into the right atrium and into the duodenum (45). In cirrhotic subjects the ratio Cv/Ca was higher with right atrial compared to duodenal infusion whereas it was similar in normal subjects. The smaller ratio when ^{85}Kr was introduced into the duodenum suggests that blood from the portal vein entered the pulmonary vascular bed of cirrhotic patients beyond the capillary bed. Confirmatory evidence for porto-pulmonary shunting in patients with cirrhosis of the liver has been obtained directly by means of splenoportography (46, 47), intrasplenic injection of diffusible or non-diffusible indicators (47 - 49) and subtraction of the pulmonary arteriovenous shunt (45) from the overall venous admixture calculated with the classical shunt equation during 50% oxygen breathing (50). The results suggest that porto-pulmonary shunting expressed as a percentage of cardiac output is increased in a minority of cases of portal hypertension. The highest porto-pulmonary shunt ratios which have been reported range from 5.4% cirrhotics and 3.9% in normal subjects (50) to 14.4% in cirrhotics compared to zero in control subjects (49). Taking into account the high oxygen saturation of portal blood, these figures support the conclusion that shunting of portal blood is not large enough to account for the arterial hypoxaemia commonly found in liver cirrhosis except in a few individual cases (49, 50).

SUMMARY

In normal lung bronchial blood flow amounts to about 1 - 2% of left ventricular output and drains for the most part into pulmonary veins. The bronchial circulation is a nutrient circulation and it may also be an important route for blood-borne agents influencing effectors in the lung such as bronchial smooth muscle and glands.

In various disorders of the lung, for instance bronchiectasis, lung carcinoma and pulmonary emboli, performed bronchial arteries and newly formed bronchial, mediastinal and intercostal arteries undergo a remarkable proliferation and cause a marked increase in the collateral circulation of the lung. It should be emphasised that the latter does not participate to alveolar gas exchange as long as there is no arterial hypoxaemia.

The collateral circulation of the lung increases left ventricular output above right ventricular output and causes arterial contamination of mixed venous blood in diseased areas of the lung. Thus, measurement of cardiac output in lung diseases known to be associated with an increased collateral lung circulation is fraught with difficulties. In the presence of hypoxaemia lung collateral circulation participates to alveolar gas exchange; in fact it is the principal and in some instances the only source of pulmonary blood flow for gas exchange in certain congenital diseases with an hypoplastic or atretic pulmonary artery.

The collateral lung circulation is the most frequent source of haemoptysis in lung disease; embolisation of the enlarged systemic vessels has proved useful in treating life-threatening or repeated haemoptysis not amenable to surgical treatment.

REFERENCES

1.   I. de Burgh Daly and C.Hebb.
         Bronchial vascular system.
         in: "Pulmonary and Bronchial Vascular Systems", Edward
         Arnold Ltd., London (1966).

2.   A. A. Liebow,
         Patterns of origin and distribution of the major
         bronchial arteries in man.
         Am. J. Anat., 117, 19, (1965).

3.   J. Delarue, Ch. Sors, J. Mignot et J. Paillas.
         Lesions bronchopulmonaires et modifications circulatoires.
         Presse med., 63, 173, (1955).

4.   L. E. Fahri and H. Rahn,
         A theoretical analysis of the alveolar-arterial oxygen

         difference with special reference to the
         distribution effect.
         J. appl. Physiol., 7, 699, (1955).

5.   J. B. West.,
         Ventilation-perfusion ratio inequality and
         overall gas exchange.
         In: "Ventilation/blood flow and gas exchange".
         Blackwell Scientific Publications, Oxford (1977).

6.   H. W. Fritts,Jr., P. Harris, C. A. Chidsey, R. H. Clauss
         and A. Cournand.
         Estimation of flow through bronchial-pulmonary
         vascular anastomoses with use of T-1824 dye.
         Circulation, 23, 390, (1961).

7.   L. Cudkowicz, W. H. Abelman, G. E. Levinson,
         G. E. Katznelson and R. M. Jreissaty.
         Bronchial arterial blood flow in man.
         Clin. Sci., 19, 1, (1960).

8.   P. Aramendia, J. Martinez, L. de Letona and D. M. Aviado.
         Exchange of blood between pulmonary and systemic
         circulations via bronchopulmonary anastomoses.
         Circulation Res., 11, 870, (1962).

9.   F. H. Ellis Jr., J. H. Grindly, and J. E. Edwards.
         The bronchial artery. I. Experimental occlusion.
         Surgery, 30, 810, (1951).

10. J. Remy, A. Arnaud, H. Fardou, R. Giraud, and C. Voisin.
       Treatment of hemoptysis by embolization of bronchial
       arteries.
       Radiology, 122, 33, (1977).

11. N. L. Mills, A. D. Boyd and C. Gheranpong.
       The significance of bronchial circulation in lung
       transplantation.
       J. Thorac. Cardiovasc. Surg., 60, 866, (1970).

12. F. J. Veith, M. Torres, I. Colon, K. Pinsker,
       S. K. Koerner, R. Crane and D. Paulson.
       Transplantation of the left lung into the right
       hemithorax to facilitate immediate reconstitution of
       bronchial artery flow.
       J. Thorac. Cardiovasc. Surg., 75, 141, (1978).

13. F. G. Pearson, M. Goldberg, R. M. Stone and
       R. F. Colapinto.
       Bronchial arterial circulation restored after
       reimplantation of canine lung.
       Can. J. Surg., 13, 243, (1970).

14. S. S. Siegelman, J. W. C. Hagstrom, S. K. Koerner
       and F. J. Veith.
       Restoration of bronchial artery circulation after
       canine lung allotransplantation.
       J. thorac. Cardiovasc. Surg., 73, 792, (1977).

15. J. Y. Neveux, J. Bignon, T. Oancea, C. Rioux
       et J. Mathey.
       Devenir de la circulation arterielle bronchique apres
       auto-transplantation pulmonaire.
       Ann. Chir. thorac. cardiovasc., 7, 559, (1968).

16. A. A. Liebow.
       Recent observations on pulmonary collateral
       circulation.
       Med. thorac., 19, 609, (1962).

17. D. J. Armstrong and J. C. Luck.
       Accessibility of pulmonary stretch receptors from the
       pulmonary and bronchial circulations.
       J. appl. Physiol., 36, 706, (1974).

18. G. G. Pietra, J. P. Szidon, M. M. Leventhal and
     A. P. Fishman.
     Histamine and interstitial pulmonary oedema
     in the dog.
     Circulation Res., 24, 323, (1971).

19. E. C. Deal Jr., E. R. McFadden Jr., R. H. Ingram Jr.
     and J. J. Jaeger.
     Esophageal temperature during exercise in asthmatics and
     non asthmatic subjects.
     J. appl. Physiol. Respir. Environ. Exercise Physiol.
     46, 484, (1979).

20. J. G. Roosenburg and M. Deenstra.
     Bronchial-pulmonary vascular shunts in chronic
     pulmonary affections.
     Dis. Chest.., 26, 664, (1954).

21. P. Harris and D. Heath.
     The form of bronchopulmonary anaestomoses.
     In: "The human pulmonary circulation".
     Churchill, Livingstone, Edinburgh, London
     and New York (1977).

22. J. R. Williams and F. J. Bonte.
     Bronchial arteriography.
     Radiology, 78, 234, (1962).

23. T. H. Newton and L. Preger.
     Selective bronchial arteriography.
     Radiology, 84, 1043, (1965).

24. E. Boijsen and M. Zsigmond.
     Selective angiography of bronchial and intercostal
     arteries.
     Acta Radiologica, 3, 513, (1965).

25. Ch. Gernez-Rieux, J. Remy, C. Voisin, J. M. Rousselle
     and C: Wallaert.
     L'arteriographic bronchique selective.
     J. franc. Med. Chir. thorac., 21, 463, (1967).

26. J. Remy, P. Beguery, T. Froment and J. L. Denies.
     La vascularisation systemique du poumon: technique
     d'exploration et anatomie radiologique appliquees
     au diagnostic topographique des hemoptysies.
     Ann. Radiol., 18, 85, (1975).

27. S. F. Boushy, A. H. Helgason and L. B. North.
        Occlusion of the bronchial arteries.
        Am. Rev. resp. Dis., 103, 249, (1971).

28. J. Remy, A. Arnaud, H. Fardou, R. Giraud and C. Voisin.
        Treatment of hemoptysis by embolization of bronchial
        arteries.
        Radiology, 122, 33, (1977).

29. T. Ishihara, M. Inoue, K. Kobayashi, M. Murakami,
        T. Ikeda, K. Kikuchi, and H. Yoshimatsu.
        Selective bronchial arteriography and hemoptysis
        in non malignant lung disease.
        Chest, 66, 633, (1974).

30. M. Daussy et R. Abelanet.
        Modifications circulaoires de certains poumons
        pathologiques: Donnees hemodynamiques.
        J. franc. Med. Chir. thorac., 10, 305, (1956).

31. L. Cudkowicz and D. G. Wraith.
        A method of study of the pulmonary circulation in
        finger clubbing.
        Thorax, 12, 13, (1957).

32. A. A. Liebow, M. R. Hales and G. E. Lindskog,
        Enlargement of the bronchial arteries and their
        anastomoses with the pulmonary arteries in
        bronchiectasis.
        Am. J. Pathol., 25, 211, (1949).

33. G. G. Rowe, C. A. Castillo, G. Maxwell, R. J. Botham
        and C. W. Crumpton.
        Pulmonary wedge position as a site for injection of
        indicator-dilution substances.
        Circulation, 20, 760, (1959). Abstract.

34. E. H. Wood.
        Diagnostic applications of indicator-dilution
        techniques in congenital heart disease.
        Circulation Res., 10, 531, (1962).

35. A. Fonseca Costa, G. Noronha Andrade, Z.P. Coutinho,
        and H. E. Jouval.
        Method for evaluation of systemic to pulmonary artery
        pre-capillary shunts.
        Bull. Physiopath. resp., 6, 265, (1970).

36. W. Valladares, B. Ranson-Bitker, J. Mensch-Dechene
         et A. Lockhart.
         La circulation collaterale pulmonaire dans le cancer
         du poumon. Une cause d'errlur dans la mesure du
         debit carchaque par les indicateurs.
         Bull. europ. Physiopath. resp., 12, 715, (1976).

37. H. W. Fritts Jr and A. Cournand.
         The application of the Fick principle to the
         measurement of pulmonary blood flow.
         Proc. nat. Acad. Sci., 44, 1079, (1958).

38. A. P. Fishman.
         The clinical significance of the pulmonary collateral
         circulation.
         Circulation, 24, 677, (1961).

39. A. P. Fishman, G. M. Turino, M. Brandfonbener
         and A. Himmelstein.
         The 'effective' pulmonary collateral blood flow
         in man.
         J. clin. Invest., 37, 1071, (1958).

40. F. Herles.
         The pulmonary artery wedge pressure. Its origin and
         value in assessing pulmonary haemodynamics in
         emphysema.
         Cor Vasa, 8, 161, (1966).

41. A. Walton and M. E. Kendall.
         Comparison of pulmonary wedge and left atrial
         pressure in man.
         Am. Heart. J., 86, 159, (1973).

42. R. P. Sapru, S. H. Taylor and K. W. Donald.
         Comparison of the pulmonary wedge pressure with the
         left ventricular end-diastolic pressure in man.
         Clin. Sci., 34, 125, (1968).

43. A. Lockhart.
         Fonction du ventricule gauche dans la bronchite
         chronique.
         Bull. Physiopath. resp., 8, 1448, (1972).

44. P. Calabresi and W. H. Ablemann.
     Porto-caval and porto-pulmonary anaestomoses
     in Laennec's cirrhosis and in heart failure.
     J. clin. Invest., 36, 1257, (1957).

45. H. W. Fritts Jr., A. Hardewig, D. F. Rochester, J. Durand
     and A. Cournand.
     Estimation of pulmonary arteriovenous shunt-flow
     using intravenous injections of T-1824 dye and Kr^{85}.
     J. clin. Invest., 39, 1841, (1960).

46. S. Shaldon, J. Caesar, L. Chiandussi, H. S. Williams,
     E. Sheville and S. Sherlock.
     Demonstration of porto-pulmonary anaestomoses in
     portal cirrhosis with the use of radioactive
     krypton (Kr^{85}).
     New England J. Med., 265, 410, (1961).

47. J. H. Williams and W. H. Abelmann.
     Portopulmonary shunts in patients with portal
     hypertension.
     J. Lab. clin. Med., 62, 715, (1963).

48. K. Mellemgaard, K. Winkler, N. Tygstrup and J. Georg.
     Sources of venoarterial admixture in portal
     hypertension.
     J. clin. Invest., 42, 1399, (1963).

49. T. Nakamura, S. Nakamura, T. Tazawa, S. Abe, T. Aikawa
     and K. Tokita.
     Measurement of blood flow through portopulmonary
     anastomosis in portal hypertension.
     J. Lab. clin. Med., 65, 114, (1965).

50. A. Chiesa, G. Ciappi, L. Balbi and L. Chiandussi.
     Role of various causes of. arterial desaturation
     in liver cirrhosis.
     Clin. Sci., 37, 803, (1969).

Discussion

RIEDEL: Your proposal for a blood gas analysis for quantitative measurement is subject to error. But there is a perfect method which I would like to propose to you which measures this precisely. Simply, if you inject dye into the ascending aorta and sample it from the mitral valve by catheter then under normal conditions you get only the recirculation after let's say 15 seconds or so. With increased bronchial collateral circulation one obtains a curve which can be quantitatively measured and which represents only the bronchial collateral circulation, provided that patent ductus is excluded. So, if you measure cardiac output by dye dilution into the pulmonary artery and sampling from any peripleural artery, and you deduct this collateral flow, the output of the right and the left ventricles is obtained separately. This method can measure up to 0.5% of cardiac output, and it was found in patients with chronic pulmonary hypertension due to thromboembolic disease there is a bronchial collateral circulation as much as 50% of cardiac output.

LOCKHART: If I may have my last reserve slide, please. I think you are quite right. This is work I did some twenty years ago when I was still a cardiologist working with infants and congenital heart diseases. This is a schematic drawing of the aortic arch and arterial sampling carried out in the left brachial artery and this is a curve of congenital heart disease with no patent ductus arteriosis, as proved by subsequent surgery. Now, if one injects dye here one gets first a direct passage of blood, first that in the artery and then recirculation, early recirculation. If one injects dye here a similar pattern shows. If one injects blood here, in this artery, blood backflow takes place and blood can be sampled from the left brachial artery, which is here.   In a normal aorta, sampling from the left brachial artery, nothing is found following injection in the descending aorta and this shows the marked flow from the collateral bronchial circulation.   Now as you suggest, sampling proximally to this point in the left atrium may provide a better curve than this one, which can be used for calculation of flow. But I think you are quite right. Proper use of dye curves in rather sophisticated studies can enable one to get estimates of flow. I know this to be so by the accuracy of your method, because in my hands the reproducibility of dye output at intervals of a few minutes is not so precise perhaps plus or minus ten per cent.

DENISON: Like the previous speaker I enjoyed the clarity of your talk. Now, many of his arguments rested on the assumption that bronchial flow enters the pulmonary circulation upstream of the lung, and yet we heard from Keith Horsfield this morning that in normal lungs at least this was not provable. I m sorry to be ignorant, but is there good evidence that much bronchial flow enters the lung upstream of the capillary bed in disease? The second question concerns Fishman's estimation of shunt flow - he made one lung hypoxic in order to measure the flow to the other lung. Yet, as we all know, if you make one lung hypoxic you force blood through the other lung, so perhaps it is not an especially accurate method for measuring it and I'd like your comment on that. And the third question: you showed at the beginning of your talk dye dilution curves in which dye was injected into the pulmonary artery, but I did not hear where the blood was sampled from which produced the curves, and of course that might help you answer the first question. Thank you.

LOCKHART: The third one is the easiest one to answer; blood was sampled from the brachial artery. Now, answering the first question. I think that in most instances of abnormally developed collateral lung circulation, be it from pre-existing vessels, bronchial vessels, or new formed vessels coming in the lung from either mediastinal or thoracic wall, or even newly formed bronchial vessels from the artery as in most acquired lung diseases, there is good evidence that the blood reaches the pulmonary artery bed proximal to the capillaries. This is documented by the fact, as I have shown on the slide to which you refer, that if you inject dye distal to the balloon occluding the pulmonary artery, blood is washed away. Whereas if the blood was coming distal to the capillary bed my guess would be that it would just sit in there, and not be moved away by incoming blood. Secondly, if one samples blood from the PA in a diseased area one gets very often blood that can be as high in its oxygen content as arterial blood. And in fact it has been proposed by Liebow that inflowing blood from the collateral circulation would divert blood to non diseased areas. Third piece of evidence: bronchial arterial angiography which very often shows a back-filling of the pulmonary artery in the area of enlarged collateral arterial supply. Regarding your second question, I may have used a word I did not intend to use. I don't think Al Fishman has actually measured; he has provided some sort of estimate, because, as you rightly say, making one lung severely hypoxic would alter considerably the distribution of blood in the lesser circulation.

HEATH: Well, I would just like to say that I support Denison absolutely in what he just said. I think, for example, in portal-pulmonary anastomosis that the morbid anatomist can actually demonstrate the presence of this anastomosis by naked eye vision. Now, you can do this very easily in rats by giving them cirrhosis of the liver and the mechanism is as follows and one can see this under the microscope. It goes along the stomach wall, up the side of the oesophagus, penetrates the lung as mediastinal veins and the veins, as Liebow suspected, form anastomoses, not with arteries, not with capillaries, but with veins. So that when that blood gets into the lung it gets into the lung at the pulmonary vein at the first place.

It never gets anywhere near the capillary bed. And that's why when
I was listening to what you are saying and quoting Japanese authors,
it struck me as very odd that you were saying that the degree of
oxygen saturation was unrelated to the amount of anastomosis,
because I just can't conceive of that.

LOCKHART: Well, I tried to be very careful and separate very
sharply acquired lung diseases on the one hand, in which I believe
that most of the evidence favours precapillary anastomosis versus
cirrhosis of the liver, which I treated separately, in which I
entirely agree that anastomoses are mainly postcapillary. What the
Japanese work tends to show is either that there is no close
relationship between the amount of shunting and the unsaturation, or
that the technique of estimation of collateral blood flow which they
used is unreliable. And I think that this is what actually happens.

EVEN: Radioactive albumen shows absolutely no imaging and probably
they are drained directly in pulmonary veins and systemic arteries.
And the third situation, 'there is a retrograde flow towards
pulmonary arteries, and the microspheres are redistributed not in
the injected territory, but the other territory of the lung.

LOCKHART: May I ask what is the size of the microsphered?

EVEN: One microsphere is 50 microns.

LOCKHART: Now, 50 microns can go somewhat through a normal lung
circulation.

CUMMING: But not to the capillaries.

LOCKHART: Part of them can escape through the lung circulation.

A NEW APPROACH FOR CLINICAL STUDY OF CONTROL OF RESPIRATION

J. Milic-Emili, M. Aubier, A. Grassino, and
J.-Ph. Derenne
Department of Physiology and Meakins Christie
Laboratories, McGill University
Montreal, Canada

Most acute and chronic lung diseases are accompanied by hyperventilation, usually in the form of rapid, shallow breathing. This pattern occurs in patients with acute pulmonary vascular congestion and edema, and has been linked with increased J-receptors discharge.[1,2] However, CO_2 retention in acute pulmonary edema is not uncommon. The reasons why some patients with edema develop CO_2 retention are not clear. Arterial P_{CO_2} was found not to be correlated with roentgenographic abnormality, P_{aO_2}, or survival.[3] Further, CO_2 retention was not related to the ventilatory response to CO_2 measured after the edema had resolved.[4] In chronic pulmonary congestion due to mitral stenosis resting ventilation is high and P_{aCO_2} low, while the ventilatory response to CO_2 is lower than normal.[5] After corrective surgery, resting ventilation in two patients with mitral stenosis decreased and the ventilatory response to CO_2 increased.[5] It is not known whether lung function tests improved following surgery.

To our knowledge, this about summarizes the scanty studies of control of breathing in patients with congested lungs and pulmonary edema. Clearly, further work is needed in this relatively neglected area of respiratory physiopathology. In the present account we will review recent advances in the study of control of breathing which may usefully be applied to patients with lung congestion and edema.

Although a good number of lung function tests are now performed routinely in most hospitals, the clinical assessment of abnormalities in the regulation of breathing is in general limited to measurements of arterial blood gases. The last few years, however, have seen an explosion of interest in regulation of breathing with

a welcome clinical orientation to the subject. Indeed, two clinically applicable, simple and rapid methods for measuring the ventilatory response to carbon dioxide[6] and hypoxia[7] have been described.
Neither of these methods, however, is capable of differentiating
patients who will not breathe because of central or neuromuscular
inadequacy from those who cannot breathe because of abnormalities
of the chest, such as airways obstruction or decreased compliance
of the respiratory system. Furthermore, there has been accumulating
evidence which indicates that the assessment of the respiratory
response to acute hypoxia and hypercapnia does not always provide
an explanation for the abnormal blood gas composition observed
in many patients during room air breathing at rest. In fact, it
seems to us that in the past too much attention has been paid in
studying respiratory responses to hypoxia and hypercapnia.

In the present paper, we describe a method which focuses on
assessment of control of respiration during natural breathing at
rest, and which permits to separate patients who will not breathe
because of inadequate neuromuscular drive from patients who cannot
breathe because of altered mechanical properties of the ventilatory
pump.

Measurement of respiratory mechanical work[8,9], oxygen cost of
breathing[10] and diaphragmatic electromyograph[11] have been proposed
in the past to separate the above two categories of patients. These
measurements, however, are time consuming, technically complex and
cause patient discomfort, for they involve the use of esophageal
balloons and electrodes.

More recently, measurement of the mouth occlusion pressure
has been proposed as a useful alternative.[12] This technique has
the advantage of being non-invasive, and requires relatively simple
equipment. Coupled with a detailed analysis of the spirogram and
with measurement of the classical variables which characterize gas
exchange within the lungs (CO_2 production and physiological dead
space), the mouth occlusion pressure provides a useful tool for
assessment of the factors causing abnormal blood gas composition,
e.g.,retention of CO_2. This last point will be illustrated using
results obtained in patients with chronic obstructive lung disease
(COLD) in stable clinical and functional state[13] and in acute
respiratory failure.[19]

Control of Breathing in Chronic Phase of COLD

It has been known for a long time that some patients with COLD
develop CO_2 retention while others do not. A number of hypotheses
have been advanced in the past to explain this difference. These
include a selective depression of the respiratory center,[15] increased
inspiratory mechanical work,[16] altered function of the peripheral
chemoreceptors,[17] lower pulmonary compliance,[18] and decreased

central responsiveness to CO_2.

A more logical approach to this problem has been proposed by Šorli et al.[13] Their analysis was centered on the inverse relationship between arterial P_{CO_2} (P_{aCO_2}) and effective alveolar ventilation:

$$P_{aCO_2} = \frac{K \times V_{CO_2}}{\dot{V}_E \ (1-V_D/V_T)}$$

where $\dot{V}_{CO_2}$ is metabolic CO_2 production, $\dot{V}_E$ is minute ventilation, V_D is physiological dead space, V_T is tidal volume, and K is a constant.

In 15 clinically and functionally stable COLD patients (8 without CO_2 retention and 7 with elevated P_{aCO_2}) Šorli et al.[13]   found that the main characteristic of the patients with CO_2 retention was a significantly lower tidal volume (Table 1). Both V_D and $\dot{V}_{CO_2}$ were nearly identical in the two groups of patients, while $\dot{V}_E$ was somewhat lower in the hypercapnic group, although the difference was not statistically significant. Similar results have been described by Burrows et al.[18]

On the basis of the above results, it is logical to ask what is the nature of the decrease in V_T in the hypercapnic patients. This could be due to decreased pressure developed by the inspiratory muscles. To investigate this point, measurements of $P_{0.1}$, that is the mouth pressure developed 0.1 sec after the onset of an occluded inspiration at functional residual capacity, are most appropriate. This pressure, whose technical details are described elsewhere,[12] is an index of the rate at which pressure (or force) is generated by the inspiratory muscles. As shown in Fig.1, on the average, there is no difference in $P_{0.1}$ between hypercapnic and non-hypercapnic COLD patients. In both, $P_{0.1}$ is two to three times greater than in normal individuals. Thus, COLD patients with and without CO_2 retention appear to be "fighters," in the sense that they all increase the activity of their inspiratory muscles in an attempt to overcome the increased mechanical impedance of the respiratory system caused by their disease. This is contrary to previous notions whereby it was hypothesized that patients with CO_2 retention were "non-fighters."[20]

As $P_{0.1}$ does not appear to differ between COLD patients with and without CO_2 retention, the reduction of V_T in patients with elevated P_{aCO_2} must be explained in an alternate way. As shown in the lower panels of Fig.1, the reduced V_T in patients with CO_2 retention is due to a shortening of duration of inspiration (T_I). One also sees in Fig.1 that the mean inspiratory flow (V_T/T_I) is virtually identical in the two groups of patients, and in both slightly higher than in normal individuals.

Table 1. Comparison of respiratory variables between non-hypercapnic and hypercapnic COLD patients in stable state. (After Šorli et al.[13]).

	$\dot{V}_{CO_2}$ (ml/min)	$\dot{V}_E$ (1/min)	V_D (ml)	V_T (ml)	$PaCO_2$ (mmHg)
Non-hypercapnic	260	10.6	370	710	38
Hypercapnic	280	9.4	320	560	50
P	NS	NS	NS	<0.01	<0.005

The mouth occlusion pressure is an index of neuromuscular inspiratory drive for it represents the pressure potentially available for inspiration. The mean inspiratory flow, on the other hand, is a measure of the resulting flow. For a given rate of rise of mouth occlusion pressure ($P_{0.1}$), the mean inspiratory flow will clearly drop as lung compliance decreases and/or flow resistance increased. In fact, by dividing $P_{0.1}$ by V_T/T_I an index of inspiratory impedance is obtained, and $P_{0.1}/(V_T/T_I)$ has been termed "effective" inspiratory impedance.[13] This did not differ significantly between the hypercapnic and non-hypercapnic COLD patients in Fig.1. In both, it was markedly higher than in normal individuals. These results suggest that CO_2 retention in COLD is not related to a high value of inspiratory impedance but rather to a shortening of inspiratory duration. The latter may be caused by inspiration-inhibiting reflexes originating from the lungs [1,2,13] or chest wall.[21] Clearly, further studies are required to elucidate this phenomenon which appears to be crucial in determining CO_2 retention in COLD patients.

Control of Breathing in COLD Patients during Acute Respiratory Failure

The results obtained by Derenne et al.[14] in 20 patients are shown in Table 2. All patients had marked hypoxemia and hypercapnia. One can see that even in acute failure minute volume is not significantly different from normal. On the other hand, the acutely ill patients have a markedly reduced V_T. The reduction in V_T is not caused by decreased neuromuscular inspiratory drive as the mean inspiratory flow (V_T/T_I) is higher in patients in spite of the marked airway obstruction which characterizes acute respiratory failure in COLD. In fact, the $P_{0.1}$ values were five times greater than in the normal individuals. This implies a markedly increased central inspiratory activity, and not a central depression as commonly thought. Because ventilation is maintained at the expense of increased inspiratory muscle activity, one may expect that in the long range these patients may develop respiratory muscle fatigue. However, at the time of the study the principal cause of the reduced V_T was a shortening of inspiratory duration. One can see from Equation 1 that the smaller is V_T, the greater is Pa_{CO_2}. One can also see that with a small V_T relatively small changes in V_D will have a considerable effect on Pa_{CO_2} if the V_D/V_T ratio is high to start with.

CONCLUSION

This brief review illustrates that with the newly developed approach for clinical study of control of breathing one can better detect the causes of abnormal control of breathing than in the past. Having located the main cause of CO_2 retention in COLD, namely shortened T_I, one can better plan further experiments designed to elucidate the nature of this shortening. Thus, new

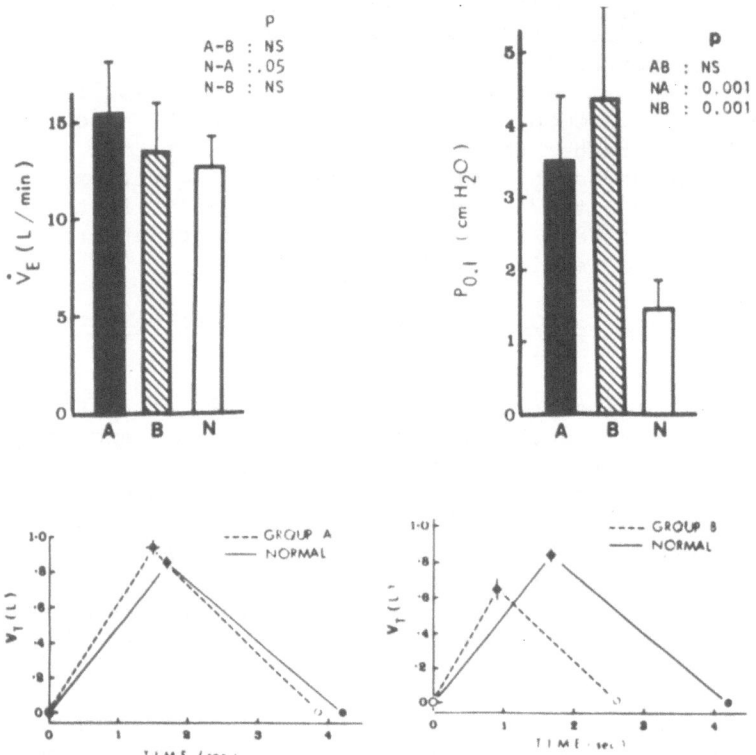

Fig. 1. <u>Above</u>: Mean values (± SD) for ventilation ($\dot{V}_E$)and $P_{0.1}$
in non-hypercapnic (A) and hypercapnic (B) COLD patients
in stable phase, and in normal individuals (N).
<u>Below</u>: Schematic spirograms. Bars indicate SEM. Mean
inspiratory flow (V_T/T_I) is represented by the slopes of
the ascending limbs of the spirograms.(From Grassino
et al.[19]).

Table 2. Comparison of respiratory variables between COLD patients in acute failure and normal individuals (After Derenne et al[14]).

	Pa_{O_2} (mmHg)	Pa_{CO_2} (mmHg)	$\dot{V}_E$ (1/min)	V_T (ml)	f (cpm)	T_I (sec)	V_T/T_I (ml/sec)
Patients	36.5	61	11.4	376	31.6	0.69	563
Normals	80.9	37.6	12.4	778	17.2	1.72	484
P	<0.001	<0.001	NS	<0.001	<0.001	<0.001	NS

progress can be made in both knowledge of the factors leading to abnormalities in control of breathing and its treatment.

REFERENCES

1. A. Guz, M.I.M. Noble, J.H. Eisele, and D. Trenchard, Experimental results of vagal block in cardiopulmonary disease, in: "Breathing: Hering Breuer Centenary Symposium," Ciba Foundation, J. & A. Churchill,London (1970).

2. A. S. Paintal, The mechanism of excitation of type J receptors, and the J reflex, in: "Breathing: Hering-Breuer Centenary Symposium," Ciba Foundation, J. & A. Churchill, London (1970).

3. A. Aberman and M. Fulop, The metabolic and respiratory acidosis of acute pulmonary edema, Ann. Int. Med. 76: 173 (1972).

4. M. Spierer,The ventilatory response to carbon dioxide in patients who have recovered from cardiogenic pulmonary edema, Clin. Sci. Molec. Med. 47: 285 (1974).

5. H. G. Pauli, F.E. Noe, and E. O. Coates, Ventilatory response to carbon dioxide in mitral disease, Br. Heart J. 22: 255 (1960).

6. D.J.C. Read, A. Clinical method for assessing the ventilatory response to carbon dioxide, Australas Ann. Med. 16: 20 (1967).

7. A. S. Rebuck, E.J.M. Campbell, A clinical method for assessing the ventilatory response to hypoxia, Am. Rev. Resp. Dis. 109: 345 (1974).

8. D. Brodovsky, J.A. MacDonell and R.M. Cherniack, The respiratory response to carbon dioxide in health and in emphysema, J. Clin. Invest. 39: 724.(1960).

9. J. Milic-Emili, and J.M. Tyler, Relation between work output of respiratory muscles and end-tidal CO_2 tension, J. Appl. Physiol. 18: 497 (1963).

10. R. M. Cherniack, The oxygen consumption and efficiency of the respiratory muscles in health and emphysema, J. Clin. Invest. 38: 494 (1959).

11. R. V. Lourenço, and J. M. Miranda, Drive and performance of the ventilatory apparatus in chronic obstructive lung disease, N. Engl. J. Med. 279: 53 (1968).

12. W.A. Whitelaw, J.-Ph. Derenne, and J. Milic-Emili, Occlusion pressure as a measure of respiratory center output in conscious man, Respir. Physiol. 23: 181 (1975).

13. J. Šorli, A. Grassino, G. Lorange, and J. Milic-Emili, Control of breathing in patients with chronic obstructive lung disease, Clin. Sci. Molec. Med. 54: 295 (1978).

14. J.-Ph.Derenne, M. Aubier, D. Murciano, M. Fournier, and R. Pariente, Hypoxic contribution to central respiratory drive in acute and chronic respiratory failure, Bull. Eur. Physiopath. Resp. 13: 130 (1977).

15. A.P. Fishman, P. Samet, and A. Cournand, Ventilatory drive in chronic emphysema, Am. J. Med. 19: 533 (1955).
16. S. S. Park, Factors responsible for carbon dioxide retention in chronic obstructive lung disease, Am. Rev. Resp. Dis. 92: 245 (1965).
17. W. Kepron, and R.M. Cherniack, The ventilatory response to hypercapnia and to hypoxemia in chronic obstructive lung disease, Am. Rev. Resp. Dis. 108: 843 (1973).
18. B. Burrows, F.B. Saksena, and C.F. Diener, Carbon dioxide tension and ventilatory mechanics in chronic obstructive lung disease, Ann. Intern. Med. 65: 685 (1966).
19. A. E. Grassino, J. Šorli, G. Lorange, and J. Milic-Emili, Respiratory drive and timing in chronic obstructive pulmonary disease, Chest, 73: (suppl.) 290 (1978).
20. E. D. Robin, and R. P. O'Neil, The fighter versus the non-fighter, Archiv. Environ. Health, 7: 125 (1963).
21. J. E. Remmers, and I. Mortilla, Action of intercostal muscle efferents on the respiratory rhythm of anesthetized cats, Respirat. Physiol. 24: 31 (1975).

Discussion

BONSIGNORE: Gordon Cumming. You discuss always when you hear
about closing volume, about the closure of peripheral airways. I
should like to stimulate you to discuss.

CUMMING: May I begin by making a comment. If breathing at
residual volume causes closure of dependent airways, then the gas
beyond comes rapidly into equilibrium with mixed venous blood, which
is hypoxemic. Is it your suggestion that because there is local
hypoxemia, that there is a shunting away of blood into the other
parts of the lung?

MILIC EMILI: Yes, that's what I am trying to say.

CUMMING: Therefore what would be the consequence - that if you
measure the arterial oxygen tension during this manoeuver, it would
first diminish and then restore itself to normal.
MILIC EMILI: Did you find that?

CUMMING: No, we did not. Perhaps I could talk about this in the
paper tomorrow, which follows on directly from your paper and shows
that there are even more difficulties than you have suggested.

LOCKHART: You described a very nice phenomenon in subjects holding
their breath at different lung volume. Now, my question is, will
such phenomenon take place in a normal breathing subject or, to word
it in a different manner, are the time constants of this phenomenon
which you described short enough for them to take place during the
cyclic changes in volume with normal breathing?

MILIC EMILI: Suppose that instead of breathing normally I breathe
a tidal volume from residual volume, for the phenomenon to be
present we must breathe in a range of lung volume where there is a
reclosure. Now, you are saying, suppose that I close some airways
during expiration and then reopen them during inspiration. What's
going to happen then? My suggestion would be that there is partial
airways closure during expiration, reopening during inspiration.
During one part of the cycle, there will be compression of the
capillaries and decreased blood flow. I think that this phenomenon
is only of academic interest. All I am trying to say is that when
you go to residual volume there is the development of a zone I in
the lower part of the lung. There is no mystery to what is
happening. So we still have the three zones as originally
described.

ZARDINI: Its not that I want to take up the defence of West since
I think that competing with Milic on this would be difficult. I do

think that zone 4 exists not out of solidarity with West, I am
convinced that it does exist and that it becomes exacerbated
especially when there is perivascular oedema and that therefore the
extra-alveolar vessels have a considerable importance. I am also
convinced that in the normal lung, the error is often the background
and is a result of the level at which one starts in order to
measure. And therefore here you are in agreement with me that at
total lung capacity the lung is in zone 2 for the most part.

MILIC EMILI: Yes, it is in Zone 2.

ZARDINI: The experiment carried out by Antoniesen which is the
measurement of the various pressures at the different degrees of
lung expansion, was also carried out by us, pretty much at the same
time. It hasn't been cited because you don't read Italian works -
they are never cited - we measured the pressure by means of a
catheter in the pulmonary artery and then measured this at the
various lung volumes before carrying out a radioscan with radio
active Xenon. Now, I agree with you as regards the increase of
pulmonary arterial pressure at total lung capacity and the more so I
am convinced, because I have measured this several times, of the
large increase in wedge pressure after forced expiration. Hence my
conviction, seen in the work published in the Italian Journal of
Experimental Biology, that at total lung capacity the lung works for
the most part in Zone 2 and that on the other hand, after forced
expiration, it works mostly in Zone 3. I find it difficult to admit
to Zone 1 in the lower part of the lung, but on the other hand, your
explanation is very convincing. As regards the distribution of
blood flow at the various degrees of expansion of the lung (and here
also I have an article published by Minervs Medica in January 1967)
where we show a distribution similar to that shown by Michael
Hughes' work in 1968. We were concerned with this problem because
at the beginning it seemed that there were irregularities in
distribution which didn't have a great significance. However, when
we repeated your experiment - in other words - when we examined how
the residual volume is distributed in the lung, we realised that the
distribution of the pulmonary blood flow is from the lower part to
the upper part. In other words, there is increased flow in the
apical areas at residual volume because the residual volume too was
distributed in this manner. In other words, if you inject
radioactive Xenon and you scan with a fixed scan method after forced
expiration, you will find that the residual volume is essentially in
the apical zones or medioapical zones of the lung.

MILIC EMILI: Yes, but this is very different.

ZARDINI: Yes, but you make it per alveolus rather than per unit of
volume. This is the problem. Therefore you also come up with the
explanation of why the blood flow must be in this direction. But
there is another, more important difference and this depends on how

you inspire.   In other words, the speed at which you inspire
influences the distribution of the inspired air. We have seen that
if you start from residual volume not doing this per alveolus but by
unit of volume, if you start after forced inspiration and inspire to
the maximum, much of the inspired air is distributed in the
middle-lower part, more so than when inspiration is slow.   In other
words, you have a more uniform distribution if you inhale slowly.
Perhaps the clue here is the mechanism of time constant of the
airways in the distribution of the inspired air at the various
levels?
MILIC EMILI: These measurements of gas distribution by perfusion
and by inhalation were obtained inhaling exactly in the same way.   I
think here that we are all more or less agreed that a subject with
pulmonary oedema - with the oedema situated in the lower part of the
lung - that there is a Zone 4 and in the subject with mitral
stenosis there is impared distribution in the lower part. We are
all agreed. Many people have measured this.

      However, the fact that breathing at residual volume produces a
diminution of perfusion in the lower part of the lung is not
relevant to the discussion of whether Zone 1 conditions prevail at
that time.

ACTIVE CONTROL OF THE PULMONARY CIRCULATION

Gwenda R. Barer

Department of Medicine
University of Sheffield
England

Introductory Survey

Chemical and nervous mechanisms influence the pulmonary circulation. Differences from the systemic circulation are related
to the prime function of the lung for gas exchange and the fact
that it has to transmit the whole cardiac output from right to
left ventricle. For efficient gas exchange there must be matching
of ventilation ($\dot{V}$) and blood flow ($\dot{Q}$) in individual lung units.
This regulation of $\dot{V}/\dot{Q}$ ratios is achieved to some extent by
changing O_2 and CO_2 tensions. There is, however, controversy as
to the importance and efficiency of these mechanisms. Pulmonary
vessels possess motor nerves which have been shown to constrict,
dilate or stiffen the vessels in animal experiments. Yet in man
we have no proof of any situation in which nerves function, nor
any evidence of nervous tone. In the systemic circulation blood
flow is switched from one organ to another according to need
through nervous activity. There is no evidence for a comparable
mechanism in the lung, which is uniform in function. Neither, so
far as we know, is the pulmonary circulation regulated by feedback reflexes from its sensory receptors in the way that the systemic circulation is regulated by baro and chemoreceptors. This
low pressure low resistance vascular bed is passively affected by
gravity, by changing cardiac output and by respiratory movements.
The relative importance of active and passive influences cannot be
settled at present. It is a difficult circulation to investigate
and problems will remain until we can study it under the varying
conditions of everyday life.

The fetal pulmonary circulation is a higher pressure system
than that of the adult. It has muscular pulmonary arterioles in a

high state of tone caused by low oxygen tension (PO_2), high CO_2 tension (PCO_2) and sympathetic nerve activity. These factors maintain low blood flow through the unventilated lung and divert most of the right ventricular output through the ductus arteriosus. It has been suggested that these constrictor mechanisms are important in the fetus but vestigial in the adult (Dawes, 1969). The adult pulmonary circulation seems less reactive than the fetal to all stimuli; this may be due to the fact that the arterioles rapidly become thin-walled after birth (Naeye, 1961). Muscular pulmonary arterioles are found in people at high altitude and patients with hypoxic diseases where they may account for some of the changed properties of this circulation in these circumstances.

Besides $\dot{V}/\dot{Q}$ ratios, other important factors could be regulated in the pulmonary circulation. These include resistance, impedance, blood volume, capillary surface area and capillary pressure. Several nervous and chemical stimuli have been shown to alter these variables experimentally but we do not know if they are actively or passively controlled in life.

The main known facts about chemical and nervous control of pulmonary vessels will be summarised and attention will be drawn to areas of ignorance and controversy. Our knowledge of mechanisms stems mainly from analytical experiments in animals but those confirmed in man will be mentioned.

Haemodynamic Measurements in the Pulmonary Circulation

Problems of haemodynamic measurements are discussed because much work on the pulmonary circulation has been spoilt through failure to control or measure important factors.

In man pulmonary vascular resistance is usually defined as the ratio of pulmonary arterial pressure (Ppa) minus wedge pressure (Pw), or left atrial pressure (P_{LA}), over cardiac output. However, changes in this ratio do not necessarily indicate active changes in resistance. It may be decreased passively when cardiac output rises and distends and opens vessels. Special techniques are necessary to detect active changes. A change in Ppa at constant flow or a change in flow at constant Ppa, if Pw or P_{LA} remain constant is a strong indication of active change; these conditions can be fulfilled by setting up controlled circuits in animals or occur by chance in man. The most convincing evidence for an active process is a change in the slope of the pressure/flow relationship which is usually linear in the physiological pressure range and in the supine position. The slope of this line is the best measure of pulmonary vascular resistance. The relationship can be measured by several techniques in animals (Barer, 1976; Szidon & Flint, 1977) which include isolated perfused lungs and open-chest preparations in vivo where a lobe of lung is perfused at a range of flow rates

while Ppa and P_{LA} are measured. In man a few points of pressure/
flow lines can be obtained by occluding one pulmonary artery.
Cardiac output, Ppa and Pw are measured. In the control state 50%
of flow is assumed to go through each pulmonary artery; during
occlusion the whole cardiac output goes through the open artery and
points can be measured both at rest and in exercise. Thus three
points are obtained and a fourth is added if pressure at zero flow
is assumed to be Pw. Changes in the pressure/flow line in several
diseases (Harris & Heath, 1977) and at high altitude (Lockhart et
al, 1976) have been shown by this method. The animal techniques
have shown active changes in resistance caused by hypoxia, hypercapnia, nerve stimulation and many vaso-active substances. Even
the above techniques do not prevent passive effects on Ppa caused
by alveolar or bronchial artery pressure; these influences can be
excluded in animal experiments (Daly & Hebb, 1966) but there is no
certain way to do this in man.

In addition to resistance, the work of the right heart must overcome the input impedance of the pulmonary vascular bed. Impedance is
the ratio of pulsatile pressure to pulsatile flow. There is a "spectrum" of values corresponding to the frequency components (harmonics)
of the complex pressure and flow waves created by the heart beat and
the properties of the pulmonary vessels. Nervous and chemical influences can alter the level of impedance, the maxima and minima of its
spectrum and the proportion it represents of the work output of the
right heart. They do this by changing the time course of ventricular
ejection, vascular compliance, resistance and volume. Compliance
affects pulse wave transmission and resistance affects reflected
waves. The subject is complex and at an early stage of exploration
but there is evidence that some active changes may minimise ventricular work and aid transmission of blood from right to left ventricle
(Reuben et al, 1971; Piene & Hauge, 1976 a,b).

Chemical Control of the Pulmonary Circulation

The lung stores and synthesises numerous vasoactive substances
and is subject to changing O_2 and CO_2 tensions. Only for the gases
have we any idea of their physiological role in the pulmonary
circulation.

Action of Hypoxia and Hypercapnia. Hypoxic pulmonary vasoconstriction has been demonstrated in every species tested including
unanaesthetised man. It is at least in part a mechanism intrinsic
to the lung as it occurs in isolated perfused lungs. Generalised
hypoxia leads to a high Ppa as in the fetus, where PO_2 in the pulmonary artery may be only 20 torr, at high altitude and in hypoxic
lung disease. Local hypoxia, which in life is caused only by hypoventilation or bronchial occlusion, leads through vasoconstriction
to a reduction in local blood flow and its diversion to better
ventilated regions. The sensitivity of lung vessels to hypoxia

has been explored by plotting the relationship between blood flow
to an area of lung against alveolar or pulmonary venous PO_2 (cats
and dogs, Barer et al, 1970; dogs, Benumof & Wahrenbrock, 1975;
the South American mammal coatimundi, Grant et al, 1976 and ferrets,
Barer et al, 1978b). All species except coatimundi gave a curvilinear relationship which resembled an O_2 dissociation curve. In
most there was a small fall in blood flow at supranormal oxygen
tensions and a steep fall within the physiological range. Thus
a substantial reduction in flow would be predicted when PO_2 falls
from arterial to mixed venous levels in unventilated lung. In
coatimundi a very small region of lung was studied and the animal
was breathing spontaneously. A linear relation was shown between
blood flow and PO_2 up to 150 torr and blood flow fell to zero at
mixed venous PO_2. In man Durand et al (1970) made one lung
hypoxic and the other hyperoxic. Blood flow, measured by a radioactive gas technique, was diverted from the hypoxic to the hyperoxic lung according to the level of hypoxia. Calculations from
their results gave a curvilinear relation between resistance in
the hypoxic lung and alveolar PO_2, with the steep part in the
physiological range (Harris & Heath, 1977).

The significance of hypoxic vasoconstriction must be assessed.
In the fetus, where the pulmonary circulation is in parallel with
other organs, hypoxic vasoconstriction is one of the main factors
which keeps pulmonary blood flow low and prevents a large shunt of
blood through the non-functioning organ (Dawes, 1968). In the neonatal period, if the infant is hypoxic and the ductus arteriosus
fails to close, hypoxic vasoconstriction may again diminish blood
flow and be deleterious. In the adult the importance of the
hypoxic mechanism has not been established in spite of clear demonstration of its presence and power. West (1969) suggested that
the mechanism might be superfluous in the healthy adult. He calculated from his studies on the vertical distribution of blood
flow and ventilation that there would be a fivefold difference in
$\dot{V}/\dot{Q}$ between base and apex of the lung but that this would cause
only a 5 torr fall in arterial PO_2. However, it is doubtful if
tests have been made when the effect of local hypoxia might be
maximal such as during inactivity and sleep. In these states
there may be hypoventilation of many lung units which might lead
to severe $\dot{V}/\dot{Q}$ inequality and arterial hypoxaemia if there was no
hypoxic vasoconstriction. We need to know the degree of hypoventilation and local hypoxia that can develop in normal man.
Yet the efficiency of hypoxic vasoconstriction may not be great.
Complete bronchial occlusion caused only a 50-70% reduction in
blood flow in dogs and cats (Barer et al, 1969). In these species
hypoventilation of a lobe led, like hypoxia, to big falls in blood
flow but these were not sufficient to prevent large decreases in
$\dot{V}/\dot{Q}$ ratio and pulmonary venous PO_2 (unpublished work). A high
gain mechanism would approximately maintain $\dot{V}/\dot{Q}$ and PO_2. Grant
et al (1976) calculated the efficiency of the hypoxic mechanism in

coatimundi by control systems theory; efficiency was only moderate
and maximal at PO_2 65–85 torr. Nonetheless hypoxia can overcome
the effect of gravity. It greatly increased the zone of low blood
flow found at the base of the upright dog lung (Hughes et al, 1968).
Also Cumming's group, as described elsewhere in this publication,
were able to divert blood flow from the base to the apex of the
human lung when the base was made hypoxic (Abraham et al, 1970).

In contrast to the normal adult hypoxia plays an important role
at high altitude and in patients with hypoxic lung disease, typically
chronic obstructive lung disease. In these states it leads to
pulmonary hypertension by causing both vasoconstriction and muscularisation of pulmonary arterioles; the anatomical change is a
contributory cause of high resistance. $\dot{V}/\dot{Q}$ inequality is a major
cause of hypoxaemia in chronic lung disease. The distribution of
$\dot{V}/\dot{Q}$ ratios in disease is being explored by a valuable new technique
in which a mixture of inert gases is given intravenously followed
by their analysis in expired air and arterial blood (West, 1977).
Abnormal distributions of $\dot{V}/\dot{Q}$ ratios and a wide range of values
was found in chronic obstructive lung disease (Wagner et al, 1977).
One may ask why $\dot{V}/\dot{Q}$ inequality is so great and hypoxaemia so severe
if hypoxic vasoconstriction is functioning. The answer may lie in
the fundamental inefficiency of the mechanism in the face of widespread hypoventilation, or in the presence of opposing dilator
substances (see below). Also high intravascular pressures may oppose
hypoxic vasoconstriction (Benumof & Wahrenbrock, 1975). By contrast, in some localised lung disease (pneumonia, collapsed lung)
there may be no hypoxaemia which suggests adequate adjustment of
blood flow in nonaerated areas. We have as yet insufficient
evidence to assess the importance of hypoxic vasoconstriction in
the normal adult at sea level. At high altitude the pulmonary
hypertension may cause a more uniform vertical distribution of
blood flow and a larger capillary area for gas exchange.

The relationship between pulmonary venous PCO_2 and local blood
flow was also curvilinear in cats and dogs (Barer et al, 1970).
It indicated that only a small fall in blood flow would occur when
PCO_2 rose from arterial to venous levels in unventilated lung.
Thus hypercapnia made a smaller contribution than hypoxia to vasoconstriction in collapsed lungs (Barer et al, 1969). It is
however, an important cause of pulmonary vasoconstriction in the
fetus (Dawes, 1968). There is also evidence that CO_2 may cause
vasodilatation (Viles and Shepherd, 1968) and it may enhance or
diminish the action of hypoxia in different species and circumstances (Barer & Shaw, 1971; Emery et al, 1977). In man CO_2
enhanced the effect of hypoxia (Durand et al, 1970). CO_2 probably
regulates ventilation to blood flow. When a pulmonary artery is
occluded in man (Even et al, 1972) or animals, ventilation to the
affected area is reduced by constriction of airway smooth muscle.
The stimulus is probably hypocapnia as the effect is prevented by

ventilation with CO_2 mixtures (Severinghaus et al, 1961).

   Mechanism of action of gas tensions. In the systemic circulation both hypoxia and hypercapnia cause vasodilatation. Their
paradoxical actions on the pulmonary circulation require explanation,
especially the action of hypoxia. One would not expect lack of
oxygen to stimulate smooth muscle activity. A comparison can be
made between pulmonary vessels and the carotid body since peripheral
chemoreceptors are the only other organs which respond positively
to hypoxia. The relationship between arterial PO_2 and the rate of
firing in a single carotid nerve fibre is also curvilinear with
sensitivity in the supranormal PO_2 range (Lahiri & Delaney, 1975).
A common biochemical mechanism is a possibility. Lahiri and
Delaney speculate that deoxygenation of a haemoglobin-like molecule
could be one step in the stimulus response sequence. Mills and
Jobsis (1972) found a low affinity cytochrome in the carotid body
which might explain sensitivity at supranormal PO_2 values. The
cytochrome P_{450} found in the lung has not this special property but
substances which inhibit it reduced hypoxic vasoconstriction in the
pig (Sylvester & McGowan, 1978). However, one cannot be sure that
this action was specific. Experiments designed to solve this
mechanism fall into two groups, those in which a mediator liberated
by hypoxia has been sought and those in which a direct action of
hypoxia on the smooth muscle cell has been investigated. The subject
has been splendidly reviewed by Fishman (1976) and will not be discussed in detail. The response to hypoxia is fragile and disappears
or may wax and wane while responses to other vasoconstrictor agents
remain stable. This could be due to variations in storage or synthesis of a transmitter. Moreover the basic response of pulmonary
vessels to hypoxia may be, as in other organs, relaxation. Relaxation occurs during hypoxia in isolated strips of pulmonary artery
except in special circumstances; also hypoxic vasoconstriction is
lost and dilatation occurs in isolated perfused lungs that have
been slowly prepared (Daly & Hebb, 1966). Yet there is at present
no evidence of a mediator common to all species. In favour of a
direct action are the observations that isolated strips of pulmonary
artery can be "trained" by special conditions to contract in hypoxia
(Bohr, 1977) and that pulmonary vascular smooth muscle loses K^+
during hypoxia (Bergofsky and Holtzman, 1967). Inhibitors of trans-
membrane Ca^{++} transport suppress hypoxic vasoconstriction in isolated rat lungs but the action need not be on the smooth muscle cell
(McMurtry et al, 1976). Any theory must take into account the high
temperature sensitivity of hypoxic vasoconstriction (Nilson & Hauge,
1968). Lastly there may exist a receptor sensitive to hypoxia which
gives a local neural or humoral response. The neuroepithelial
bodies of the respiratory tract which show cytological changes in
acute hypoxia are possible candidates (Lauweryns & Cokelaere, 1973).

   The mechanism of action of CO_2 has been less studied although
it is also a local mechanism present in isolated perfused lungs.
The constrictor action is attributed to formation of carbonic acid

(Bergofsky et al, 1962; Barer et al, 1967) although this has been
disputed. Certainly acids constrict and alkalis dilate cat pulmonary
vessels (Barer et al, 1971) although large changes are required.
The smaller changes in pH caused in man were not effective (Harris &
Heath, 1977). No mediator has been found for the vasoconstrictor
action of CO_2; the vasodilator action was abolished by large doses
of β adrenoreceptor inhibitors in isolated rat lungs but it is not
certain that this action was specific (Emery et al, 1977).

    Action of non-gaseous vasoactive substances. Many substances
stored or formed in the lung or present in circulating blood have
profound effects on pulmonary vessels but for none do we know its
normal role. Pulmonary vascular tone is low in the healthy adult
so that dilator compounds have small effects. Yet a fall in Ppa
of 1 or 2 torr may be significant in a vascular bed across which
the total pressure difference is so low. All the dilator agents
have increased effects during vasoconstriction. Several vasoactive agents, in addition to CO_2 have a dual action on pulmonary
vessels. This may be manifested as constriction when tone is low
and dilatation when it is high; it could therefore be a dual action
on the same vessels. Alternatively the two actions could be at
different sites such as pre and postcapillary vessels. In no case
do we yet know if this is so. It is an important point to investigate as a differential action on arteries and veins would alter
pressure and volume in alveolar capillaries and affect gas exchange
and fluid balance.

    α and β adrenoreceptor agonists cause constriction and
dilatation respectively; these actions are abolished by α and β
inhibitor drugs. Noradrenaline has a mainly constrictor action
though dilatation may be seen after α blockade. Dopamine is a
constrictor stored in large quantities in the lung in some species.
Adrenaline has both α and β actions while isoprenaline, not a
natural substance, has a wholly β action, best seen during hypoxic
vasoconstriction. In cats and dogs α and β adrenoreceptor antagonists respectively dilate and constrict pulmonary vessels; this
suggests that a balance between α and B agonists might maintain
pulmonary vascular tone. These actions have been shown in animals
and mostly confirmed in man. In cats and fetal lambs α adrenoreceptor antagonists inhibited hypoxic vasoconstriction but this
was not confirmed in other species (Howard et al, 1975).

    Histamine is present in large quantities in lung mast cells,
many of which are perivascular. It has an H_2 pulmonary dilator
action reduced by H_2 inhibitor drugs and an H_1 vasoconstrictor
action abolished by H_1 inhibitors. Dilatation occurs with smaller
doses than constriction in cats (Barer et al, 1978a) and has been
shown in man. Constriction affects mainly pulmonary veins but the
site of dilatation is unknown (Glazier & Murray, 1971; Brody &
Stemmler, 1968). However, Thompson et al (1976) showed that
histamine could contract and relax the same pulmonary artery strip.

Histamine has an H_1 constrictor action on peripheral airway smooth muscle but recently an H_2 relaxant action has been described (Chand & Eyre, 1978). An H_2 action also inhibits mast cell discharge, perhaps through an action on adenyl cyclase. Thus when antigen-antibody reactions in the lung cause mast cells to release histamine (among other substances), histamine release and H_1 effects on bronchi and vessels may be limited by H_2 action (Austen & Orange, 1975). Hauge (1968) found good evidence for histamine as a mediator of hypoxic vasoconstriction in the rat but similar evidence was not forthcoming for other species and histamine actually causes dilatation during hypoxia in the rat (Shaw, 1971). However, mast cells increase in number in rat lungs during chronic hypoxia (Kay et al, 1974; Mungall, 1976).

Serotonin causes large increases in vascular resistance in animal lungs. It affects pre and post capillary vessels (Brody & Stemmler, 1968). It may be released from platelets in emboli and be stored in neuroepithelial bodies. Part of its action may be due to causing small temporary aggregates of blood cells in small vessels. In spite of its potency in animals no effect on pulmonary vessels has been shown in man, even in carcinoid syndrome (Harris & Heath, 1977). Serotonin has probably been excluded as a mediator of hypoxic vasoconstriction.

The lung is a major site for synthesis of prostaglandins (PGs) and related substances (Hyman et al, 1977). Synthesis follows numerous stimuli which include hyperventilation, handling the lung, emboli, anaphylaxis, hypoxia, histamine and other chemicals. Many types of PG compounds are formed. Some cause vasoconstriction and bronchoconstriction, others vasodilatation and bronchodilatation; they might regulate $\dot{V}/\dot{Q}$ ratios. Dilator compounds may predominate and have a tonic effect on pulmonary vessels; they may be important in dilating vessels at birth and in the neonatal period (Tyler et al, 1977). Unstable intermediate endoperoxides may be more potent than the stable later products such as the vasoconstrictor PGF2α and the dilator PGE1. Some PGs may increase pulmonary vascular resistance through platelet aggregation and vascular obstruction. Thromboxane is a platelet aggregator and prostacyclin (PGI_2) a disaggregator. PGI_2 is generated in the lungs and released into the systemic circulation (Gryglewski et al, 1978) and may play an important part in preventing intra-arterial thrombosis. It resolves the pulmonary hypertension caused by platelet aggregation in dogs (Hyman et al, 1977). PGs are released following antigen-antibody reactions in the lung. Dilator PGs stabilise mast cells, like H_2 histamine action, probably through an action on adenyl cyclase (Austen & Orange, 1975). Hypoxic vasoconstriction persists in the presence of PG synthetase inhibitors and may be increased through loss of dilator PG action. Thus these compounds are not responsible for but may modulate the action of hypoxia (Weir et al, 1976).

Adenosinetriphosphate constricts pulmonary vessels but dilatation has been seen during hypoxia. Adenosine is a dilator which reverses hypoxic vasoconstriction (Mentzner et al, 1975).

Angiotensin II is formed from angiotensin I by the peptidase "converting enzyme" on pulmonary endothelium (Junod, 1977). It has a relatively weak pulmonary vasoconstrictor action in man and animals compared with its powerful systemic vasoconstrictor action, although large doses cause constriction in isolated perfused lungs. It cannot be the mediator of hypoxic vasoconstriction because this action survives when the effect of angiotensin II has been suppressed by the specific inhibitor saralasin (rats, McMurtry et al, 1975). It may however, play a supporting role by maintaining muscular reactivity. Berkov (1974) found its presence in subpressor quantities necessary to maintain the hypoxic response in rat lungs perfused with artificial fluid. Alexander et al (1976) found it revived the failing hypoxic response in dogs, while doses of angiotensin II enhanced the hypoxic response in some species (Barer et al, 1977). Bradykinin, which is inactivated by the same "converting enzyme" in the lung is a powerful dilator when tone is high in both man and animals and reverses hypoxic vasoconstriction (Howard et al, 1975). However, vasoconstriction has been demonstrated from the control state in some animals. Bradykinin is released in antigen–antibody reactions in the lung.

Acetylcholine has a dual action causing both vasoconstriction and dilatation, both abolished by atropine and independent of bronchoconstriction. Dilatation occurs with smaller doses in cats and is well demonstrated during hypoxic vasoconstriction in both animals and man (Daly & Hebb, 1976; Harris & Heath, 1977). Atropine does not affect the hypoxic response.

Reversal of hypoxic vasoconstriction by dilator compounds might lower arterial PO_2 by increasing blood flow through unventilated areas of the lung. The fall in PO_2 sometimes seen clinically following isoprenaline or aminophylline has been attributed to this cause. Adrenal discharge reduced hypoxic vasoconstriction in cats (Howard et al, 1975), an observation which could be important because catecholamines circulate at increased levels in hypoxia.

The lung is active in altering or absorbing many substances which it receives from the venous circulation. These activities were studied by Vane and colleagues who showed by continuous biological assay that there were big concentration differences for certain amines and peptides between mixed venous and pulmonary venous blood (Vane, 1969; Bakhle & Vane, 1977). Thus the lung determines which vasoactive substances pass through it to affect the systemic circulation. Noradrenaline and serotonin are absorbed by active transport in the lung while adrenaline and histamine pass through. Some PGs are retained and others pass. The formation in

the lung of the systemic vasoconstrictor angiotensin II and inactivation of the systemic dilator bradykinin by the same enzyme could
be a mechanism for regulating systemic blood pressure (Junod, 1977).

Pulmonary vessels become more reactive in chronic hypoxia
probably because of more muscular arterioles. The isolated perfused
pulmonary vessels of chronically hypoxic rats responded more strongly
than controls to both dilator and constrictor stimuli, including
several degrees of hypoxia (Emery et al, 1979). However, McMurtry
et al (1978) found pulmonary vessels of similar rats less responsive
than controls to hypoxia. The difference is not explained; there.
may in some circumstances be a metabolic adaptation to chronic
hypoxia. Changes in reactivity can be expected in hypoxic patients
and people at high altitude.

The lung receives the full impact of drugs given intravenously.
It is therefore extremely important to test the reaction of this
circulation to drugs and this is rarely done.

Nervous Control of the Pulmonary Circulation

Pulmonary vessels are extensively innervated though less so
than systemic vessels. In animals adrenergic and cholinergic fibres
have been demonstrated by histochemical methods (Hebb, 1969). There
are more nerves on arteries than veins and more adrenergic than
cholinergic endings. There are species differences in their distribution. In some species intrapulmonary fibres are few or absent
while in others both types of fibre extend down to small arteriolar
vessels (30–40 μ diameter) and are found on large or medium-sized
veins. In man Spencer and Leof (1964), who used non-specific staining methods, showed that motor nerves supply all arteries and veins
down to those 30 μ in diameter.

The best evidence for nervous control of pulmonary vessels
comes from experiments on fetal lambs by Dawes and colleagues
(Colebatch et al, 1965). They showed that blood flow to one lung
was doubled by vagal stimulation and reduced nearly to zero by
sympathetic stimulation; neither effect was due to pressure changes.
Also sympathectomy greatly reduced pulmonary vascular resistance
while vagotomy had no effect. Thus, in contrast to the adult,
there is sympathetic vascular tone in the fetus which helps to
maintain a low blood flow through the fetal lung.

Nerve stimulation has caused changes in vascular resistance,
impedance and compliance in adult lungs. In isolated perfused
dog lungs de Burgh Daly (Daly & Hebb, 1966) showed that sympathetic
stimulation constricted both arteries and veins and increased inflow
impedance. There was also a sympathetic dilator mechanism observed
occasionally and a vagal dilator mechanism observed rarely.

Kadowitz et al (1976) confirmed the sympathetic vasoconstrictor action on pulmonary arteries and veins by an ingenious technique in intact dogs. One lobe of lung was perfused with the animal's own blood at constant flow through a balloon-tipped catheter impacted in a lobar artery. Piene (1976a) recorded pulsatile pressure and flow in the cat pulmonary artery. Sympathetic nerve stimulation caused increases in vascular resistance and impedance and decreases in compliance. Impedance was more affected than resistance so that pulsatile work of the right heart increased relative to total work. However, the effect on impedance grew less as cardiac output rose. Thus when cardiac output rises in exercise sympathetic activity could stiffen pulmonary vessels with little extra load on the right heart.

Fishman and his group think that sympathetic nerves control the compliance of large pulmonary arteries and have no effect on resistance. In dogs Ingram et al (1970) plotted the change in diameter of the main pulmonary artery against the simultaneous change in Ppa with each heart beat. Thus they obtained a diameter/ pressure line whose slope was a measure of compliance. Sympathetic stimulation reduced this slope so that the vessels became stiffer. The same reaction could be elicited centrally by stimulating an area of the hypothalamus. Noradrenaline slightly reduced compliance but also increased resistance, so that the effects of nerve stimulation could not be attributed to adrenal discharge. The α adrenoreceptor inhibitor phenoxybenzamine, increased compliance which suggests that sympathetic activity may maintain constant tension in the main pulmonary artery.

Szidon and Flint (1977) described an important sympathetic reflex which affects the pulmonary artery during systemic hypoxia. When dogs were given 8-10% O_2 to breathe compliance of the pulmonary artery, measured by the method of Ingram et al (1970) was reduced. The effect was abolished by cutting pulmonary sympathetic fibres or by cutting the vagus and glossopharyngeal nerves; it was mimicked by injecting the chemoreceptor stimulant lobeline into the root of the aorta. They deduced that systemic hypoxia stimulated peripheral chemoreceptors and lead to a reflex with its efferent arc in pulmonary sympathetic fibres. In other dogs hypoxia restricted to one lobe moved its pressure/flow line in the direction of increased resistance. This change, not abolished by sympathectomy, vagotomy or adrenalectomy, was the well-known local effect of hypoxia. Hypoxia therefore has two actions on pulmonary vessels, the chemoreflex which stiffens large arteries and the local constrictor action shown to affect mainly small arteries (Bergofsky, 1969). These two actions can be expected in patients with chronic hypoxic lung disease and residents at high altitude. Stiffening of the vessels might account for the large rises in Ppa sometimes seen on exercise in hypoxic patients.

Additional reflex and central actions on pulmonary vessels have been described. Reflex changes in resistance followed stimulation of the carotid body and carotid sinus. They cannot yet be interpreted because the direction of change depended on the state of the bronchial circulation (Daly & Hebb, 1966). Stern and Braun (1966) observed pulmonary vasoconstriction, possibly venous, when they stimulated aortic chemoreceptors in dogs. Lloyd and Schneider (1970) observed complex changes in pulmonary artery pressure when they raised the pressure in the left heart in dogs which were in part due to a sympathetic reflex. Malik (1977) showed that raised intracranial pressure caused intense pulmonary vasoconstriction in dogs, probably of sympathetic origin.

The pulmonary circulation is an important reflexogenic zone. There are mechanoreceptors in the main pulmonary artery which respond to pressure changes in the physiological range (Coleridge et al, 1961). The J receptors, believed to be near the alveoli and the stretch and irritant receptors of the respiratory tract can be stimulated chemically through the pulmonary circulation, while the J receptors also respond to pulmonary congestion and oedema (Widdicombe, 1974). True chemoreceptors have not with certainty been demonstrated in this circulation (Daly & Hebb, 1966). One might predict their presence because large changes in gas tensions occur in mixed venous blood on exercise. However, Grodins (1967) has argued from control engineering theory that they should be situated on the arterial side where these values are closely regulated. Intrapulmonary reflexes causing hypoxic vasoconstriction have not been excluded. At present no pulmonary receptor is known to cause feedback adjustment of the pulmonary circulation. Instead they affect systemic vessels, heart rate, bronchial tone and breathing. Recent work on the mechanoreceptors (Ledsome, 1977) may indicate that they are part of the blood volume control system and that they might affect breathing during exercise. There are many untraced sensory fibres from the lungs and many proposed reflexes for which conclusive evidence is lacking (Daly & Hebb, 1966).

In spite of much work we are ignorant as to the physiological role of pulmonary vascular nerves. No function can be assigned to the vagal fibres or the sympathetic vasodilator fibres. The sympathetic vasoconstrictor fibres are active in the fetus but it is not certain that they function in the adult. If sympathetic stiffening of large vessels occurs during excitement and exercise it may prevent pooling of blood in the lung, ensure a more uniform vertical distribution of blood flow and aid synchronisation of the two ventricles through increased pulse wave transmission (Szidon & Fishman, 1969). Piene (1976b) showed that increased pulse wave transmission improved the performance of the left ventricle. Decreased compliance increases the impedance load on the right ventricle but this effect is diminished if there is a simultaneous increase in cardiac output (Piene, 1976a). A function for

sympathetic vasoconstriction is not evident but two studies showed
that a combination of increased resistance and decreased compliance
might have a "useful" result. In both vasoactive substances rather
than sympathetic stimulation were used but the principle is the same.
Piene and Hauge (1976 a&b) showed that moderate vasoconstriction
reduced input impedance in rabbit lungs in spite of decreased compliance. Reuben et al (1970) showed that when resistance increased
and compliance decreased in dog lungs, as a result of hypoxia and
serotonin, the time constant of the pulmonary vessels (resistance x
compliance) remained constant. The result was that the pattern of
pulsatile blood flow reaching the alveolar capillaries for gas
exchange was unaltered. In adult man there is no evidence for
sympathetic vasomotor tone; drugs which blocked sympathetic ganglia
and nerve terminals caused no change in pulmonary vascular resistance
(Harris & Heath, 1977). We need to look for evidence of nervous
activity in the whole animal at rest and during exercise but the
task is formidable.

The Pulmonary Circulation in Exercise

We do not know whether active mechanisms intervene or whether
changes in the pulmonary circulation are purely passive during
exercise. Cardiac output rises and causes a rise in Ppa which may
open up the vascular bed in a passive manner. If sympathetic
stimulation occurs it may increase pulse wave transmission and assist
the performance of the left heart. Increased heart rate, also a
sympathetic effect, may bring the chief harmonic of the pulse wave
near to the impedance minimum which is near 3 c.p.s. and thus
reduce the phasic work of the right heart. In pulmonary venous blood
decreased PO_2 and pH, increased PCO_2 and released hormones could
all affect pulmonary vessels. Hypoxic vasoconstriction which affects
vessels accessible to alveolar air probably does not take place if
ventilation is adequate (Hauge, 1969). The overall result, as far
as evidence goes at present, is that vascular resistance is not
altered in normal man; points measured during exercise lie on approximately the same pressure/flow line as those measured at rest
(Harris & Heath, 1977).

Conclusions

Pulmonary vessels are affected by nervous activity and vasoactive substances, especially the respiratory gases. These influences are probably of vital importance in the fetal and neonatal periods. They are retained in adult life where some of them
are important in lung disease and at high altitude. Their role
in normal daily life, particularly in exercise and sleep, relative
to the passive effects of gravity and changing cardiac output,
still awaits critical assessment.

REFERENCES

Abraham, A. S., Cumming, C., Horsfield, K. and Prowse, K., 1970,
    Regional hypoxia and distribution of blood flow, Scand.
    J. resp. Dis., 51:33-36.
Alexander, J. M., Nyby, M. D. and Jasberg, K. A., 1976, Effect of
    angiotensin on hypoxic pulmonary vasoconstriction in iso-
    lated dog lung, J. appl. Physiol., 41:84-88.
Austen, K. F. and Orange, R. P., 1975, Bronchial asthma: The pos-
    sible role of the chemical mediators of immediate hyper-
    sensitivity in the pathogenesis of subacute and chronic
    disease, Am. Rev. resp. Dis., 112:423-436.
Bakhle, Y. S. and Vane, J. R., 1977, Metabolic functions of the lung,
    in: "Lung biology in health and disease", C. Lenfant, ed.,
    Marcel Dekker Inc., New York and Basel.
Barer, G. R., 1976, The physiology of the pulmonary circulation and
    methods of study, Pharmac. Ther. B., 2:247-273.
Barer, G. R., Emery, C. J., Mohammed, F. H. and Mungall, I. P. F.,
    1978a, H_1 and H_2 histamine actions on lung vessels: their
    relevance to hypoxic vasoconstriction, Q. J. exp. Physiol.,
    63:157-169.
Barer, G. R., Howard, P. and McCurrie, J. R., 1967, The effect of
    carbon dioxide and changes in blood pH on pulmonary vas-
    cular resistance in cats, Clin. Sci., 32:361-376.
Barer, G. R., Howard, P., McCurrie, J. R. and Shaw, J. W., 1969,
    Changes in the pulmonary circulation after bronchial oc-
    clusion in anaesthetised dogs and cats, Circulation Res.,
    25:747-764.
Barer, G. R., Howard, P. and Shaw, J. W., 1970, Stimulus-response
    curves of the pulmonary vascular bed to hypoxia and hyper-
    capnia, J. Physiol., 211:139-155.
Barer, G. R., McCurrie, J. R. and Shaw, J. W., 1971, Effect of
    changes in blood pH on the vascular resistance of the nor-
    mal and hypoxic cat lung, Cardiovasc. Res., 5:490-497.
Barer, G. R., Mohammed, F. H. and Suggett, A. J., 1977, Angiotensin,
    hypoxia, verapamil and pulmonary vessels, J. Physiol.,
    270:43-44P.
Barer, G. R., Mohammed, F., Suggett, A. J. and Twelves, C., 1978b,
    Hypoxic pulmonary vasoconstriction in the ferret, J.
    Physiol., 281:40-41P.
Barer, G. R. and Shaw, J. W., 1971, Pulmonary vasodilator and vaso-
    constrictor actions of carbon dioxide, J. Physiol., 213:
    633-645.
Benumof, J. L. and Wahrenbrock, E. A., 1975, Blunted hypoxic vaso-
    constriction by increased lung vascular pressures.
    J. appl. Physiol., 38:846-850.
Bergofsky, E. H., 1969, in: "The pulmonary circulation and inter-
    stitial space", A. P. Fishman and H. H. Hecht, eds.,
    University of Chicago Press, Chicago and Basel.

Bergofsky, E. H. and Holtzman, S., 1967, A study of the mechanism
        involved in the pulmonary arterial response to hypoxia,
        Circulation Res., 20:506-519.
Bergofsky, E. H., Lehr, D. E. and Fishman, A. P., 1962, The effect
        of changes in hydrogen ion concentration on the pulmonary
        circulation, J. clin. Invest., 41:1492-1502.
Berkov, S., 1974, Hypoxic pulmonary vasoconstriction in the rat.
        The necessary role of angiotensin II, Circulation Res.,
        35:256-261.
Bohr, D. R., 1977, The pulmonary hypoxic response – state of the
        field, Chest, 71 Supplement: 244-246.
Brody, J. S. and Stemmler, E. J., 1968, Differential reactivity in
        the pulmonary circulation, J. clin. Invest., 47:800-808.
Chand, N. and Eyre, P., 1978, Spasmolytic action of histamine in
        airway smooth muscle, Agents and Action, 8:191-198.
Colebatch, H. J. H., Dawes, G. S., Goodwin, J. W. and Nadeau, R. A.,
        1965, The nervous control of the circulation in the fetal
        and newly expanded lungs of the lamb, J. Physiol., 178:
        544-562.
Coleridge, J. C. G., Kidd, C. and Sharp, J. A., 1961, The distri-
        bution connections and histology of baroreceptors in the
        pulmonary artery with some observations on the innervation
        of the ductus arteriosus, J. Physiol., 156:591-602.
Daly, I. de B., and Hebb, C., 1966, "Pulmonary and bronchial vascu-
        lar systems", Arnold, London.
Dawes, G. S., 1968, "Fetal and neonatal physiology", Yearbook
        Medical Publishers, Chicago.
Dawes, G. S., 1969, in: "The pulmonary circulation and interstitial
        space", A. P. Fishman and H. H. Hecht, eds., University of
        Chicago Press, Chicago and London.
Durand, J., Ladurie, M. L. and Ranson-Bitker, B., 1970, Pulmonary
        circulation, in:"Progress in respiration research",
        J. Widimsky and S. Daum, eds., Karger, Basel, Munchen,
        Paris, New York.
Emery, C. J., Bee, D. and Barer, G. R., 1979, Mechanical properties
        and reactivity of the rat pulmonary circulation in chronic
        hypoxia. A possible model of human hypoxic disease.
        Proc. Pulmonary Circulation III, Prague, Bull. eur. Physio-
        path. resp. (in press).
Emery, C. J., Sloan, P. J. M., Mohammed, F. H. and Barer, G. R.,
        1977, The action of hypercapnia during hypoxia on pulmonary
        vessels, Bull. eur. Physiopath. resp., 13:763-776.
Even, P., Duroux, P., Caubarrere, I., Ruff, F., Butez, J. and
        Bronet, G., 1972, Respiratory effects induced by pulmonary
        artery occlusion, Bull. Physiopath. resp., 8:467-473.
Fishman, A. P., 1976, Hypoxia on the pulmonary circulation. How and
        where it acts, Circulation Res., 38:221-231.
Glazier, J. B. and Murray, J. F., 1971, Sites of pulmonary vaso-
        motor activity in the dog during alveolar hypoxia and sero-
        tonin and histamine infusions, J. clin. Invest., 50:

2550–2558.

Grant, B. J. B., Davies, E. E., Jones, H. A. and Hughes, J. M. B.,
1976, Local regulation of pulmonary blood flow and ventilation–perfusion ratios in Coatimundi, J. appl. Physiol.,
40:216–228.

Grodins, F., 1967, Some simple principles and complex realities of
cardiopulmonary control during exercise, Circulation Res.,
Supplement 20 & 21:1.171–1.178.

Gryglewski, R. J., Korbut, R. and Ocetkiewicz, A., 1978, Generation
of prostacyclin by lungs in vivo and its release into the
arterial circulation, Nature, 273:765–767.

Harris, P. and Heath, D., 1977, "The human pulmonary circulation",
2nd Edition, Churchill Livingstone, Edinburgh, London and
New York.

Hauge, A., 1968, Role of histamine in hypoxic pulmonary hypertension
in the rat. I. Blockade or potentiation of endogenous
amines, kinins and ATP, Circulation Res, 22:371–383.

Hauge, A., 1969, Hypoxia and pulmonary vascular resistance. The
relative effects of pulmonary arterial and alveolar PO_2.
Acta. physiol. scand., 76:121–130.

Hebb, C., 1969, in: "The pulmonary circulation and interstitial
space", A. P. Fishman and H. H. Hecht, eds., University of
Chicago Press, Chicago and London.

Howard, P., Barer, G. R., Thompson, B., Warren, P. M., Abbot, C. J.
and Mungall, I. P. F., 1975, Factors causing and reversing
vasoconstriction in unventilated lung, Resp. Physiol.,
24: 325–345.

Hughes, J. M. B., Glazier, J. B., Maloney, J. E. and West, J. B.,
1968, Effects of extra–alveolar vessels on the distribution
of blood flow in the dog lung, J. appl. Physiol, 25:701–712.

Hyman, A. L., Spannhake, E. W. and Kadowitz, P. J., 1977, Prostaglandins and the lung, Am. Rev. resp. Dis., 117:111–136.

Ingram, R. H., Szidon, J. P. & Fishman, A. P., 1970, Response of
the main pulmonary artery of dogs to neuronally released
versus blood borne norepinephrine, Circulation Res., 26:
249–262.

Junod, A. F., 1977, Metabolism of vasoactive agents in the lung,
Am. Rev. resp. Dis., Comroe Symposium, 115:51–57.

Kadowitz, P. J., Knight, D. S., Hibbs, R. G., Ellison, J. P.,
Joiner, P. P., Brody, M. J. and Hyman, A. L., 1976, Influence of 5 and 6 hydroxydopamine on adrenergic transmission and nerve terminal morphology in the canine
pulmonary vascular bed, Circulation Res., 39:191–199.

Kay, J. M., Waymire, J. C. and Grover, R. F., 1974, Lung mast cell
hyperplasia and pulmonary histamine forming capacity in
hypoxic rats, Am. J. Physiol, 226:178–184.

Lahiri, S. and Delaney, R. G., 1975, Stimulus interaction in the
responses of the carotid body chemoreceptor single afferent fibres, Resp. Physiol., 24: 249–266.

Lauweryns, J. M. and Cokelaere, 1973, Hypoxia-sensitive neuro-
        epithelial bodies. Intrapulmonary secretory neuroreceptors
        modulated by the C.N.S., Z. Zellforsch. mikrosk. Anat.,
        145:521-540.
Ledsome, J. R., 1977, Reflex role of pulmonary arterial barorecep-
        tors, Am. Rev. resp. Dis., Comroe Symposium, 115:245-250.
Lloyd, T. C. and Schneider, A. J. L., 1970, Reflex pulmonary vascular
        responses to distension of the lungs and left heart, J.
        appl. Physiol., 29:318-322.
Lockhart, A., Zeller, M., Mensch-Dechene, J., Antezano, G.,
        Paz-Zamora, M., Vargas, E. and Courdet, J., 1976, Pressure-
        flow-volume relationships in pulmonary circulation of
        normal highlanders, J. appl. Physiol., 41:449-456.
McMurtry, I. F., Hiser, W. W., Reeves, J. T. and Grover, R. F.,
        1975, Dissociation of hypoxia and angiotensin II-induced
        pulmonary vasoconstriction by saralasin, Fed. Proc., 34:
        438.
McMurtry, I. F., Davidson, I. B., Reeves, J. T. and Grover, R. F.,
        1976, Inhibition of hypoxic pulmonary vasoconstriction by
        calcium antagonists in isolated rat lungs, Circulation Res.,
        38:99-104.
McMurtry, I. F., Petrun, M. D. and Reeves, J. T., 1978, Lungs from
        chronically hypoxic rats have decreased pressor response
        to acute hypoxia, Am. J. Physiol., H105-H109.
Malik, A. B., 1977, Pulmonary vascular response to increase in intra-
        cranial pressure:role of sympathetic mechanisms, J. appl.
        Physiol. Respirat. Environ. Exercise Physiol., 42:335-343.
Mentzner, R. M., Rubio, R. and Berne, R. M., 1975, Release of adeno-
        sine by hypoxic canine lung tissue and its possible role in
        the pulmonary circulation, Am. J. Physiol, 229:1625-1631.
Mills, E. and Jobsis, F. F., 1972, Mitochondrial respiratory chain
        and chemoreceptor response to changes in oxygen tension,
        J. Neurophysiol., 35:405-428.
Mungall, I. P. F., 1976, Hypoxia and lung mast cells: influence of
        disodium cromoglycate, Thorax, 31:94-100.
Naeye, R. L., 1961, Arterial changes during the neonatal period,
        Archs. Path., 71:121-128.
Nilson, K. H. and Hauge, A., 1968, Effects of temperature changes
        on the pressor response to acute hypoxia in isolated rat
        lungs, Acta. physiol. scand., 73: 111-120.
Piene, H., 1976a, The influence of pulmonary blood flow rate on
        vascular input impedance and hydraulic power in the sym-
        pathetically and noradrenaline stimulated cat lung, Acta.
        physiol. scand., 98:44-53.
Piene, H., 1976b, Improved left ventricular performance by the
        transmission of pulse waves through the pulmonary vascular
        bed, Acta. physiol. scand. 98:450-456.
Piene, H. and Hauge, A., 1976a, Reduction of pulsatile hydraulic
        power in the pulmonary circulation caused by moderate
        vasoconstriction, Cardiovasc. Res., 10:503-516.

Piene, H. and Hauge, A., 1976b, Influence of moderate vasoconstriction on the wave reflection properties of the pulmonary arterial bed, Acta. physiol. scand., 98:37-43.

Reuben, S. R., Gersch, B. J., Swadling, J. P. and Lee, G. de J., 1970, Measurement of pulmonary arterial distensibility in the dog, Cardiovasc. Res., 4:473-481.

Reuben, S. R., Swadling, J. P., Gersch, B. J. and Lee, G. de J., 1971, Impedance and transmission properties of the pulmonary arterial system, Cardiovasc. Res., 5:1-9.

Severinghaus, J. W., Swenson, E. W., Finley, T. N., Lategola, M. and Williams, J., 1961, Unilateral hypoventilation produced in dogs by occluding one pulmonary artery, J. appl. Physiol., 16:53-60.

Shaw, J. W., 1971, Pulmonary vasodilator and vasoconstrictor actions of histamine, J. Physiol, 215:34-35P.

Spencer, H. and Leof, D., 1964, The innervation of the human lung. J. Anat., 98:599-609.

Stern, S. and Braun, K., 1966, Effect of chemoreceptor stimulation on pulmonary veins, Am. J. Physiol., 210:535-539.

Sylvester, J. T. and McGowan, C., 1978, The effect of agents that bind to cytochrome P-450 on hypoxic pulmonary vasoconstriction, Circulation Res., 43:429-437.

Szidon, J. P. and Fishman, A. P., 1969, in: "The pulmonary circulation and interstitial space", A. P. Fishman and H. H. Hecht, eds., University of Chicago Press, Chicago and London.

Szidon, J. P. and Flint, J. F., 1977, Significance of sympathetic innervation of pulmonary vessels in response to acute hypoxia, J. appl. Physiol. Respirat. Environ. Exercise Physiol., 43:65-71.

Thompson, B., Barer, G. R. and Shaw, J. W., 1976, The action of histamine on the pulmonary vessels of cats and rats, Clin. & exp. Pharmac. & Physiol., 3:399-414.

Tyler, T. L., Leffler, C. W. and Cassin, S., 1977, Effects of prostaglandin precursors, prostaglandins and prostaglandin metabolites on pulmonary circulation of perinatal goats. Chest, 71 Supplement:271-273.

Vane, J. R., 1969, The release and fate of vasoactive hormones in the circulation, B. J. Pharmac., 35:209-242.

Viles, P. H. and Shepherd, J. T., 1968, Evidence for a dilator action of carbon dioxide on the pulmonary vessels of the cat, Circulation Res., 22:325-332.

Wagner, P. D., Dantzker, D. R., Dueck, R., Clausen, J. L. and West, J. B., 1977, Ventilation-perfusion inequality in chronic obstructive pulmonary disease, J. clin. Invest., 59:203-216.

Weir, E. K., McMurtry, I. F., Tucker, A., Reeves, J. T. and Grover, R. F., 1976, Prostaglandin synthetase inhibitors do not decrease hypoxic pulmonary vasoconstriction, J. appl. Physiol., 41:714-718.

West, J. B., 1969, in: "The pulmonary circulation and interstitial
        space", p 302, A. P. Fishman and H. H. Hecht, eds.,
        University of Chicago Press, Chicago and London.
West, J. B., 1977, State of the art. Ventilation-perfusion re-
        lationships, Am. Rev. resp. Dis., 116:919-943.
Widdicombe, J. G., 1974, in: "Recent advances in physiology",
        p.p. 239-278, R. J. Linden, ed., Churchill Livingstone,
        Edinburgh and London.

Discussion

HAUGE: First I'd like to say that this was a very admirable survey
of a large and difficult theme. I have a few questions and
comments. When I see the nerve stimulation results presented in
many people's work, it appears that the frequency of stimulation is
almost always higher than normal. I think in one of your slides you
showed 30 Hz, and I wonder if there is evidence that stimulation of
the sympathetic nerves at normal frequencies causes vasoactive
responses. I have also a suggestion. It may be that an additional
role for the regulation of the vascular tone in the lung could be
that the pulsatile hydraulic power of the right ventricle contains a
large fraction of Kinetic energy, much larger than in the systemic
circulation. It's a bigger flow compared to the pressure. And
there will be pulse wave reflexions in the lung and it's not
unimportant when pulse wave reflexions return from points in the
vascular bed back to the ventricle. This may be a regulator system.
As Fishman has suggested, there may be a regulation of compliance of
the vessels, but as far as I remember they just considered pulse
wave transmission through the lung and not pulse wave reflexions,
and it is of some importance when pulse wave reflexions return.
That's only a suggestion that this may be regulated also in the
vascular bed. I also wonder, that I found myself many times and I
do not have the answer, why do denervated lungs react qualitatively
opposite to so many vasoactive drugs? It is not a matter of dosage,
because you can give the very same dosage of a vasoactive substance
and when the lung is denervated you get a qualitatively opposite
effect: dilataion in the denervated and constriction in the
re-innervated.

BARER: Will you give an example?

HAUGE: Yes, acetylcholine is the most powerful constrctor in the
denervated rabbit lung, whereas it is a very potent dilator in the
intact lung. And bradykinin, as you mentioned yourself, constricts
in the isolates lung and dilates in the innervated.

BARER: Is there any difference in the resistance relative to dose?

HAUGE: Not measured in the conventional way, as pressure divided
by flow. And it is not a difference of dosage either.

BARER: The question of the action of such drugs as acetylchholine
is very interesting. You can get it on the same strip of vessel.
If you take a strip of pulmonary artery you can get constriction and
dilatation by histamine on the same preparation.

RIEDEL: Not all the patients with chronic hypoxia have pulmonary hypertension even if their hypoxia is of long standing and similarly severe. My question is - are there patients that differ in individual reactivity to the pressure stimuli, or perhaps are there animals that you have tested some of them reacting very much to the same stimuli and the other not. Perhaps that could be of clinical importance. We could identify patients who are liable to develop chronic pulmonary hypertension.

BARER: There are certainly differences between species. I think I mentioned serotonin, which even in carcinoid syndrome does not seem to have any action in man. Until we knew of prostaglandins we thought it was the strongest vasoconstrator we had in animals.

RIEDEL: This is not what I asked. I mean is there any test with people or animals by some constant stimulus and find whether vasoconstrctor activity is higher in some of them than in the others?

BARER: I am sorry, I don't know of any evidence for that, but I think that Denolin may be able to help.

DENOLIN: It has been very well demonstrated in the papers of the group from Denver that there are large differences in different species of animals and very large differences in individuals. When you consider people living at high altitude, pulmonary pressure is quite different from one to another.

BARER: Yes, there is the question of the differences in response to hypoxia. Also, it was shown by the Australian group, and the difference may affect the prognosis.

LOCKART: Denolin has answered the question that Riedel raised. In some normal subjects at high altitude a disproportionate rise in pressure with exercise occurs and also a disproportionate rise in pressure when hypoxia is superimposed on the basal level of hypoxia due to altitude. I don't know any study suggesting that this is a genetic trait in man. However, the fact that it is carried as a genetic trait has been extensively documented, as Denolin said, in cattle by Drover's group in Denver. I think they have now reached the fourth generation of inbred cattle - those that have brisket disease and those that do not have it. And the fourth generation get a disproportionate increase in pressure at altitude when they come from parents with brisket disease, whereas those that are offspring of normal cattle don't get the brisket at altitude. I don't know any further data suggesting how this genetic trait is mediated into a disproportionate vasoconstrictive response. I think also there is a paper from the Denver group which suggests that not only they are hyper-responsive to exercise and hypoxic stimuli, but also to some drugs.

BARER: Yes that's right. We had some argument about that last week.   There is also the observation that the mean pressure in people in India is higher for the same altitude than people in South America, which might suggest that there has been some genetic selection in South America.

HEATH: Dr. Barer, I wonder, could I ask you what do you think is the function of the pulmonary argyrophil cells, the cells which look like little carotid bodies in the bronchial tree? What relation do they have to the chemical control of the pulmonary circulation? I imagine that as you are all physiologists you must be terribly knowledgeable about this.

BARER: Well, we don't know which the receptor is to hypoxia or even if there is one, but the argyrophil cell is a good candidate. That's all I can say.

MORPURGO: A very short question. What is your opinion about the vasodilating effect of calcium antagonists?

BARER: Well, we confirmed it in rats, which the Denver group did first of all, and we confirmed it also in cats. We did it in live animals as well as isolated lungs and we found that it abolished the vasoconstrictor response only for a few minutes. When you tried another hypoxic test ten minutes later it was unaltered. Some people in England are trying it clinically now.

CORRIN: I've recently seen demonstrated (and I refer to work being done at the Hammersmith Hospital in London), nerves in the lung which are neither adrenergic nor cholinergic. These are the peptidergic nerves, a third peripheral nervous system which is well developed in the gastrointestinal tract. The peptides include the general inhibitor stomatostatin, and a stimulator. They act neither as neurotransmitters, nor as endocrines, but as a paracrine function. They would be secreted locally to modulate the secretion of further cells and an anatomical structure which suggests itself as a paracrine structure in the lung is not the isolated argyrophil cell which seems to be devoid of nerve supply, but neuroepithelial bodies as their name implies are innervated and could bring together very nicely the neural control of blood flow together with local chemical action of a paracrine system.

BARER: Yes, it is very interesting and I think that quite a lot of work has been done with reference to the bronchial tree. But as far as I know no work has been done on it yet with reference to the pulmonary arteries except the suggestion that the neuroepithelial bodies could be the receptor.

HEATH: If I could make just one comment. It is very interesting that in fact there is an increased number of neuroepithelial bodies in the lungs of rabbits.

BARER: They are believed to contain serotonin, are they not? Which is one of the transmitters which has really been quite in doubt.

LOCKART: I just want to make a short comment about Morpurgo's question about the calcium antagonist. In my hospital at the present time some of the clinicians are studying the effects of Adalat in relatively acute respiratory failure. It turns out to be the most potent vasodilator of the pulmonary circulation I have ever come across. However, in such cases it causes extraordinary fall of arterial PO_2 as any vasodilator will do, and this may be a very important drawback for anyone who would like to use it as a vasodilator. This suggests that this common final pathway for hypoxic vasoconstriction is an increase in intracytoplasmic concentration of calcium in smooth muscle and that's all. It does not tell us anything about the mechanics whereby hypoxia causes vasoconstriction.

DENISON: In Lockart's comment this morning and in your own, it's implicit that in hypoxic vasoconstriction you will be looking for the increase in concentration of a substance. It was certainly true of his. I wanted to draw attention to the possibility that the actual hypoxia could result in the reduction of the synthesis of the catechol amines. There is increasing interest now, and Bakhle I think knows much more about this than I do, in the group of reactions that are mediated by the oxygenase enzymes, that have a lower oxygen affinity. And one of the important discoveries that has come out of their study in the nervous system and the effect of hypoxia on the central nervous system, is that the effect of hypoxia is not to change the concentration of the mediator in a given amount of brain, but to change the turnover, because both the synthesis and the ·destruction of the biogenic amines is controlled by these enzymes. There can be more than one which is affected by hypoxia, and so it can both reduce the production and at the same time reduce the destruction. It may be misleading simply to look at concentration. It may be very important, if the contral nervous system is any guide, to look at turnover. I'd be very glad to hear Bakhle's comment.

BARER: I am not personally committed now, though I was ten years ago, to the transmitter theory of some substance being increased. I think the subject is completely wide-open at the moment.

HAUGE: I just wanted to comment to the last speaker. It is a peculiar observation about the pressure response to hypoxia that it is extremely temperature sensitive. If you compare the effect of an injected vasoconstrictor agent and plot it against the fall in temperature, the constrictor effect stays constant from 38 down to 28°. Whereas if you look at constrictor response to hypoxia, it falls down to zero within the same temperature range, which may suggest it's far away from pointing out any enzymatic action, but may suggest that there is a metabolic mechanism involved.

CONGENITAL MALFORMATIONS OF THE LUNG: ANATOMICAL VIEW-POINT

Antonio Blasi

Professor of Respiratory Diseases
Naples University
Ospedale "V. Monaldi"
Camaldoli
Naples 80131, Italy

This lecture is concerned only with congenital malformations of the lung due to anatomical defects; the following aspects will be discussed:-

1. Definition
2. Classification and personal clinical material
3. Anatomical components of the lung with anatomical malformation
4. Problems concerning the remaining lung.

1. DEFINITION

Lung malformations due to anatomical defect: a definitive arrest of the developing lung at different levels of the bronchial tree.

Stages of Organogenesis and Development of the Lung

22nd - 24th day of embryonal life: formation of the primitive pouch (laryngotracheal groove).

25th - 26th day: cranio-caudal descent of the primitive pouch, separating from the ventral surface of the cephalic intestine.

27th - 28th day: appearance, at the base of the pouch, of a sulcus with two lateral evaginations.

29th - 30th day: formation of the earliest rudiments of
the stem bronchi and the right and left
lung buds.

31st - 34th day: appearance of 3rd order bronchial divisions.

35th - 40th day: formation of 4th and 5th order bronchi.

3rd - 5th month: formation of distal bronchi and bronchioles.

2a. CLASSIFICATION

There are four types of malformation of the lung
due to anatomical defect, which correlate with arrest
during development of the bronchial tree.

1st degree: arrest at one side of the tracheal bifurcation
(agenesis of the lung).

2nd degree: arrest after the formation of one of the
principal bronchi.

3rd degree: arrest at lobar, segmental or subsegmental
bronchi, with absence of bronchiolo-alveolar
development; one or more segments, a lobe or
the entire lung may be involved.

4th degree: arrest at the distal bronchi with partial
bronchiolo-alveolar development.

2b. CLINICAL MATERIAL

We have studied 159 cases in our Clinic, subdivided
as shown in the Table.

TABLE. Clinical Material

Type of malformation	Total N° of cases	Male	Female	Right lung	Left lung
1st degree	5	3	2	2	3
2nd degree	15	6	9	3	12
3rd degree	127	59	68	35	92
4th degree	12	8	4	6	6

There is a markedly greater incidence of 3rd degree malformations (127 cases), which include 56 cases involving the entire lung (total 3rd degree malformation), 59 cases of lobar 3rd degree malformation and 12 cases of segmental 3rd degree malformation. The left lung is affected more frequently than the right in the ratio of

right to left = 1: 3.5.

3. ANATOMICAL COMPONENTS OF THE LUNG WITH ANATOMICAL MALFORMATIONS

In first degree anatomical malformations there is complete agenesis of the lung. Second, third and fourth degree malformations have the following anatomical defects on the side of the malformation:-

Bronchopathic Component

Bronchial branches up to the level of arrested development are involved: at the principal bronchus (2nd degree); at lobar, segmental or subsegmental bronchi (3rd degree); at peripheral bronchi (4th degree). There is bronchiectasis to a greater or lesser extent, with hyperplasia of the mucus-secreting apparatus and the occurence of infection.

Parenchymal Component

No bronchiolo-alveolar structural differentiation takes place, but fibro-connective or dense fibro-elastic tissues develop, giving rise to massive fibrosis (primary massive fibrosis of the lung).

Vascular Component

Development of the pulmonary circulation is absent or poor, with overdevelopment of the bronchial circulation.

4. PROBLEMS CONCERNING THE REMAINING LUNG

The condition of "single lung" arises in both 1st and 2nd degree anatomical malformations. Functionally a total 3rd degree malformation presents as a single lung syndrome.

The single lung must compensate both anatomically and functionally. Thus it develops a greater parenchymal mass than normal, which extends towards the opposite side, occupying the upper part of the half of the thoracic cavity belonging to the site of agenesis. With time, hyperdistension and emphysema develop, giving rise to a progressive syndrome of respiratory insufficiency.

Discussion

CUMMING: This paper is now open for discussion and comments.
Perhaps I may take the chairman's perogative and make both a comment
and ask a question. Blasi has shown great clarity of thought in his
diagnostic procedures. Because in defining disease it is usual for
a clinician to erect a defining characteristic. Now, the defining
characteristic has many forms. It may be aetiological, anatomical,
biochemical, anything at all. Blasi selected for his defining
characteristic an anatomical definition, and that was the defect in
the bronchus. Now, when he came to make a diagnosis he said the
only diagnostic form that would give the defining characteristic was
an anatomical one, and one which defined the defining
characteristic. So I compliment him on an unusual clarity of
thought about making a defining characteristic and selecting that
particular diagnostic tool which would demonstrate it with clarity.
From this comment rises my question. If the lung in first and
second degrees is absent during the time of development, what
adaptation is made by the remainder for taking over its function.
You mentioned, sir, that the number of orders or divisions
increased. Could I ask some very simple questions like: was the
lung volume approaching that of the two lungs? Was the volume of
blood approaching that of the two lungs? And was the ability to
transfer CO equal or not equal to the normal values when two lungs
are concerned?

BLASI: Certainly not in a proportional manner to the two lungs.
In other words, the increase of volume of the surviving parenchymal
mass is perhaps one third or one fourth over and above one normal
lung.

SPINA: I would like to ask you for an explanation of a problem
which has always somewhat perplexed me. You have talked of third
and fourth degree and in the figure you showed and in the case
material, you gave us a very small number of fourth degree cases.
(By way of differentiating you established the development of a
functioning part of the lung - to differentiate between the two
degrees). It is obvious that in the most peripheral part of the
lung which is malformed we do not have the development of
ventilating lung. How do we distinguish, in practice the extremely
peripheral malformation of the fourth degree from the third degree
malformation?

BLASI: From the radiological point of view there is no
differentiation. On the bronchograph the third degree is relatively
proximal be this a defect of the upper area at the level of the
segmentary lobe or in the lower part; it is always a defect of the
sub-segmentary bronchial branches of the fifth or sixth order and

not beyond that. Whereas in the fourth degree we have distal branches proper and even the differentiation of bronchioles. So, while the third degree is an homogeneous category - either the whole lung or lobe has this anatomical defect in which there is no differentiation in the lung tissue - the fourth degree, in some aspects, does show differentiation between bronchiol and alveolar territory and in other areas remains at the level of bronchi and bronchioles which dilate and take on cyst like formation. This is the configuration as presented by radiographic and bronchographic pictures. But we also have the functional aspect which clearly shows the difference.

In defects of the third degree, there is very small movement without any consumption of oxygen. It is completely absent. In the fourth degree defect there is a very small movement upwards which signifies that there is some oxygen consumption; even if slight it nonetheless exists and varies according to the extension of the 4th degree defect which in fact is a very non-homogeneous type of defect but which does manifest some bronchio-alveolar differentiation.

CARRATU: Blasi has asked me to go further into the functional aspects. I go back to the question put by Cumming as regards the functional behaviour. We have studied this from many points of view, from the morphological, angiographic, scintifigraphic and also haemodynamic standpoint. We have evaluated parameters such as pressure and we have evaluated them by means of radiocardiography. Cardiac output is unchanged, but it goes through the pulmonary circuit at a higher velocity. Therefore we have reduced circulation time since there is a reduction of vascular volume and only by increasing the speed can we maintain volume/minute. As regards anastomoses, mentioned by Blasi in his slides and histological data, we have used two methods: selective radiocardiography as developed by Monasteri and Donato which provides for the introduction of macromolecules into the system which are stopped at the lung capillaries and give just one peak when recorded at the precordium. If there is a real anatomical shunt these molecules of 40 - 50 microns in size (they are gold on carbon or macroaggregates of albumin) pass through these anastomoses and are found in the systemic system. We have found this by assessing the radioactivity, of the systemic blood. In the normal subject there is no radioactivity in these subjects the number of counts per minute was very much increased. As regards the functional aspect, at first there is compensation by as much as 30%, but subsequently there is hyperdistention, and then emphysema. Hyperdistention confers no functional benefit. Thus we have an increased resistance in the lesser circulation which increases on exercise. Why is this? Because of the employment of those reserve vascular areas which are over developed and called upon to work in the case of a single lung - when we have the first or second or even the total third degree and because of the absence of these reserve vascular areas and because of the phenomenon of hyperdistension we have an increased resistance in the lesser circulation with pulmonary hypertension and evolution to cor pulmonale.

GUNELLA: I wanted to ask you in the light of these functional investigations whether there are any surgical indications in these patients, obviously because I suppose that there might be cases of hypoxaemic subjects of the second and third degree - probably also hypercapnic too - with pulmonary hypertension who could benefit from surgery.

BLASI: What Gunella says is perfectly right. Excision of a malformed process especially of the second and third degree gives rise to infection but prevents those anatomical short circuits which are intrinsic to the substratum of malformed tissue. Now, in the third degree we have gone ahead and we still carry out excision, and we have a whole series of resected lungs from patients with total third degree defect. A case of total third degree is always a tricky question, especially since if we free the cavity on one side of the chest, we accentuate the phenomenon of mechanical adaptation in the surviving viscera which tends to develop towards emphysema. The indications are clear and positive and no time should be lost in partial defects of the third degree. There are many patients in this category. For example, in the last case we saw a woman of 57 years - we haven't yet decided to operate - we must tread very carefully but in the case of partial third degree of a lobular or segmentary nature the indication for surgery is very clear. In the case of total third degree there is some indication and this must be evaluated case by case and especially during diagnosis - whether the patient is young or old. In the very last diagnosis we carried out, we saw in fact a woman of 57 years who had been previously considered a bronchitic patient. She is a housewife and yet she has an anatomical defect of the whole of the lower lobe, and there is indication for surgery. Where we have been more cautious and we have had a couple of cases - is in the second degree, because the second degree signifies a problem for the surgeon with the small bronchial stump and of what happens to that stump once it has been resected and sutured. There is the risk that a fistula forms at the suture line, especially if very proximal. I have said and this is a difference which we have drawn up recently in agreement with my colleagues Carratu, Barriffi, Marzio and Olivieri, that is between proximal and distal cases in the second and third degree, the main bronchus is of about 2 or 3 cms, especially on the left - a good 3 cms. The bronchus may terminate immediately after its emergence and here the surgical problems are considerable. The surgeon is hard put to resect that small sac which is the source of very bad and abundant secretion and also to suture effectively for the long term. This perhaps is easier if the sac is distal, if the peduncleis a little longer by a couple of cms. and as in the second or third cases I showed you. The second degree then, presents these difficulties for the surgeon with the possibility of a post operational fistula on that small sutured stump. From the clinical pathophysiological point of view, surgery would always be indicated but this must always be weighed against the risks of the operation itself and its consequences afterwards.

UNIDENTIFIED LADY: I wanted to ask Blasi whether in some of his anatomical and histological findings in 1959 of malformations especially of the third and fourth degree, there was evidence of cell movement of an inflammatory nature almost as an outcome of processes which had taken place during foetal life?

BLASI: In the bronchial structure there may be inflammatory processes but there are consequences - in other words they take place in patients who manifest a hypersecretion with inflammation - which leaves its histological mark on the bronchial branches, but I don't think that these can be attributed to the prenatal period.

RECENT DEVELOPMENTS IN THE PHARMACOKINETIC FUNCTION OF LUNG

Y.S. Bakhle

Department of Pharmacology
Royal College of Surgeons
Lincoln's Inn Fields
London WC2A 3PN   England

INTRODUCTION

Since the late 1960's, interest in a non-respiratory function of lung, the pharmacokinetic function, has been growing with the exponential rate apparently inherent in scientific research. This function, which in spite of its name, is chiefly involved with vasoactive hormones and other endogenous substrates, is usually expressed as the change in biological activity of the substrate as it passes through the pulmonary circulation. This field of research, perhaps above all others, has emphasised the importance of cellular environment on enzymic activity by providing many examples of differences between results from broken cell preparations and those from perfused lungs either in isolation or in vivo (see Bakhle and Vane, 1974).

The results of the past 10 years' work, apart from increasing the sum of our knowledge of the lung's functions, have at least three important general implications. First, the research has emphasised that the transfer of substrate from the vascular space to the enzyme is a crucial step and is often rate-determining in the overall metabolic capability of lung. Second, several of the metabolic reactions studied take place in endothelial cells and this has contributed to the renaissance of interest in endothelial cells, for long considered to be biochemically uninteresting and pharmacologically unimportant. Thirdly, it has given much support to the belief that this pharmacokinetic function is an important physiological control mechanism because of the combination of the pulmonary circulation's anatomical

position and its manifest enzymic activities.   If this belief is
well-founded, then we would expect that changes in the lung's
environment, either physiological or pathological, would change
the pharmacokinetic properties of the lung.   Some work on this
aspect has been done and will be reviewed here, along with the
effects of some more iatrogenic changes in the environment of
lung.

OESTROUS CYCLE AND PREGNANCY

Lung contains monoamine oxidase (MAO) which is probably the
most important enzyme in regulating monoamine levels in vivo.
Pulmonary MAO activity is in vitro identical in many respects,
substrate and inhibitor specificity, pH optima etc. to that in
liver and brain (Bakhle and Youdim, 1979).   However in the
perfused lung and in vivo a highly selective uptake system controls
access to MAO such that 5-hydroxytryptamine (5-HT), noradrenaline
and phenylethylamine (PEN) are metabolized and thus inactivated
on passage through the pulmonary circulation, whereas the
equivalently good substrates of MAO, adrenaline and dopamine,
are not metabolised or inactivated (Ginn and Vane, 1968; Nicholas
et al, 1974).

We have recently investigated the variation of MAO activity in
lung homogenates and, in perfused lungs, amine metabolism and
uptake during the various stages of the oestrous cycle in rats
(Bakhle and Ben-Harari, 1979a, b) using 5-HT and PEN as substrates.

During the oestrous cycle in rats, the activity of monoamine
oxidase was found to vary in uterus, ovary and in parts of the
brain (Holzbauer and Youdim, 1973).   Although liver, heart and
kidney MAO did not vary during the cycle (Holzbauer and Youdim,
1973), we were able to show that rat lung MAO activity, measured
in homogenates with either 5-HT or PEN as substrates, did change
significantly over the 4 day oestrous cycle (Bakhle and Ben-Harari,
1979a, b).   For both substrates, activity peaked at met-oestrus
and was lowest at pro-oestrus.   A kinetic analysis of the
reactions showed that, for 5-HT, the major effect was on Km,
suggesting a change in affinity, whereas for PEN, the major effect
was on Vmax, suggesting a change in the amount of catalytic
protein present.

However, for both substrates, metabolism in perfused isolated
lungs was not correlated with the changes observed in vitro.   Thus,
in perfused lungs, for 5-HT, metabolism at met-oestrus was less
than that at pro-oestrus, the reverse of findings in vitro and for
PEN, metabolism at met- and pro-oestrus were the same in spite of
a five-fold difference in vitro.   This discrepancy was due to

the overriding effect of the uptake step which varied independently
and was better correlated with the metabolism in perfused lung.
For 5-HT, uptake was highest at pro-oestrus and for PEN uptake at
met- and pro-oestrus was similar and higher than at the other two
stages.

We have drawn two general conclusions from these results.
First that, unlikely as this may seem, the lung is a "target"
organ for sex steroids with both an intracellular site of action
on MAO activity and a membrane site of action on the uptake
system for the amines.   The finding that the metabolism of
endogenous amines is susceptible to the changes brought about by
a physiological change in the body, the oestrous cycle, strengthens
our belief that we are dealing with a physiologically important
function.   Second, the importance of the uptake step in lung
pharmacokinetics is demonstrated yet again.   Predictions of
activity in the whole organ based on in vitro results would have
been totally misleading.

If amine uptake is affected by the oestrous cycle, then this
suggests an effect on the endothelial cell membrane, the locus of
the uptake system.   Another important pulmonary enzyme, the
peptidase angiotensin converting enzyme is also located on the
endothelial cell membrane (Ryan and Ryan, 1977).   Measurement of
the conversion of angiotensin I in isolated perfused lungs from
rats over the oestrous cycle showed that this activity also varied.
Conversion was highest at pro-oestrus and low during met-oestrus
and oestrus (Bakhle and Ben-Harari, 1979c).

Allied to this presumably steroid-mediated change in lung
metabolism of monoamines and peptides is the change in metabolism
of prostaglandins (PGs) during pregnancy in rabbits.   In cell-free
systems (Bedwani and Marley, 1975; Sun and Armour, 1974) and
in vivo (Egerton-Vernon and Bedwani, 1975), pulmonary metabolism
of PGs in the mothers increased towards term with a maximum at
parturition.   It seems therefore that the pharmacokinetic function
of lung is susceptible to the physiological changes occurring
during the oestrous cycle and pregnancy.

COMPOSITION OF VENTILATING GASES

The pharmacokinetic properties of the lung are not dependent
on ventilation for their proper expression as non-ventilated
perfused lungs are comparable in these properties to the lung
in vivo.   However, changes in the ventilating gas mixture do
affect some of those properties.   Thus the addition of halothane
to the ventilating gas in pentobarbital-anaesthetized dogs almost
abolished the inactivation of noradrenaline across the pulmonary
circulation but not that of PGE_2 (Bakhle and Block, 1976).

The content of oxygen in the ventilating gas is also a determinant of enzymic activity. Hypoxia has been studied both as chronic and acute insults. Chronic hypobaric hypoxia - as a model of high altitude conditions - increased the components of the renin-angiotensin system including lung converting enzyme (Molteni et al, 1974). Analogies have been drawn between these results and the hypoxia in neonatal respiratory distress states to explain the increase in serum converting enzyme found in infants with respiratory distress (Mattioli et al, 1975).

Acute hypoxia is known to cause pulmonary vasoconstriction and in 1974 Berkov proposed, with later support from Alexander et al (1976), that angiotensin II was involved in the mediation of this vascular response, perhaps via an increase in converting enzyme activity.

Recently, however, Leuenberger et al (1978) found the converse. Using dogs and assessing the conversion of angiotensin I by its pressor effect, they showed that conversion was directly related to arterial pO_2, this value being decreased by changing from room air to hypoxic (21-8% O_2; N_2) gas mixtures. Thus conversion fell to 40% at a pO_2 of 30mm from 94% at a pO_2 of 84mm, suggesting that the pulmonary hypertension observed was not simply related to increased production of angiotensin II. Another remarkable feature of this work was the rapidity of the changes. As the oxygen in arterial blood fell so did angiotensin conversion and as the animal was returned to room air and arterial oxygen increased, so the conversion returned to normal. These rapid changes have been attributed to a physical change in the endothelial cell membrane (the locus of converting enzyme) rather than changes in enzyme amount or affinity.

The toxic effects of hyperoxia - exposure to 90-100% oxygen atmospheres - are usually correlated with alveolar epithelial cell damage. However, in early stages, capillary endothelium is damaged (Kistler et al, 1967) and this should lead to alterations in the fate of substrates metabolised in these cells. Block and Fisher (1977) found a small decrease in 5-HT metabolism in isolated lungs from rats after only 18 hr to exposure to 97% O_2 and this fell further to 65% of control levels after 48 hr exposure. Metabolism of PGE_2 was also decreased following a similar regime of oxygen exposure (Klein et al, 1978). We have recently studied 5-HT, PGE_2, angiotensin I and bradykinin metabolism in isolated lungs from rats exposed to atmospheres containing 95% O_2 (Bakhle et al, 1979a). In our experiments metabolism of all substrates was decreased after 60 hr O_2 exposure but 5-HT was not affected before this time. Angiotensin conversion was decreased after 48 hr and the earliest changes were seen with PGE_2 after 36 hours. The latter effect was completely reversed after 48 hr in room air.

From all these experiments it appears that exposure to high concentrations of oxygen will damage the pharmacokinetic potential of lung and, in some instances, will do so at a time earlier than damage to epithelial cells and consequent impaired gas exchange occurs.   Although Fisher's group have suggested 5-HT metabolism might provide an "early warning" of oxygen toxicity, we feel that PGE_2 metabolism might prove to be a better test variable.

Another pulmonary insult commonly offered via the airways is tobacco smoke.   Most work with tobacco exposure has concentrated on the metabolism by lung tissue of carcinogenic polycyclic hydrocarbons present in cigarette smoke.

The immediate effects of inhaled cigarette smoke on metabolism of $PGF_2\alpha$ and of angiotensin I were studied in isolated rabbit lung (Hagedorn & Kostenbauder, 1977, 1978).   The ventilating gas (room air) was replaced by cigarette smoke for 4 x 2 sec puffs and this single short and acute exposure had no effect on metabolism.

At the same time we were studying this question (Bakhle et al, 1979b), using a regime of smoke exposure known to increase metabolism and binding of benzo-(a)-pyrene (Cohen et al, 1977) and to affect testosterone metabolism (Hartiala et al, 1978) in rat lung.

After 1 day's exposure (1 hr per day), the conversion of angiotensin I was doubled and the inactivation of PGE_2 was decreased but metabolism of bradykinin and of 5-HT was unchanged. After 10 days' exposure, the angiotensin conversion returned to normal, bradykinin and 5-HT metabolism were still unchanged and PGE_2 metabolism appeared to be further decreased.   From these initial experiments some interesting conclusions can be drawn. The selectivity of the effects seen argues against a non-specific "poisoning" of the lung cells.   Furthermore, the different types of enzymic activity affected one membrane-bound peptidase (converting enzyme) and one intracellular dehydrogenase (PG dehydrogenase), do not suggest a common mode of action of cigarette smoke.   Our experiments do however suggest that the alteration of the normal control function of the pulmonary circulation by smoke exposure may be a mechanism for the initiation of the cardiovascular changes associated with cigarette smoking.

DRUG TREATMENT

The two last examples of altered pulmonary pharmacokinetics are iatrogenic in nature.   First, pulmonary inactivation of $PGF_2\alpha$ (Bito and Baroody, 1975) and PGE_2 (Bakhle et al, 1978) in rat

isolated lung was decreased by infusion of an indicator dye,
bromcresol green.   Other indicator dyes - bromcresol purple and
thymol blue - were also effective (Bakhle et al, 1978).   This
apparently general efficacy of dyes as PG inactivation inhibitors
led to the testing of clinically used dye molecules as inhibitors
of PGE_2 inactivation in rat lung (Bakhle, 1978).   The most potent
(on a molar basis) was indocyanine green followed by bromsulphalein,
phenol red, Evans blue and methylene blue.   Preliminary experiments
in human isolated lung suggest that, in this tissue also, these dye
molecules are effective inhibitors of PG inactivation.   These
results imply that the assumption usually made that these dye
marker substances are physiologically inert is no longer valid and
that these dyes may alter the system they are used to monitor.

The second example is of true pharmacokinetics.   Passage
through the pulmonary circulation leads to the extensive and
rapid binding of many basic drugs like imipramine (Junod, 1972),
amphetamine (Anderson et al, 1974), propranolol (Dollery and Junod,
1976) and lignocaine (Post et al, 1978).   This binding is not
followed by metabolism.   Junod (1972) had shown displacement of
bound ^{14}C-imipramine by chlorpromazine in rat isolated lungs.   In
a recent series of papers, lignocaine binding to lung in both pigs
(Bertler et al, 1978) and man in vivo (Jorfeldt et al, 1979) had
been demonstrated to be extensive.   More important, nortriptyline
bound to pig lung in vivo was displaced by a bolus injection of
lignocaine with a subsequent decrease in cardiotoxicity (Post and
Lewis, 1979).   Although in this particular case the improvement
in the ECG could be due to the lignocaine itself, this result does
suggest that displacement of tricyclic antidepressants could be
achieved with other basic drugs with no intrinsic cardiac effect,
thus relieving the cardiotoxic effects of tricyclic antidepressant
overdosage.

CONCLUSIONS

In this brief review of the pharmacokinetic function of lung,
I have emphasised alterations in this function brought about by
physiological and pathological interventions.   Of particular
importance is the general inference that changes in ventilating
gases can change the metabolism of blood-borne substrates.   The
mechanisms by which insults originating in the airways are
transferred to the endothelial cells of the pulmonary capillaries
are not yet known but their existence means that our environment
can have a direct influence on the circulating level of
physiologically important vasoactive hormones.

It is also very relevant to this meeting to emphasise the
importance of the lung in pharmacokinetics of basic drugs.   We
shall be hearing more about this later (Geddes, this vol.) but it

seems to me that we may see the binding of drugs to lung providing
as many interactions between basic drugs as those we are more
familiar with between acidic drugs bound to plasma proteins.

It is very clear to me that investigations into the biochemical
properties of the lung as a whole and particularly those expressed
towards endogenous vasoactive substances will add to our knowledge
of systemic homeostatic mechanisms.   Furthermore such investigations may also provide a greater understanding of the lung's own
response to alterations in its internal or external environment.

REFERENCES

Alexander, J.M., Nyby, M.D. and Jasberg, K.A. 1976, Effect of
    angiotensin on hypoxic pulmonary vasoconstriction in
    isolated dog lung. J.appl.Physiol., 41: 84.
Anderson, M.W., Orton, T.C., Pickett, R.D. and Eling, T.E. 1974,
    Accumulation of amines in the isolated perfused rabbit
    lung. J.Pharm.exp.Therap., 186: 456.
Bakhle, Y.S. 1978, Clinically used dyes are inhibitors of
    prostaglandin E_2 inactivation in rat isolated lung.
    Br.J.Pharmac., 64: 386P.
Bakhle, Y.S. and Ben-Harari, R.R. 1979a, Effects of oestrous
    cycle and exogenous ovarian steroids on 5-hydroxytryptamine
    metabolism in rat lung. J.Physiol., 291:11.
Bakhle, Y.S. and Ben-Harari, R.R. 1979b, Effects of the oestrous
    cycle and exogenous ovarian steroids on metabolism of
    β-phenylethylamine in rat lung. Br.J.Pharmac. (in press)
Bakhle, Y.S. and Ben-Harari, R.R. 1979c, Metabolism of
    angiotensin and bradykinin in rat isolated lungs during
    the oestrous cycle. J.Physiol. (in press)
Bakhle, Y.S. and Block, A.J. 1976, Effects of halothane on
    pulmonary inactivation of noradrenaline and prostaglandin E_2
    in anaesthetized dogs. Clin.Sci.mol.Med., 50: 87.
Bakhle, Y.S., Hartiala, J. and Toivonen, H. 1979, Exposure to
    oxygen inhibits metabolism of vasoactive hormones in rat
    isolated lung. J.Physiol. (in press)
Bakhle, Y.S., Jancar, Sonia and Whittle, B.J.R. 1978, Uptake and
    inactivation of prostaglandin E_2 methyl analogues in the
    rat pulmonary circulation. Br.J.Pharmac., 62: 275.
Bakhle, Y.S. and Vane, J.R. 1974, Pharmacokinetic function of
    the pulmonary circulation. Physiol. Rev., 54: 1007.
Bakhle, Y.S. and Youdim, M.B.H. 1979, The metabolism of 5-hydroxy-
    tryptamine and β-phenylethylamine in perfused rat lung and
    in vitro. Br.J.Pharmac., 65: 147.
Bedwani, J.R. and Marley, P.B. 1975, Enhanced inactivation of
    prostaglandin E_2 by the rabbit lung during pregnancy or
    progesterone treatment. Br.J.Pharmac., 53: 547.

Berkov, S. 1974, Hypoxic pulmonary vasoconstriction in the rat;
        the necessary role of angiotensin II. Circ. Res., 35: 256.

Bertler, A., Lewis, D.H., Löfström, J.B. and Post, C. 1978,
        In vivo lung uptake of lidocaine in pigs. Acta anaesth.,
        Scand., 22: 530.

Bito, L.Z. and Baroody, R.A. 1975, Inhibition of pulmonary
        prostaglandin metabolism by inhibitors of prostaglandin
        bio-transport (probenecid and bromocresol green).
        Prostaglandins, 10: 633.

Block, E.R. and Fisher, A.B. 1977, Depression of serotonin
        clearance by rat lungs during oxygen exposure. J.appl.
        Physiol., 42:33.

Cohen, G.M., Uotila, P., Hartiala, J. Suolinna, E.M., Simberg, N.
        and Pelkonen, O. 1977, Metabolism and covalent binding of
        ^{3}H benzo(a) pyrene by isolated perfused lungs and short-term
        tracheal organ culture of cigarette smoke-exposed rats.
        Cancer Res. 37: 2147.

Dollery, C.T. and Junod, A.F. 1976, Concentration of ($\pm$)
        propranolol in isolated, perfused lungs of rat. Br.J.Pharmac.,
        57: 67.

Egerton-Vernon, J.M. and Bedwani, J.R. 1975, Prostaglandin 15-
        hydroxydehydrogenase activity during pregnancy in rabbits
        and rats. Eur.J.Pharmacol., 33: 405.

Ginn, R. and Vane, J.R. 1968, Disappearance of catecholamines
        from the pulmonary circulation. Nature, 219:740.

Hagedorn, B. and Kostenbauder, H.B. 1977, Studies on the effect
        of tobacco smoke on the biotransformation of vasoactive
        substances in the isolated perfused rabbit lung. I -
        prostaglandin $F_2\alpha$.   Res. Commun. Chem. Pathol. Pharm.,
        18: 495.

Hagedorn, B. and Kostenbauder, H.B. 1978, Studies on the effect
        of tobacco smoke on the biotransformation of vasoactive
        substances in the isolated perfused rabbit lung. II -
        Angiotensin I conversion. Res.Commun.Chem.Pathol.Pharm.
        20: 195.

Hartiala, J., Uotila, P. and Nienstedt, W. 1978, The effects
        of cigarette smoke exposure on testosterone metabolism in
        the isolated perfused rat lung. J.Steroid Biochem.,9:365.

Holzbauer, M. and Youdim, M.B.H. 1973, The oestrous cycle and
        monoamine oxidase activity. Br.J.Pharmac., 48: 600.

Jorfeldt, L., Lewis, D.H. Löfström, J.B. and Post. C. 1979,
        Lung uptake of lidocaine in healthy volunteers. Acta.
        anaesth.scand. (in press)

Junod, A.F. 1972, Accumulation of ^{14}C-imipramine in isolated
        perfused rat lungs. J.Pharm.exp.Ther. 183:182.

Kistler, G.S., Caldwell, P.R.B. and Weibel, E.W. 1967,
        Development of fine structural damage to alveolar and
        capillary lining cells in oxygen poisoned rat lungs.
        J.cell.Biol., 33:605.

Klein, L.S., Fisher, A.B., Soltoff, S. and Colburn, R.F. 1978,
    Effect of oxygen exposure on pulmonary metabolism of
    prostaglandin E_2. Amer.Rev.resp.Dis., 118:622.
Leuenberger, P.J., Stalcup, S.A. Mellins, R.B., Greenbaum, L.M.
    and Turino, G.M. 1978, Decrease in angiotensin I
    conversion by acute hypoxia in dogs. Proc.Soc.exp.Biol.Med.
    158:586.
Mattioli, L. Zakheim, R.M., Mullis, K. and Molteni, A. 1975,
    Angiotensin I converting enzyme activity in idiopathic
    respiratory distress syndrome of the newborn infant and in
    experimental alveolar hypoxia in mice. J.Pediatrics.,87:97.
Molteni, A., Zakheim, R.M., Mullis, K.B. and Mattioli, L. 1974,
    The effect of chronic alveolar hypoxia on lung and serum
    angiotensin I converting enzyme activity. Proc.Soc.exp.
    Biol.Med., 147:263.
Nicholas, T.E., Strum, J.M., Angelo, L.S. and Junod, A.F. 1974,
    Site and mechanism of uptake of ^{3}H-l-norepinephrine by
    isolated perfused rat lungs. Circ.Res., 35:670.
Post, C., Andersson, R.G.G., Ryrfeldt, A. and Nilsson, E. 1978,
    Transport and binding of lidocaine by lung slices and
    perfused lung of rats. Acta.pharmacol.toxicol., 43:156.
Post, C. and Lewis, D.H. 1979, Displacement of nortriptyline
    and uptake of ^{14}C-lidocaine in the lung after administration
    of ^{14}C-lidocaine to nortriptyline in intoxicated pigs.
    Acta.pharmacol.toxicol. (in press)
Ryan, J.W. and Ryan, U.S. 1977, Pulmonary endothelial cells.
    Fed.Proc., 36:2683.
Sun, F.F. and Armour, S.B. 1974, Prostaglandin 15-hydroxydehydro-
    genase and Δ^{13} reductase levels in the lungs of maternal,
    fetal and neonatal rabbits. Prostaglandins, 7:327.

Discussion

CUMMING: When you spoke of the diminution in activity of lung converting enzyme related to the endothelial cell, you concluded that there was a change in the geometry of the endothelial cell and you mentioned invagination as one of the mechanisms. When you showed us the slide which showed a diminution in converting enzyme due to hyperoxia you did not draw the same conclusion. Can you tell us why?

BAKHLE: Because I have not done the recovery experiment for hyperoxia.

CUMMING: Thank you.

HEATH: I wonder if I can just make a point, chairman, as a morbid anatomist, about endothelial cells. It is very interesting in a conference of this sort to have morbid anatomists and physiologists sitting together. In Bakhle's very interesting paper he talked about the endothelial cell and of course I realise that the complexities of trying to find out which endothelial cells he is referring to are extremely profound. But it would be an enormous advance if we knew this because the interesting thing is that from the point of view of a morbid anatomist the endothelial cells which you find, say, in the pulmonary trunk are quite different in shape and surface area to those in the pulmonary vein. And they, again, are different in size and shape from the endothelial cells in the systemic veins or the endothelial cells of the aorta. When Bakhle talks about morphological changes in cells resulting in disturbances of the functions of these enzymes, I could well believe that this is within the realm of possibility, because even to somebody using such a crude technique as morbid anatomy you can actually see changes in these endothelial cells. For example, we have done some work on feeding rats on the Crotellaria Spectabilis alkaloids. Now, if you do that the endothelial cells of the pulmonary trunk change in size and area. We are not even talking here about minute, ultrastructural differences on the cell membrane, which almost certainly will occur; you actually get a change in the gross configuration of the cell. So my message is: there are large differences, I am sure, there are different sorts of endothelial cells in the pulmonary circulation and even now we know that they do change in type under different sorts chemical and physical conditions.

CUMMING: Would you like to comment on that, Bakhle.

BAKHLE: Yes. The evidence that is so far available suggests that, as far as the amines are concerned, if you believe autoradiography at EM level (and some people just don't believe it) the silver stains in EMs, when you give a rat lung radioactive noradrenalin or 5-hydroxy tryptamine, seem to be down amongst the alveolar capillary endothelial cells. Now, this may be merely a statistical thing, and that is where most of the blood is anyway, but I wouldn't like to go too far in that. The second thing is: you can demonstrate angiotensin converting enzyme immunohistochemically and you can also use it to demonstrate it again at EM level by coupling it in various subtle ways. Now, when you do that, again you can see the staining down at the alveolar capillaries. So all I can say is that at least you can demonstrate it at the alveolar capillary. What, as I am sure you know, is very difficult to do is to make a quantitative assessment of this sort of staining things and say "yes, 50% is there and 25% is there". One sees a spot here and another spot there, so that it is essentially an inaccurate art. The other thing is of course many people use cultured endothelial cells. Most people have been driven to use it from the pulmonary artery, merely because of the size of the vessel. There are people who say you can get capillary endothelial cells by perfusing the lung with dilutions of trypsin or something like that. Maybe. But I don't know anybody who has done the comparison between pulmonary arterial endothelial cells and others. I agree that would be interesting. There is one last thing to say: there have been published photographs which suggest that the endothelial cells in the lung, have projections almost like villi, on their surface. If those projections (which must increase surface area enormously) disappear, that may do it - no - that probably wouldn't do it because you somehow have to remove the total area. The trouble with your Crotellaria is that it takes time. This stuff is almost like a switch. That's what I find so fascinating.

CUMMING: Bahkle said that the activity is likely to be in the alveolar capillary membrane because that is where most of the blood is. That is not a true statement. Most of the blood is not in the alveolar capillary membrane.

BAKHLE: O.K.

CUMMING: Of the 150 ml. in the pulmonary artery, 145 ml. is in the large branches and about 5 ml in the distal branches. There is a similar situation in the pulmonary vein. Depending how you measure it, there may be 100 ml, so you are talking about 30% only. I think there was another problem involved - a rate of change of transfer. Now, here it is important that the flow shall be slow, and it is in this area that the flow is slow.

LEE: I have two questions. One: what happens to the circulating platelets with hypoxia and hyperoxia? And two: what hapens to the flow of lymph.

BAKHLE: Well, my answer must be very quick. I am told that
chronic hypoxia leads to an increased aggregability of platelets.
Whether this is something that happens specifically in lungs or it
will happen anywhere, and the reason perhaps that you see it in
lungs is because there the capillaries are smaller. It is a better
filter than perhaps in the periphery. That may be so. Your second
question was about the lymph. One knows absolutely nothing about
the lymph changes under these conditions.

LEE: Because if one went to an appropriate animal one could do
acute experiments and look at the lymph drainage contents which
would tell you something about the interstitial environment, which
you can't get at any other way.

BAKHLE: Indeed.

LEE: The other thing is that if the platelets are involved then
there will be a change in distribution of substrate because the
platelets will be full of vasoactive amines which would then start
forcing the reaction.

BAKHLE: I suspect that the lung has an enormous capacity for
handling these substrates. One experiment in a dog lung put the
blood flow up five times and they got exactly the same percentage
conversion of angio 1 as they had under normal circumstances. So,
as far as that is concerned we can say that a lung can handle at
least five times normality. That may not be what you are trying to
say, but I suspect that there is an incredible capacity in the lung
to handle an awful lot of stuff.

HORVATH: As far as I understook in your excellent exciting
lecture, the data relates to lung homogenates, after washing free of
blood.

BAKHLE: Yes, the perfused lungs are blood free.

HORVATH: Blood free, that is very important. What is the
situation when blood remains in the lungs? Have you control
experiments, for example, on the effect of platelets.

BAKHLE: I am in the lucky position that the experiments were first
done many years ago in vivo. So that the conversion of angio, the
metabolism of 5-HT, the metabolism of bradykinin, have all been done
in vivo first. What surprises me is that when you take something as
artificial as perfused lungs, that they give you the same answers as
the lungs in vivo, with platelets, leukocytes, blood, dirt,
everything.

BARER: First of all the place of angiotensin II as a transmitter of hypoxic vasoconstriction. The ferret lung is extremely reactive to hypoxia, but shows no constriction whatsoever to angiotensin II. Secondly, the question of the antidepressants. We have recently shown that imipramine and amitryptaline give large rises in pulmonary artery pressure when given acutely. Now, these effects are somewhat delayed and we suspected that they were releasing other substances from the lung. Could you suggest what these might be?

BAKHLE: It is the delay that worries me. If you had got a more or less instantaneous effect I would assume that what you were doing is interfering with the normal metabolism, say of 5-HT. It's the delay I don't understand. I am not sure what natural product drugs like amitryptaline could displace from the lung. They will interfere, as you know, with amine uptake, but the amine must be there in the first place. It may be that the amitryptaline is slowly diffusing perhaps to a sympathetic nerve ending. And changing some reaction there, which of course it could do, because as we know, amitryptaline does potentiate the effects of ordinarily released catecholamines. But I don't know of any naturally occurring material which is made in the lung which could be released in that way by amitryptaline.

BLASI: There is a general disease with a possible excessive involvement of the lung which produces an increase in angiotensin convertase. This is sarcoidosis, how does this come about?

BAKHLE: In the normal lung, it is difficult to find staining for angiotensin converting enzyme except in endothelial cells. Some people now use angio converting enzyme as a marker for endothelial cells, and in a carcinoma it is impossible to see what they are. The change in serum converting enzyme which you see in sarcoid, is now reasonably well established. It has taken some time but we can agree that that happens. When Silverstein tried biopsy of lungs, he said if you took unaffected lung there were practically no changes. If he managed to take a piece of sarcoid it had much higher angiotensin converting enzyme activity? But the unaffected lung didn't seem to have any such increase. Now, this could be because sarcoid is a focal disease. But I suspect this is what I would call an epiphenomenon. I don't think it's causative. It does seem to reflect the course of the disease, and its treatment. As it is treated with steroids, with radiological improvement, so the activity in the serum returns to normal. But I don't think it is directly a cause.

HAUGE: In many of the studies you have told us that you have looked at the difference between arterial and venous blood and from this difference drawn conclusions on what is happening within the lung tissue chemically. Wouldn't it in some instances be even more advantageous to look at the difference between arterial blood and lung lymph, since the dilution effect then would be much less. If

you look at the amount of lung tissue compared to the blood going
through, there must be quite a large dilution. Whereas if you
collect the lymph coming from the lung you might benefit from doing
that type of study.
  BAKHLE: Indeed.   The difficulty that I have is that in a way my
primary interest in the lung is as a control mechanism for the rest
of the body. In a way I don't care what happens to the lung itself.
It is a very reactionary thing to say in this audience, but my
interest really is as a control function. Therefore to me what is
important is that AV difference. And since the lymph has got to
come back anyway into the venous side of the circulation - if I am
seriously looking for a transmitter, for a mediator of the hypoxic
vasoconstriction, then that is a sort of experiment which I must do.
I agree with you there.

HEATH: I'd just like to make another morbid anatomical point and I
wonder if Bakhle would like to comment on it. In constriction in
vessels, say in pulmonary veins, as I hope to show tomorrow, when
the smooth muscle cells contract they tend to get shorter and
thicker with evaginations on them. And from the morbid anatomical
point of view it is very interesting that when muscle cells
constrict they get very very close association with the overlying
endothelial cells. And I am wondering if that is entirely
fortuitous and mechanical pressure on the endothelial cells, or is
there some deeper functional significance?

BAKHLE: I was very struck by my first electron microscope
pictures, where there was an incredible sort of pseudopodia sticking
right into the endothelial cells, which clearly belonged to the
underlying smooth muscle. One hope that I had, which now seems to
have been eliminated, was that since we have eliminated the
endothelial cells at the site of prostaglandin inactivation the
question remains where else does this happen. Now, the obvious
second place is smooth muscle cells. And I thought this is probably
where it happens. Unfortunately cultured muscle cells from the
pulmonary artery did not metabolise either. So we do not know where
it happens. I feel that structures like that mean something, but I
am not sure what this is.

LEE: Would you like at this stage to draw on the blackboard a
scheme for a working hypothesis to enable the rest of us to have a
feeling for how you think about the process? Because you suggested
that there are changes in the endothelial surface, that there are
changes in the rate limiting phenomena, there are other cells within
the interstitium, there are muscle cells in the alveolus. Would you
just like in this intimate audience where nobody will repeat
anything you are going to say give us an idea. (laughter).

BAKHLE: Well, I must say that you ask me a lot, because the last
time I said something about the physiology and how much blood there

was around I got my fingers slapped. So, you are asking me now to put my head in Heath's mouth. However a unifying hypothesis - I am not sure that at the moment if is worth my while to make such a hypothesis. All I can say is that most of the functions seem to lie in the endothelial cells, one big exclusion from this being the prostaglandins business. Metabolism and synthesis probably takes place where I would call distally. I don't think anybody else has any idea. In terms of the factors which may affect this sort of metabolism I am really just guessing what may happen or what may not happen. The changes we see in the estrous cycle, the changes we see in pregnancy, I have no idea what the physiological significance of these are. But the question is if you like one of faith, that is to say if I were God would I make such a change if it were not purposeful? Now, this is a very dangerous thing to say, but it keeps me happy for some time. I am really giving you some results which I hope may wake some response in somebody who has done other experiments or has seen a patient in certain conditions and thinks perhaps in this patient this may be happening. I don't think I am giving you a unifying hypothesis and I think it would be wrong, at this stage, even to attempt that. Mr. Chairman, if I might ask a question to the audience, which I am sure contains more respiratory physicians than I have seen for many years; would it be of any value to your clinical treatment to have an early warning of oxygen toxicity, before gas exchange became compromised? Would it make any difference to you, or would it make no difference?

CUMMING: Can I begin by trying to attempt an answer to that question? It has in it an assumption, and that is that oxygen toxicity occurs in some people and not in others. And it is in the people in whom it occurs that you wish to identify it at an early stage. I would guess that most clinicians now using oxygen do so in a way that would avoid oxygen toxicity in the patients whom they are treating. I think maybe with one exception, and that's the difficult exception of treating the premature neonates. A premature neonate exposed to high oxygen tensions can develop retrolental fibroplasia. The neonate who is not exposed to high oxygen tension in the inspired gas dies from anoxemia. And in fact the statistics suggest that for every one case of retrolental fibroplasia that is prevented ten deaths occur from hypoxemia. Now in that case it might be of advantage to know that you are dealing with someone who is sensitive to oxygen. Whether it would be possible, given that knowledge, so to change one's action as to avoid the difficulty, to sail between Scylla and Charybdis, I don't know.

BAKHLE: That is essentially the question, you know. Whether it would be of any value clinically and I don't know.

CUMMING: Would any other clinician like to give an opinion too? I think that most opinions are now drifting towards replacing the water loss which all of this hot air has generated here. And I

think we should now therefore retire to have our coffee break. Let
me point out two important facts; we shall be back here by eleven,
and if you have not arranged to collect your packed lunch I suggest
that you do it now and the time the bus leaves at about twelve
fifteen. Try not to do it after the meeting because this would
delay the departure of the bus and those wise virgins who have taken
the precaution of getting it early would be delayed by the foolish
ones who have not done so. Thank you.

THE BIOCHEMICAL FUNCTION OF THE PULMONARY CIRCULATION

D.M. Geddes

London Chest Hospital   Brompton Hospital
Bonner Road   Fulham Road
London   London

The majority of studies on the biochemical properties of the pulmonary circulation have concentrated on substances with short circulating half lives. This is partly a reflection of the physiological importance of pulmonary inactivation of compounds such as catecholamines, prostaglandins and 5-hydroxytryptamine and angiotensin-I, but is also due to the technical difficulties encountered when hormones with longer circulating lives are studied. This is because the lung receives the whole cardiac output, and so only very small arterio-venous differences will occur across the lung unless considerable metabolism takes place. This section concentrates on compounds with circulating half lives much longer than those of the vasoactive amines and in particular on polypeptide hormones and drugs. It is important to emphasise that the techniques are difficult and that much of the data presented is preliminary and needs confirmation by other workers before it can be fully accepted.

Polypeptide Hormones

The pulmonary conversion of angiotensin-I to angiotensin-II, and the breakdown of bradykinin into inactive fragments are catalysed by converting enzyme which is present on the luminal surface of the capillary endothelial cells. This enzyme is active on a wide range of peptide substrates and so other poly-peptides may be altered during passage through the pulmonary circulation. Korman et al,[1] investigated the fate of human gastrin in dogs and concluded that the lung was the major site of breakdown of this peptide. Their findings could not be confirmed by Dent et al,[2] and these different results may be due to different specificities of the immuno assays used by the two groups.

Furthermore, the immunoactivity of gastrin in these assays does not
correlate well with the bioactivity of the hormone and so the role
of the lung in inactivating gastrin remains uncertain. However, it
is reasonable to conclude that some alteration of the polupeptide
takes place during passage through the pulmonary circulation.
Lockett,[3] has demonstrated a renally active peptide influencing
renal sodium exchange, which is formed in the lung from α_2 globulin.
These interesting observations have not, however, been followed up
by other workers. Other polypeptides have been little studied.
Substance-P and physalaemin appears to be unaffected by passage
through isolated perfused lungs, while the effect on blood pressure
of vasopressin and oxytocin are the same when the hormones are
infused into the aorta or the right ventricle. Vasoactive
intestinal polypeptide similarly does not appear to be inactivated.

Insulin is altered be converting enzyme in vitro and
preliminary reports suggested considerable inactivation of the
hormone during passage through pulmonary circulation in man.[4] In
an attempt to confirm and extend these observations, blood samples
were taken simultaneously from the pulmonary artery and aorta from
men undergoing diagnostic cardiac catheterisation, and a number of
polypeptide hormones were estimated, as well as, free amino acids.
The results are summarised in Table I.

Table I.   Mixed Venous ($\overline{V}$) and Aortic (A) Levels of Hormones
            and Free Amino Acids in Fasting Man.

		$\overline{V}$		A	
		Mean	SD	Mean	SD
Luteinising Hormone u/l		31.20	42.40	30.30	40.70
Follicle Stimulating Hormone u/l		19.40	23.70	19.30	23.80
Thyroid Stimulating Hormone mu/l		1.80	0.70	1.80	0.50
Growth Hormone µg/l	**	1.65	1.79	1.17	3.19
Prolactin µg/l		7.97	3.50	7.98	4.70
Insulin mu/l		6.65	3.70	7.76	5.80
Glucagon pm/l	*	2.30	3.45	1.74	2.60
Glycine µm/l	*	196.40	63.90	202.20	65.90
Phenylalanine µm/l	*	56.00	11.10	58.60	11.60
Serine µm/l	*	116.60	36.30	124.00	38.80
Aspartic Acid µm/l	**	10.75	7.26	12.70	8.30

Levels of 15 other amino acids showed no significant difference.

$*p < 0.05$; $**p < 0.01$ (Wilcoxon's rank sum test for paired samples).

This suggested some effect of the pulmonary circulation of glucagon and growth hormone, and these hormones, as well as, insulin were further studied in ambulant dogs with indwelling catheters. The catheters were placed in the pulmonary artery, aorta and jugular vein, and the ends passed under the skin and brought out on the dogs back between the scapulae. Each hormone was injected as a bolus into the jugular catheter and then frequent paired aortic and pulmonary arterial blood samples were taken at timed intervals, and the hormone estimated by radio immuno assay. These studies showed significant low grade clearance of glucagon by the lungs but demonstrated no significant effect on human growth hormone. For insulin the findings were more complex: there was a significant increase in immunoactivity as a result of passage through the lungs for the first 15 minutes after injection followed by a small but significant drop in immunoactivity for the next 30 minutes by which time the measured insulin approached basal levels. These experiments are discribed in detail elsewhere (see Geddes et al 1979).[5]

In summary these studies provide some evidence of hormone breakdown by the pulmonary circulation with release of free amino acids. This is unlikely to be of any importance to the overall clearance of hormones from the blood, but may indicate a relatively non specific property of the lungs in the breakdown of circulating polypeptides.

Drugs

Many drugs accumulate in the lungs following oral or intra- venous administration. Although, some such as imipramine and noradrenaline, may have relatively specific uptake mechanisms the majority of drugs do not and uptake appears to be predominantly a reflection of the physiochemical properties of the compound. Most of these compounds are basic lipophilic amines and the drugs come from many different pharmacological families. Some examples are listed in Table II, for a complete review, see Brandenberger Brown 1974.[6] Although the site of uptake is not known, an association between some of these compounds and cell membrane fractions has been demonstrated in vitro and so it may be that drugs attach to the endothelial cell surface. However, this important fact needs to be established. A few compounds may be metabolised following uptake, for example, 5-hydroxytryptamine, imipramine, but the majority of drugs are probably unaffected by absorption into the lung and are subsequently released into the blood unchanged with little or no metabolism.

Table II.   Distribution of Compounds to the Lung.

Drug	Time After Administration	Concentration in Blood (B) or Plasma (P) Relative to Lung (Lung = 100)
Noradrenaline	2 minutes	P 16
Adrenaline	2 minutes	P 62
Promazine	24 hours	B 1
Morphine	90 minutes	B 22
Methadone	3 hours	B 1
Medazepam	2 hours	B 26
Propranolol	30 minutes	B 8
Imipramine	45 minutes	P 1

Taken from: Brandenberger Brown[6] 1974.

Since this accumulation is interesting in itself, and may also have practical implications the process has been studied in detail[7] for a few drugs and in particular propranolol. Dollery and Junod, showed that uptake of propranolol by an isolated perfused rat lung was partly saturable and that there was no appreciable metabolism. The accumulation was inhibited by some drugs such as chlorpromazine, but unaffected by 5-hydroxytryptamine and interestingly enhanced by lignocaine. [8]Propranolol uptake by the lung in man has recently been demonstrated[8] by a modification of the single pass indicator dye dilution curve method using indocyanine green. Singlr pass lung uptake of propranolol was 75% for a 0.5 mg dose. Three patients who were already taking oral propranolol were also studied and in them uptake was only 33%. This shows that uptake is very rapid, occuring predominantly in a single circulation and also suggests that the uptake is at least partially saturable by normal therapeutic doses. Similar studies have recently been done in ambulant dogs with indwelling catheters and rapid uptake confirmed. The single pass uptake was about 60% and this was constant over a bolus dose range of 0.02 - 2 mg. The lung uptake also appears to be unaffected by changes in cardiac output.

This property of the pulmonary circulation may have practical applications. It is possible that the large quantities of drug held up in the lung may be responsible for some drug side effects and interactions, for example, one drug may displace another from binding sites in the lung, so that an intravenous injection of drug A may result in a sudden increase in circulating levels of drug B, which has been previously given. [9]There is some evidence for this with lignocaine and nortriptylene. A second application is the possible protection of the lung from the lung from the toxic effects of drugs or poisons. d-propranolol has been given to patients following paraquat injection in an attempt to displace the poison and so limit lung damage. A similar approach to drugs which are toxic to the pulmonary circulation may be possible. We set out to measure lung uptake of bleomycin in the hope that this might be blocked by prior administration of propranolol with resulting protection against bleomycin induced pulmonary fibrosis. Using the technique discribed above, single pass lung uptake of bleomycin was measured in eight patients receiving regular treatment with the drug for different neoplastic disorders. There was no significant uptake of the drug and it is, therefore, unlikely that the lung is damaged by lung accumulation leading to high local concentrations. Nevertheless, the approach remains valid and it may well be that some other lung damaging drugs accumulate in the pulmonary circulation and that propranolol may be useful in limiting this accumulation. Finally, the pulmonary uptake of propranolol or some other substance might be a valuable measure of the size or function of the pulmonary circulation. This could be used to estimate the extent of damage to the vascular bed in pulmonary embolism or emphysema and might be a predictor for conditions such as shock lung or oxygen toxicity. These are at present no more than speculations, but indicate the need for more research into this intriguing aspect of pulmonary circulation.

REFERENCES

1. Korman M G, Hansky J, Soveny C (1973)
        Aust J Exp Biol Med Sci 51 679.
2. Dent R I, Levine B, James B H (1973)
        Am J Physiol 225 1038.
3. Lockett M F (1972)
        J Physiol London 224 187
4. Rubenstein A H, Zwi S, Miller K (1968)
        Diabetologia 4 236.
5. Geddes D M, Blackburn J P Muller J (1979)
        J Applied Physiol 46 593.
6. Brandenberger Brown E A (1974)
        Drug Metab Rev 3 33
7. Dollery C T, Junod A F (1976)
        Brit J Pharmacol 57 67.
8. Geddes D M, Nesbitt K, Triall T (1979)
        Thorax.
9. Andersson R G G, Lewis D H, Post C (1979)
        Brit J Pharm 66 440P.

Discussion

BARER (Robert):   I apologise for speaking because of course I am
here as a wife and not as a contributor. What has struck me, as an
interested onlooker, is that no-one, I believe, so far has mentioned
the possible role of a very important structural element in the
lung, and that is the basement membrane. Now, around your blood
vessels, around every blood vessel, particularly capillaries, you
have a basement membrane. Similarly, at the bottom of an epithelial
surface, you also have a basement membrane. What is particularly
striking in the lung is that these two basement membranes
essentially fuse together. That is your capillary with endothelial
cells, you then have an epithelium with cells that in many ways are
indistinguishable, and you have a basement membrane here. And very
frequently these two are fused together. Now, here you have air,
here you have blood. I will only remind you that anything in the
air passage that has to get into the blood has to pass through the
epithelial cells, a double layer of basement membrane, then the
endothelial cells. Similarly, anything that gets out of the
capillary finds itself in this basement membrane material. Well,
the basement membrane is a very special sort of material. It is
composed largely of mucopolysaccharides, and these
mucopolysaccharides have some very peculiar properties. You can
liken them almost to a sort of gel (of course they are charged);
they have the ability to take up a whole host of different types of
molecules; they have these special properties with regard to water,
and in fact I think one of the earliest papers was to demonstrate
that one of the effects of pure oxygen was to cause oedema in this
region. Now, what I would like to suggest is the possibility that
this sponge, highly charged and very variable, can be affected by
pH, probably by oxygen tension and so on. This sponge can act as a
sort of reserve where molecules can be stored, so to speak, for some
time. And I think particularly it's interesting that these
molecules, small molecules, seem to be just the sort of things that
might very well be taken up by material of this sort. Now, Bakhle
referred to the effects of the oestrus cycle on the uptake of
various substances. Again, may I remind you that the
mucopolysaccharides are very much affected by the sex hormones and in
particular the perfect example of this is what happens to the sexual
skin of monkeys during pregnancy and the oestral cycle. You get
enormous changes and these have been shown to be due basically to
changes in the mucopolysaccharides. So I think, what I would like
to suggest is that people working on this field should think in
terms not merely of endothelial and epithelial cells, but of this
very potent substance that lies between them, and one would like for
example to know what is the composition of this material; is it
constant or does it change in hypoxic conditions? We know that
there are many many types of mucopolysaccharides, mucoproteins, some

are positively charged, some are relatively neutral. It is not necessary that these things remain the same in health and disease, or under normal or hypoxic conditions. So in short, I would like to suggest that people begin thinking about this material as well as the other components of the lung.

CUMMING: Thank you Robert, a very wifely contribution. Would you like to comment on that, Duncan?

GEDDES: I think one only has to agree and to say that as far as I know, nobody has really established for any of these processes where they go on. The closest that they get to it is to isolate endothelial cells from a different site and show that it doesn't happen there or it does happen there. So we don't even know that they go on in the capillaries, let alone what cell in the capillaries. As far as drugs are concerned there is little evidence to show that chlorpromazine is bound to phospholipids cell membranes, regardless of which cell and also to mitochondrial surface membrane. That doesn't prove that that is the site in the lung and I think that any suggestion that takes attention away from any specific cell must be a good one.

BARER (Robert):   May I just add one point? I think you mentioned this effect of removal of drugs or hormones. I put forward this general idea some ten years ago with regard to the release of polypeptide hormones in the neurohypophysis. In the neurohypophysis you have very powerful hormones which if they were released directly into the blood stream might well have a damaging effect. Now, I suggested that if you have a sponge surrounding the glandular cells, that the hormones could be released into this sponge and stored there to be released slowly into the blood stream over a matter of minutes or possibly even hours. Now, the same sort of thing may well happen here, and in fact it fits in rather with your idea of something being dissolved or saturated and thereby preventing the access of other molecules. Similarly, I think it would be quite compatible with the idea of potentiation. It depends on the particular type of molecule. So, I think you have a whole new area, very theoretical perhaps, but a new region for investigation.

CUMMING: Thank you Robert. I wonder if I could seek clarification on two small points. What kind of distance are we talking about in perfused membranes and what would the mass be of this sponge in a normal lung?

BARER (Robert):   Well, the second question first. It is highly aqueous. There is virtually no solid mucopolysaccharide there, and yet it gives this extreme viscosity. The thing really is a mass of holes. So that when you fix it and look through electron microscopy you may see practically nothing, it seems just a thin area. So I can't give you actual figures as regards mass, but the solid mass is probably very small. With regard to distance, this varies; in some places you can get a width of double basement membrane that is perhaps of the order of ten microns or more, but in other places they are condenced and the epithelial and the endothelial layers are just separated by a narrow barrier of the order of one or two micrometers.

MEYER: You have clearly demonstrated the kinetics of propanolol uptake from the lung and you have suggested several implications that may be drawn from these experiments. My question is concerned with the mechanism of uptake of these substances. Is there any evidence for passive uptake of this substance according to concentration differences, or is there some indication for an active or carrier-mediated, facilitated uptake. Your last slide suggests that there is some concentration dependence of uptake in the dog. Furthermore, you have presented evidence for saturation kinetics of uptake of this substance, and it appears to me that there was some evidence for either induction or inhibition of uptake of propranolol by other durgs. Taking these three observations together, it appears that they can be taken as evidence for a facilitated, maybe carrier-mediated transfer or uptake of these substances. What is your view?

GEDDES: I have no direct evidence from our own studies on this. Others have shown that metabolic inhibitors did not affect the uptake, but it did not appear to be dependent upon sodium. I don't remember all the blockers that they used, but their conclusion was that there was a passive uptake without any active or facilitated transfer mechanism. As far as saturation is concerned, it is a little more complicated because they showed that partial saturation occurred. I am not competent to know what is going on, but it would seem to be purely concentration dependent. As far as competition with other drugs is concerned, the interactions are complicated and basic lipophilic amines seem to compete. Lignocaine enhances uptake and that I do not understand at all.

BAKHLE: If I could perhaps add a little bit to that answer, people in America have studied Amphetamine also which has the same sort of uptake as propranolol. Now, that sort of uptake picture results and has been analysed into two components consisting of a saturable component which would saturate about 20 to 40 micromolar and a linear component which is purely passive. So that at a low concentration there is some sort of facilitated uptake which then transforms into a linear uptake. Imipramine according to Junot, shows a pure saturated uptake. It does not have a linear component. It may be that with amphetamine, propranolol, probably lignocaine, there is that sort of mixed kinetics, but with imipramine a simply saturated kinetics. That means that the interactions between the two will become very difficult indeed. When I referred to the pigs which had a lot of nortriptyline in them, they were saturated with nortriptyline, but the lignocaine uptake in the nortriptyline saturated pigs was exactly the same as lignocaine uptake in untreated pigs. So, although lignocaine could displace nortriptyline, its own uptake was unaffected.

CUMMING: Any other questions? Perhaps I can ask one very quickly of the audience. I am intrigued by this suggestion that the lung contains a large sponge, whose mass we cannot determine because of the method of preparation. Does anybody who is an expert in double indicator dilution technique know whether the gel phase of lung structure is accessible immediately to tritiated water or not?

LEE: I can partially answer that question by saying that it is partially available. In the single path methods involving tritiated water it is uncertain whether you get total distribution, and so some of the steady state methods may be better.

CUMMING: And do these steady state methods give higher values than the single path methods?

LEE: They tend to but it is still very rudimentary.

A THEORETICAL COMPARISON OF SINGLE BREATH AND REBREATHING METHODS OF STUDYING SOLUBLE GAS EXCHANGE IN THE LUNG

D.M.Denison, N.J.H.Davies and D.J.Brown

Lung Function Unit, Brompton Hospital
London SW3 6HP, U.K.

Humphrey Davy (1800) was the first to show that lung volumes could be estimated from the degree to which alveolar gas was diluted in an inert and insoluble marker, hydrogen.   He also measured the absorbtion of the soluble gas, nitrous oxide, and realised that its uptake would depend on "the velocity of the circulation". Since then, other workers (e.g Bornstein, 1910; Krogh and Lindhard, 1912; Grollman, 1929a & b; Asmussen and Nielsen, 1953) have taken advantage of the solubility of biologically inert gases to measure pulmonary blood flow, and later, pulmonary tissue volume (Cander and Forster, 1959; Sackner et al, 1975).   Many of these authors have used various combinations of soluble and insoluble gases to determine lung volume, ventilation, perfusion and tissue content, by various manoeuvres usually involving rebreathing or rapid exhalations after a series of breatholds of known durations.   Both these techniques sacrifice much of the potential information about the inhomogenous distribution of blood and gas flows, in order to obtain a reasonably reliable functional staement about the lung as a whole.

In this paper we wish to analyse the extent to which the rules underlying the rebreathing method of measuring pulmonary blood flow and tissue volumes, developed by Cander and Forster (1959), as used for example by Peterson, Petrini and Hyde (1978), can be applied to individual slow expirations.'   Single breath methods have an advantage over rebreathing techniques, since they can also be used to compare the functional characteristics of one part of a lung with another, during fibre-optic bronchoscopy in conscious man, (Williams et al, 1979). As Figure 1 shows, they are potentially capable of giving the same information as rebreathing procedures, and indeed were used first, for the estimation of blood flow (Krogh and Lindhard, 1912).

The concepts underlying the measurements of gas volume, blood

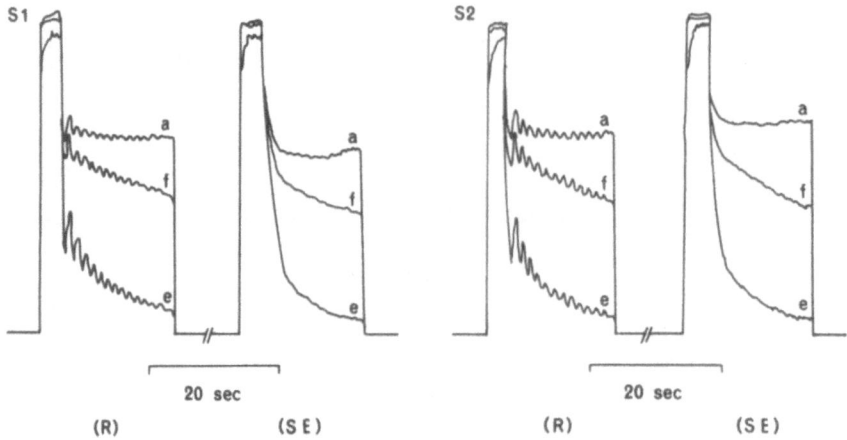

Fig. 1. Respired argon (a), freon 22 (f) and di-ethyl ether (e)
concentrations, seen in two subjects (S1,S2) during a
rebreathing (R) and single slow-exhalation (SE) manoeures.

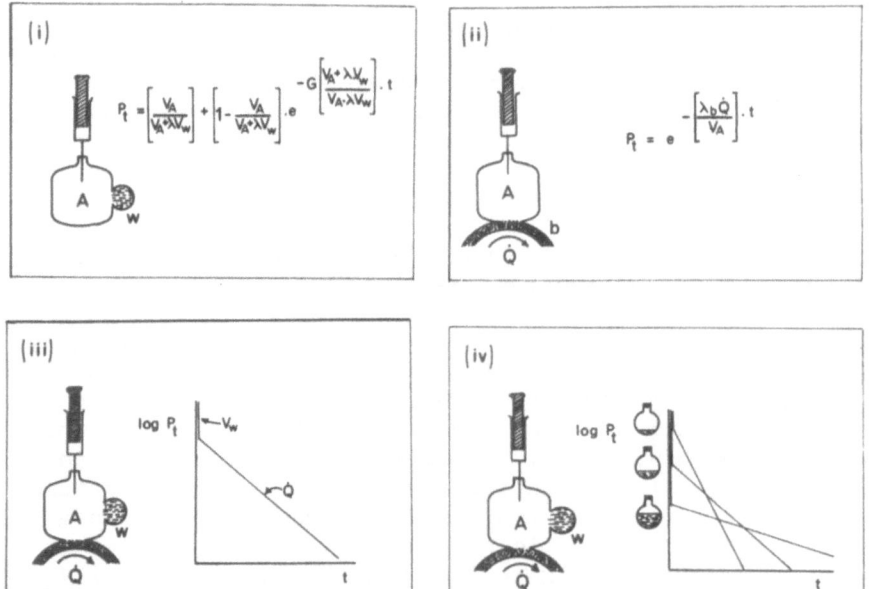

Fig. 2. A pictorial summary of the rules underlying gas exchange
between alveoli and; (i),tissue water alone, (ii), blood
flowing through a 'dry' lung, (iii),blood flowing through
a 'wet' lung, and (iv),through increasingly 'wet' lungs.

flow and tissue content from soluble gas exchange, summarised in
Figure 2, are well known, namely that any gas abruptly introduced
into an alveolar compartment A communicating with tissue fluid w,
is redistributed according to the equation in panel (i), and at the
same time is removed by circulating blood ($\dot{Q}$) as indicated in panel
(ii). If the entry into lung water is rapid, the processes of
solution in tissue and removal by flowing blood can be distinguished,
as shown by panel (iii). The immediate fall in alveolar pressure
P of the gas is a measure of lung water, and the exponential drop
that follows is a measure of blood flow. However, the volume of
lung water must be determined before blood flow can be calculated
since it, too, affects the rate of exponential decay,(panel iv).

   Although these influences affect all respired gases, their
relative effects vary with the fluid/gas partition coefficient, λ ,
of the individual gases for tissue and blood. In principle, an
insoluble marker gives the shape of the dead-space front, and the
degree of alveolar dilution; a moderately soluble one shows a
further and progressive fall in concentration, due to pulmonary
blood flow; and a very soluble gas shows a precipitous early fall
due to solution in lung water. Since the physical bases of these
processes are largely understood, mathematical models can help to
define the conditions under which one process can be distinguished
from another by gas analysis alone, at the lips or in the bronchial
tree. In this paper, we wish to contrast the rebreathing and single
breath procedures, using mathematical models to analyse some of the
complications which are introduced into the interpretation of both
types of record by the changes of lung volume on expiration, by the
uneveness of ventilation and perfusion, and by the presence of lung
water.

METHODS

   Model lungs were constructed by arranging a number of similar
units in various ways. The basic element, illustrated in Figure
3a, presents the lung unit as a series of compartments which can be
described by their effective volumes (i.e. the product of actual
volume and partition coefficient, λV), and the conductances, G, of
the interfaces that join them. In the models, the volumes and
partition coefficients of the compartments, the conductances of the
windows, and the blood flow through the alveolar compartment, could
be varied at will in each element, and the elements could be arranged
in any array desired. The models were constructed on a digital
computer (Prime 300) using an analogue simulator. Some details of
the equations used are given in the Appendix. Many studies were
conducted on the single element shown in Figure 3a, and on the
parallel array shown in Figure 3b. In the latter, the fluid
filled compartment w and d were often deleted for simplicity.

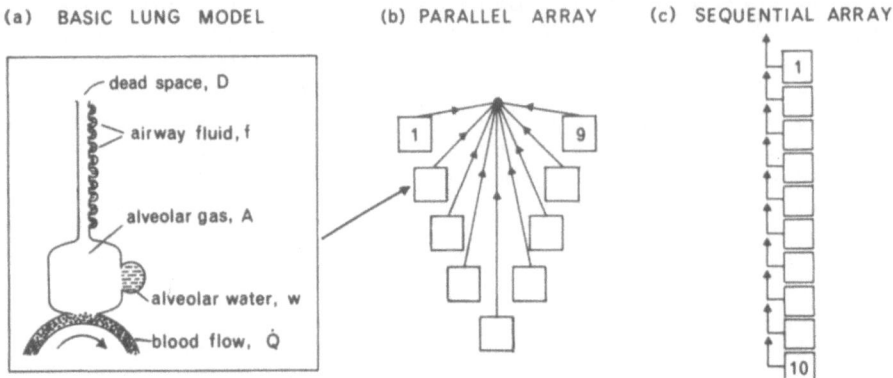

Fig. 3.   A pictorial summary of the models used for this study.

RESULTS

The results of these studies will be described in three sections, concerning the effects of diminishing lung volume, of lung water, and of regional inhomogeneity respectively.

The effects of diminishing lung volume

The basic equation in the top left panel of Figure 2;

$$PA_{x_t} = \left[\frac{V_A}{V_A + \lambda V_w} \right] + \left[1 - \frac{V_A}{V_A + \lambda V_w} \right] e^{-G\left[\frac{V_A + \lambda V_w}{V_A \cdot \lambda V_w} \right] t}$$

which describes the passive transfer of an inhaled marker from alveolar gas A to alveolar water w, can be thought of in three parts.   The first bracketed term shows the asymptote of the equilibration process, the second bracketed term is the initial deviation from that asymptote, and its exponent is the reciprocal of the time constant for solution.   The equation shows that the process is a complex function of instantaneous alveolar volume VA.   The nett effect of expiration, i.e of diminishing lung volume, is to speed equilibration.

As is well known, the equation also describes the equilibration of alveolar gas with circulating blood, (Fig 2,ii).   If the blood leaving the capillary is completely equilibrated with alveolar gas, the alveolar-capillary window can be regarded as having infinite conductance.   Similarly, until a back-pressure develops as recirculation occurs, the capillary compartment can be treated as one of infinite capacitance.   The rate of removal of marker from the alveolar compartment by the circulation is equal to the product of blood flow $\dot{Q}$ and the quantity of marker dissolved in each unit of blood volume. The effective conductance of this process is $\dot{Q}$ Thus, for a single alveolar compartment of gas volume VA and zero tissue volume, exposed to blood flow $\dot{Q}$, the basic equation simplifies to that shown in Figure 2, ii,

$$PA_{x_t} = e^{-\left[\frac{\lambda_b \dot{Q}}{VA} t\right]} \qquad \text{where } PA_o = 1$$

The time constant of this process is $VA/\dot{Q}\lambda$ Thus, this process too, is accelerated by expiration.   Since the asymptote of the simplified equation is zero the logarithm of marker concentration falls linearly with time if VA is constant,(until recirculation occurs), but must curve downwards if VA diminishes.

The combined effects of tissue fluid and blood flow upon the composition of alveolar gas(panels iii and iv of Figure 2) cannot be expressed by a simple equation but can be determined using the elementary model shown in Fig 3a and will be illustrated by the calculated fates of three particular gases that we use in practice.   They are argon, Freon-22 and di-ethyl ether, and have fluid/gas partition coefficients taken to be 0.03, 0.73 and 13.4 respectively.   The results of the calculations, assuming the gases had instant access to lung water, are given in Figure 4.   The graph on the left of the figure compares the fates of argon, freon and ether inhaled into a 5 litre alveolar space in contact with 500 ml of tissue fluid and 5 lites/min of flowing blood, firstly with the alveolar volume essentially constant, as in rebreathing, and secondly if alveolar volume diminished at a constant rate of 125ml/sec until a residual volume of 1.25 litres was reached,(solid lines).   Time is on the abscissa and the logarithm of gas concentration is on the ordinate.   The latter is expressed as a fraction of the concentration created in the alveolar compartment at the end of a sharp inspiration.

The accelerating effect of diminishing lung volume upon the falls in alveolar concentrations of the soluble gases is obvious and would lead to errors in the calculation of $\dot{Q}$ unless VA, $\dot{V}E$ and Vw were known.   This presents a problem, in practice, since the distortion of the curves by expiration also leads to an error in the determination of Vw.   Fortunately, as Overland et al (1975) showed,

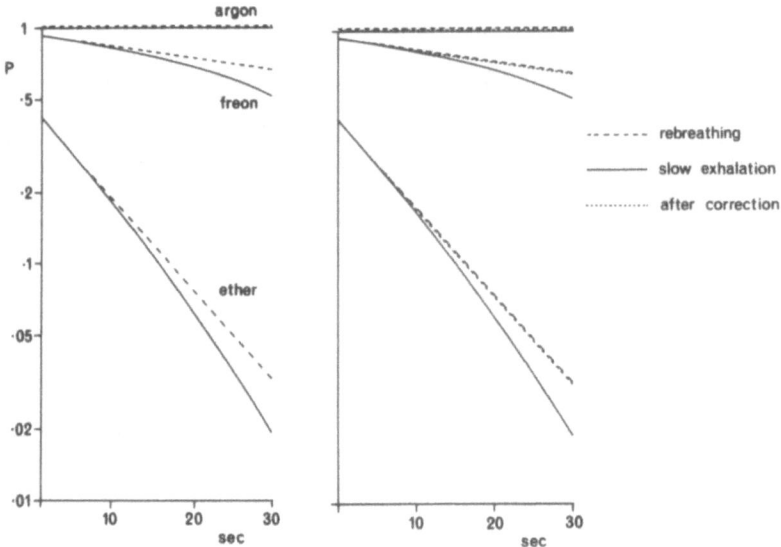

Fig. 4.   The calculated changes in argon, freon and ether pressures
          during rebreathing, and during a single slow expiration in
          a 'normal' lung. (see text for details)

it is possible to calculate Vw in another way, which enables us to
correct the observed curves for the effect of diminishing lung volume.
They pointed out that, since the log-concentration versus time curves
for any soluble gas had a decay slope that was proportional to:
$$\dot{Q}. \lambda /(Va + \lambda Vw)$$
Vw could be obtained from the ratios of simultaneously recorded
slopes for the two soluble gases.   ($\dot{Q}$ and VA are common to both and
the partition coefficients are known).

     Using this approach it is possible to apply a running correction
to single breath traces, which reverses the effect of diminishing
lung volume and restores the curves to the form they would have had
if the alveolar compartment had been held constant at its end-
inspiratory volume.   Details of this correction, which is lengthy
to describe but easy to apply, are given in the Appendix.   The
graph on the right of Figure 4 shows identical curves to that on the
left but superimposed on these are the single breath argon, freon
and ether traces after correction for diminishing lung volume.   This
correction, like that of Overland et al (1975) on which it is based,
assumes that equilibration between alveolar gas and lung water is
very rapid and that there is no accessible fluid in the airways.
Later it will be shown that gases as soluble as ether are affected
by the presence of quite small quantities of water in the bronchial
tree.   This reservation has to be kept in mind.   Gases that are
less soluble will be less affected but are also less useful for
making this correction.

Effects due to the volume and distribution of lung water

In the basic element shown in Figure 3a, the alveolar water compartment (w) is placed in parallel, rather than in series, with the
capillary space transmitting the blood flow Q̇.   Many arguments favour
this parallel position.   In the normal lung the layer of fluid lining
the alveoli fills the crevices <u>between</u> the capillaries which alt-
ernately expose thin <u>respiratory</u> and thick <u>non-respiratory</u> surfaces
to the alveolar gas, (Gil, 1978).   In the early stages of pulmonary
oedema fluid accumulates in the <u>non-respiratory</u> areas, at alveolar
junctions, (Hauge, this volume);   endothelial blisters of oedema
fluid obstructs capillaries (Brigham 1978), and fluid collects between the unfused basal laminae on the <u>non-respiratory</u> surfaces of
the capillaries.   Only terminally does it intrude between alveolar
gas and the fused basal laminae of the thin <u>respiratory</u> surface of
the capillaries.   These findings help explain why gas exchange is
preserved even in severe oedema (Hogg, 1978), a point first noticed by
Barcroft in 1920.

Cander and Forster, and subsequently many other workers, e.g
Sackner et al(1975), found that during rebreathing manoeuvres in
normal lungs, soluble gases appeared to equilibrate with lung water
in 1.5 sec or less, implying a time-constant for solution of no more
than 1 sec, which was much shorter than the time-constant for removal
of the same gases by blood flow.   This is an essential condition for
separating the two processes.

The determinants of the time-constant of solution are illustrated in Figure 5 which represents the conductance G of the air/fluid
interface as a window between the two compartments A and w.   The
ease of transfer of material is inversely proportional to the thickness of the window (d) and is directly proportional to its area 'A',
and also to the partition coefficient of the marker in the medium of
the window, (which determines the number of particles available for
transfer), and the nett linear velocity (v) of the particles in the
axis A-w.   When transfer is by diffusion alone $v=k\sqrt{mol.wt.}$, where k
is a property of the medium.   Therefore the equilibration of marker
between alveolar gas A and the sheet of stagnant water w can be described by inserting the expression for G, shown in Figure 5, into
the equation, formally derived in the Appendix, which is to be found
at the tope of Figure 2.   The time-constant of solution implicit in
that equation and shown at the bottom of Figure 5, is inversely related to the partition coefficient and is a complex function of the
geometry of the sheet of fluid and the ratio Vw/VA.

This is best presented graphically, (Fig 6).   The figure shows
how the time-constant of solution varies with the volume and geometry
of the sheet of water w, and with the partition coefficient λ .   Both
graphs plot the time constants of five imaginary gases of the same
molecular weight but differing partition coefficients (λ=0,0.1,1,10
and 100) expressed as multiples of the time-constant that would exist

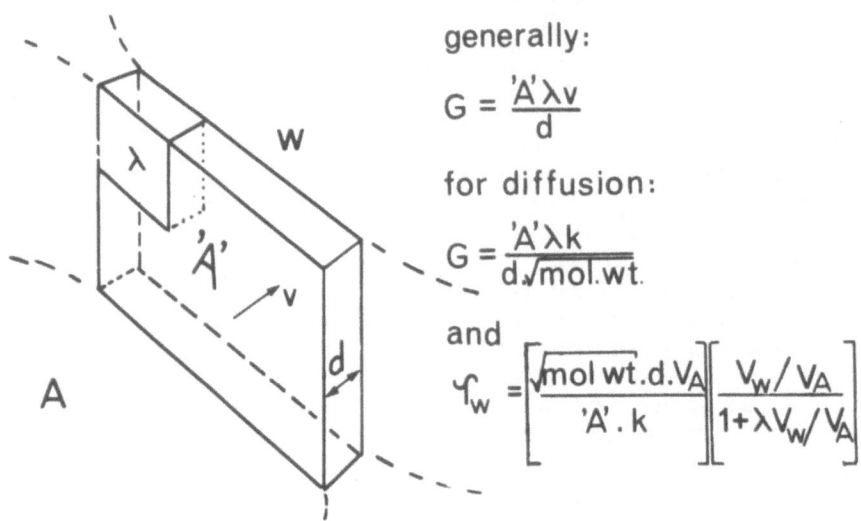

generally:

$$G = \frac{{}'A'\lambda v}{d}$$

for diffusion:

$$G = \frac{{}'A'\lambda k}{d\sqrt{mol.wt.}}$$

and

$$\mathcal{T}_w = \left[\frac{\sqrt{mol\,wt.}\,d.V_A}{{}'A'.k}\right]\left[\frac{V_w/V_A}{1+\lambda V_w/V_A}\right]$$

Fig. 5. A pictorial summary of the factors determining transfer of
gas between alveolar compartment A and tissue water compartment w, which present a surface area 'A' and has a depth d.
w is the time constant of solution (other symbols in text).

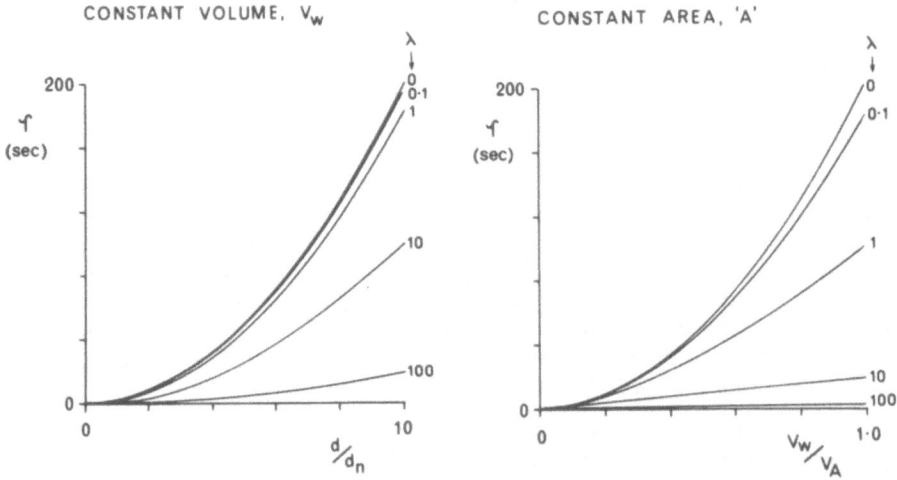

Fig. 6. The effects on the 'time constant of solution' of varying
the shape and volume of tissue water(see text for details).

in a 'normal' lung for the gas with a partition coefficient of 10 equilibrating with tissue fluid equivalent to 10% of lung volume.

The graph on the left of Figure 6 shows how these time-constants vary when the geometry of a normal quantity of fluid ($Vw/VA=0.1$) is altered by reducing its area A and thus increasing its thickness d, shown on the abscissa. The time-constants rise with the square of film thickness, as can be inferred from Figure 5, but the effects are much more marked on the insoluble than on the soluble gases. The graph on the right shows how the time-constants vary when the volume of water is increased while its area of contact with the gas phase is held constant. The ratio Vw/VA forms the abscissa. Here too the steep increases in time-constants with film thickness are more marked in the insoluble than the soluble gases. The conclusions to be drawn from these graphs are that the speed of equilibration of inhaled gas with lung water is critically dependent on the volume and geometry of the fluid present, especially for less soluble gases. The more soluble gases always equilibrate faster than poorly soluble markers but the differences in time constants are by no means as wide as the ratios of their partition coefficients would suggest. Inspection of the lowermost equation in Figure 5 explains why this is so. Although the more soluble gases do present more particles for transfer, many more are required to develop a given level of back-pressure in the fluid compartment.

We have used the model of Fig 3a to calculate how the concentrations of Freon-22 and ether would be affected by the presence of fluid in the lung, which(as in actual lungs) is not instantly accessible to such gases. Cander and Forster found the initial falls in the concentrations of nitrous oxide and acetylene ($\lambda=0.47$ and 0.77 respectively), to be complete within 1.5 sec. We have calculated the changing alveolar concentrations of freon and ether in a series of model lungs in which the time-constant for the solution of nitrous oxide in a normal quantity of lung water ($Vw/VA=0.1$), was varied between 0.15 and 1.5 sec by adjusting the conductance between A and w. The time-constants of solution for freon and ether were calculated from the nitrous oxide values using the equation of Fig.5. All models had a common alveolar volume (5 litres) and blood flow(5 litres /min) but differing quantities of alveolar water (Vw/VA ratios of 0, 0.1, 0.2 and 0.4).

Figure 7 shows the results of these calculations for the two extreme conditions. One had a time-constant for nitrous oxide solution of 0.15 secs(a) and the other had one of 1.5 sec (b). In each case the left-hand graphs plot concentrations (as a fraction of their initial values) against time, while their logarithms are shown against time on the right. Although the linear plots are superficially similar in (a) and (b), considerable differences are revealed by the logarithmic plots which emphasises the advantage of seeing the information in this form. The initial falls, most

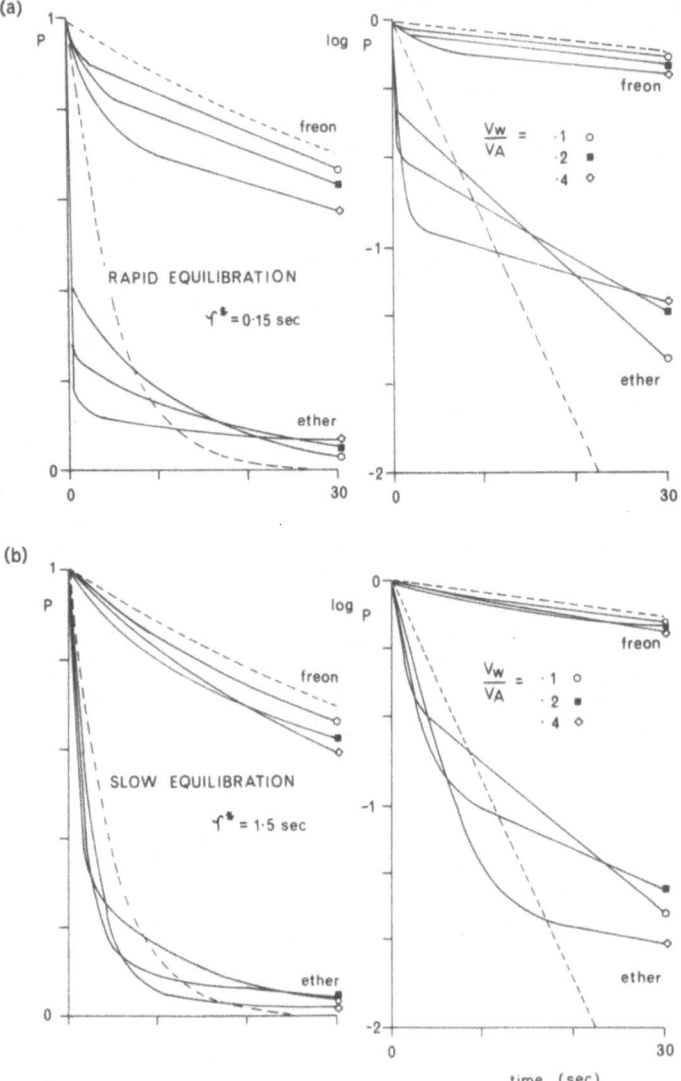

Fig. 7.   Arithmetic and logarithmic plots of the changes in argon
          freon and ether concentrations in model lungs with a time
          constant of solution of (a) 0.15 sec and (b) 1.5 sec
          (see text for further details).

evident in the ether curves, are due to relatively fast solution in
lung water and the different slopes illustrate the extent to which
Vw modifies removal of gas by the circulation.   The slopes for a
dry lung, shown as dotted lines, give the time-constants for the
circulation only, which are 5 sec for ether and 82 sec for Freon-22
(and would be 2000 sec for argon).

     Several conclusions can be drawn from this figure.   When the
time-constant of solution in lung water is much shorter than that of
removal by the circulation their individual effects are easy to distinguish and blood flow can be estimated from the slope of the
linear portion of the log plot after lung water has been determined
by extrapolating this line to time zero, as suggested by Cander and
Forster.   However, when the time-constant of the solution is comparable with that of removal by the circulation, Vw is over-estimated by
extrapolation since a significant amount of ether is removed by the
circulation before equilibration with lung water is achieved.   As a
result blood flows calculated from the final slope and the assume Vw
are also too high.   If the time-constant of solution is much longer
than that of circulation the effects of lung water are hardly seen
at all.

     In practice the time-constants of solution cannot be determined
but the time taken for the log plot to become linear is readily seen.
Figure 8 plots the errors introduced into the calculations of $\dot{Q}$ and
Vw, when lung water is not immediately accessible, against this time
as judged from the trace for ether.   It shows that intercepts can be
used with less than 20% error for estimates of Vw or $\dot{Q}$ if the ether
trace is linear within 3 seconds or so.

     In the models discussed above it has been assumed that all the
lung water lies in the alveolar compartment, however as Cander and
Forster pointed out, this is not so and account must be taken of the
fluid on and in the walls of the airways.   In rebreathing manoeuvres
the rapid flows of gas over this surface will minimise its influence,
but in slow expiration it exerts a marked effect.   This is illustrated in Figure 9, which shows the argon, freon and ether concentrations that would be expected on slow expiration following air containing equal concentrations of all three markers.   The figure is of
a 5 litre lung with 5 litre/min blood flow and a normal alveolar
water content (Vw/VA=0.1) expiring to a residual volume of 1.25 litre
at a constant rate of 125 ml/sec.   The broken line shows the behaviour of that lung with no water in the airway, and the solid line
shows that of the same lung with a total of 50 ml of water distributed along the length of the bronchial tree in proportion to airway
volume.   Gas concentrations are expressed as fractions of those
created in the alveolar space at the moment of inspiration from RV
to TLC.

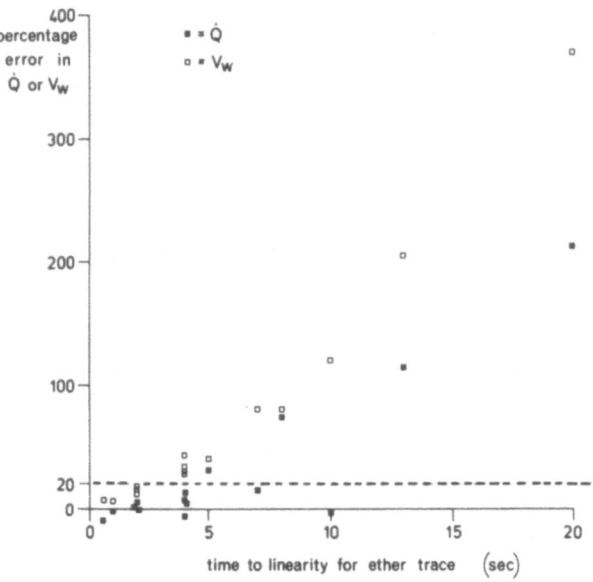

Fig. 8. Errors introduced into soluble gas estimates of $\dot{Q}$ and Vw
         when the time constant of solution is slow. The latter
         cannot be measured directly but can be judged in practice
         from the 'time to linearity' of the ether trace (shown on
         the adscissa).

     This graph shows that the expired concentrations of the insol-
uble gas argon are unaltered, and those of the moderately soluble
marker freon are barely affected by the presence of fluid in the airway, but those of the very soluble gas ether are changed in a paradoxical way.   The presence of airway water leads to an underestimate
of the total volume of fluid in the alveoli, but this effect should
be readily detected since the concentrations of the soluble marker
exceeds those of argon for a discernible time once the dead space
front appears.

     Quite small amounts of fluid in the airways are sufficient to
cause marked deformities in the concentration-time curves of very
soluble gases. In this regard, Landahl and Herrman (1950)have shown
that, during nasal breathing, up to 75% of inhaled acetone, alcohol,
or ammonia, is retained in the nose, and more recent studies suggest
that as much as 99.8% of highly soluble gas, such as SO_2, are retained there (Morgan and Frank, 1977).   As anticipated by Cander and
Forster and by Sackner, this phenomenon imposes a serious limitation

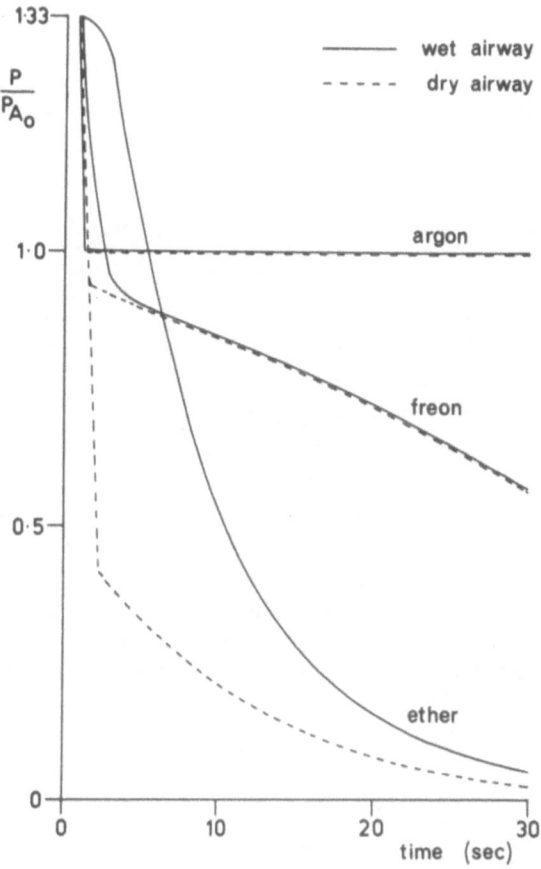

Fig. 9.   The effects of 50 ml of rapidly equilibrating fluid in the
          airway upon the gases expired from a 'normal' lung.

upon soluble gas estimates of lung water.   However, it is possible
to imagine a spectrum of soluble gases from the relatively poorly
soluble which arrive in the lung and can distribute themselves in a
finely spread film of fluid which is rapidly accessible, to gases
like SO_2 which do not arrive at all.   Some intermediate members
might be used to measure the volume of accessible water in airways.

Effects of uneven ventilation and perfusion

       It is well known that, even in the normal lung, ventilation and
perfusion are unevenly distributed, and it follows that the delivery
of soluble gases by ventilation, and their uptake by the circulation
will vary from part of the lung to another.   Figure 10 gives an il-
lustration of this.   On the left of the figure is a model of the
normal lung divided into nine horizontal slices, which is obtained
by combining the model data of West (1962), Sutherland et al(1968)

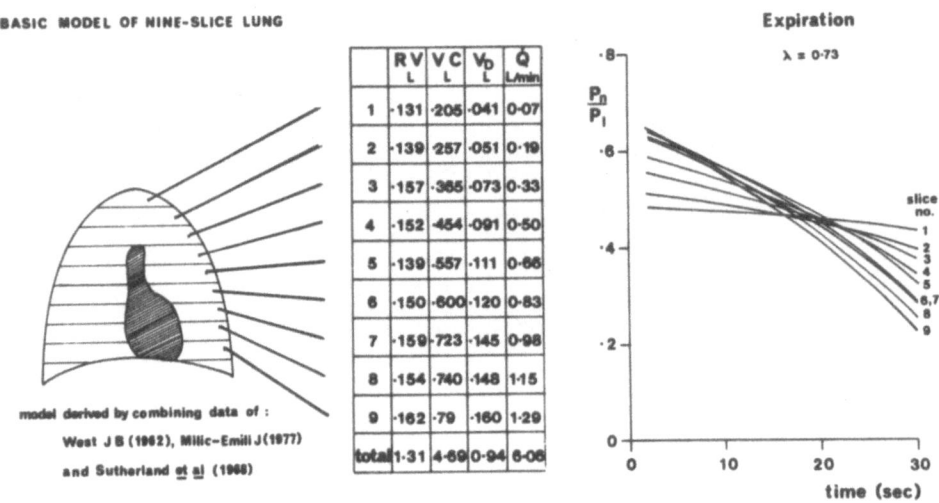

Fig. 10.   A summary of the principal feature of a 9 compartment
           model used to study some effects of regional inhomogeneity.
           The graph on the right shows how freon concentration would
           change in each 'slice' during a slow expiration from TLC
           to RV.

and Milic-Emili (1977).   Details of the residual volume, vital
capacity, dead-space volume and blood flow of each slice are given
in the figure.   An analogue of this model was constructed from the
lung elements of Figure 3a, using the parallel array of Figure 3b
The features shown in the central panel of Figure 11, the timing of
inspiration and the start and end of expiration, could be varied for
each slice independently.

     The graph on the right of the figure illustrates the freon con-
centration curves to be expected in the alveolar compartments of each
slice during an expiration at a constant rate, from TLC to RV over
the 30 seconds following a sharp vital capacity inspiration of marked
gas.   It shows that the upper slice, which is poorly ventilated and
perfused, received little gas but this was removed slowly.   By contrast the lowest slice, which was well perfused and ventilated, received more gas but this was removed rapidly.   It is interesting to
note that in this model one would expect cardiogenic oscillations in
the concentration of a soluble marker in the expired mixture to dim-

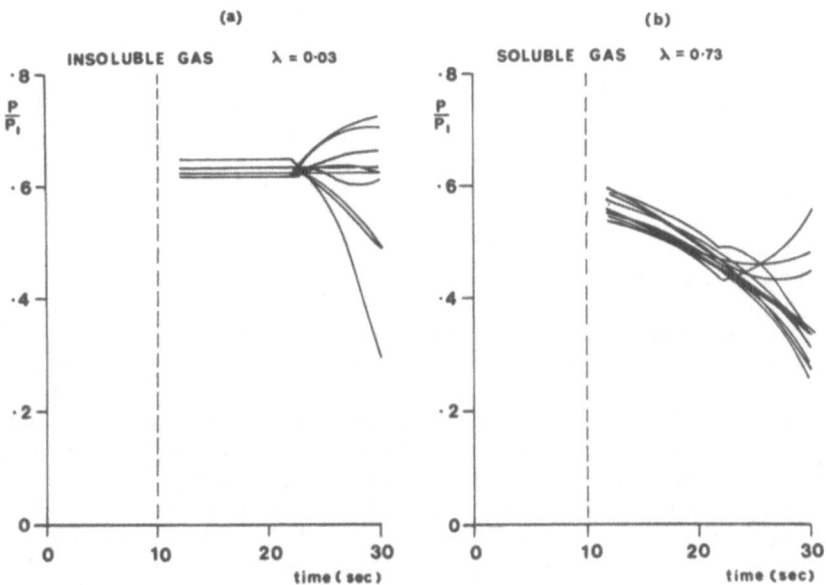

Fig.11.   Expired argon and freon concentrations that would be seen
          during a single slow expiration from a '9 slice' model of
          the lung (see text for details).

-inish, reverse their phase and increase, as expiration proceeds.

     Many experiments have been conducted with this analogue of West's
9-slice model, simulating a wide variety of ventilation/perfusion inequalities and closing volume phenomena, during the same single-
breath manoeuvre from RV to TLC and slowly back again.   The total
ventilation, blood flow and lung capacity were kept constant throughout, and the presence of fluid in the alveolar and dead-space compartments were ignored, (i.e. the lung models were 'dry').   Ten of
the trials are illustrated in Figure 11. In these, all 9 slices began
to expire at individual but constant rates, 10 sec after a sharp inspiration of air marked with helium and freon.   The slices ceased to
empty, in various sequences, from the 21st second onwards.   The expected composition of the mixed expirate at the mouth, seen after a
dead-space transit delay of 2 sec, is shown in the figure.   Concentration-time curves for helium are on the left and for freon on the
right.

     These trials, which were conducted to help us interpret single-
breath traces of soluble gas exchange, suggested the following conclusions.   The concentration of insoluble marker in expired air at
the mouth, (Fig 11a), will remain constant, providing proportional
contributions from each compartment do not change, regardless of the
degree of spatial inhomogeneity of ventilation in the lung.

Similarly, if there were no spatial inhomogeneity it would remain
constant throughout, regardless of any variations in the propor-
tionate contributions from each compartment with time.   Therefore
any departure of the insoluble marker trace from a horizontal line
cannot be attributed to spatial or temporal unevenness of ventilation
alone but must reflect that the two are present together.   For as
long as the insoluble marker trace is horizontal, the trace of the
soluble marker (Fig.11b), provides a reasonably accurate estimate of
total blood flow.   Thereafter it reflects temporo-spatial variations
of ventilation and perfusion combined.

      Although single-breath traces of insoluble gas concentrations
are commonly horizontal in normal subjects this is not so in patients
with lung disease, in whom the single-breath test of lobar or segmental function at bronchoscopy is of greatest interest.   Obviously
there are many possible patterns of temporal and spatial inequality
of ventilation and blood flow, and consequently several pitfalls of
interpretation.   One of these is illustrated in Figure 12.   The
left-hand graph shows the argon, freon and ether concentrations expected at the mouth of a particular analogue model.   The record is
similar to many we see in practice clinically (Williams et al, 1979).
It shows a gross degree of temporo-spatial inhomogeneity of ventilation, and poor separation of the argon and freon traces, suggesting
little effective blood flow.

      This trace can be analysed using the following arguments.   At
any point in the expiration the trace of the insoluble gas argon pre-
dicts the concentrations that the soluble gases freon and ether would
have had if they had not dissolved in blood and lung water.   The
effects of uneven ventilation, and, in practice, of variations in
water vapour content and mass spectrometer sensitivity, can be removed by dividing the traces by the instantaneous argon concentration,
i.e. normalising the record for argon.   It is convenient to set the
inspired ratios to one.   If the traces shown in Figure 12a are
treated in this way one obtains the normalised traces of Figure 12b
and the log of normalised concentration plot of Figure 12c.   The
latter show that the ratio of blood flow to alveolar volume in the
lung model are normal and the apparently poor separation of the argon
and freon traces in Figure 12a can be entirely explained by uneven
ventilation.   In fact the series model used for these traces,(Fig 3c)
consisted of 10 identical 500 ml compartments with blood flows of
500 ml/min,with diminishing ventilation from the top to the bottom
of the tree.   It would be incorrect to assume from Figure 12a that
pulmonary blood flow was abnormal, but it would be equally incorrect
to infer from Figure 12c that it was normal.   The practical interpretation is that the effective pulmonary blood flow is low (from
Fig 12a) but this can be attributed entirely to malventilation(from
Fig 12c).   The concept of effective blood flow, that is that part
of total flow which contributes to gas exchange, has been used previously, for example by Cotton et al (1971) and Cotton (1976).

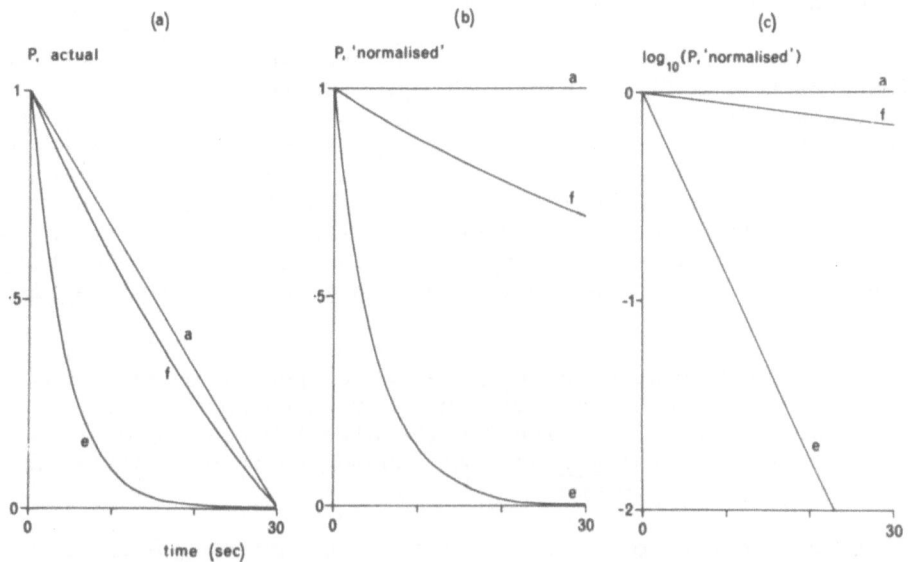

Fig. 12. Graphs of argon (a), freon (f), and ether (e) concentration
          during a single slow exhalation from a model lung with
          gross maldistribution of ventilation but evenly distributed
          blood flow.

CONCLUSIONS

The purpose of this study was to determine the extent to which the
well established methods of determining pulmonary blood flow and
fluid volumes from soluble gas exchange during rebreathing could be
extended to single breaths.   This could provide a method of comparing the function of one part of the lung with another in people
undergoing fibre-optic bronchoscopy, and would be of particular
interest in patients with diseased lungs in whom the distribution of
ventilation, perfusion and lung water could be quite abnormal.   The
study, of mathematical models of the lung, suggests the following
conclusions:

   1). The effects of diminishing lung volume could introduce large
   errors into the calculation of blood flow and water content of the
   lung but,providing the initial lung volume and the expiratory rate
   are known, these effects can be reversed precisely, by applying a
   correction which is given in the Appendix.

   2). The estimations of blood flow and water content are critically dependent upon the volume and distribution of lung water.
   If this is grossly abnormal, which can be determined from the
   apparent 'time constant of solution' by inspection of the traces,
   it is wiser to base the calculations solely on the concentration

curve of a moderately soluble marker.

3). Studies of single slow expirations are especially vulnerable
to the presence of fluid in the airways. Quite small amounts of
fluid are sufficient to cause marked deformities in the concentration-time curves of very soluble gases. These lead to under-
estimates of lung water and over-estimates of blood flow. The
present study suggests that in single breath manoeuvres this
phenomenon ought to be detected by delays in the initial falls in
concentration of the very soluble, relative to the least soluble,
of the expired markers, and might be used to determine airway fluid
content.

4). Unlimited degress of purely spatial or purely temporal uneveness of ventilation can exist without them being apparent in the insoluble marker trace. A slope to the alveolar plateau of this
marker implies temporal and spatial inhomogeneity of ventilation
relative to alveolar volume.

5). It is possible to remove the effects of uneven ventilation,
and of variations in analyser sensitivity by normalising the concentrations of soluble and very soluble markers to those of the
least soluble gas.

6). This procedure can be used to distinguish between the apparent
blood flow of the lung, (effective pulmonary blood flow) and the
total flow to the ventilated part, that would be available if
ventilation was well distributed.

ACKNOWLEDGEMENTS

We are indebted to the Research and Development branch of the
Deprtment of Health and Social Security, to the Clinical Research
Committee of the National Heart and Chest Hospitals, and to
Centronics Ltd; all of whom have very generously supported the
research programme of which this work is a part .

APPENDIX

1). Formal derivation of the equation at the top of Figure 2

In the model shown in the first panel of Figure 2, the rate of
transfer of a marker gas (x) from the alveolar compartment A to the
fluid w is described by the equation:

$$\frac{dMA_x}{dt} = G\left[PA_x - Pw_x\right] = G\left(\frac{MA_x}{V_A} - \frac{M_{TOT} - MA_x}{\lambda Vw}\right)$$

where MAx is the mass of marker present in the alveolar compartment at any instant, Mx(tot) is the total amount present in A and w, and G is the conductance of the interface between them.   Integration of this equation, as it stands, leads to a cumbersome expression that is much simpler if the effective volumes of the compartments are replaced by their reciprocals, i.e. elastances, (E=1/ .V), so

$$\int \frac{d\,MA_x}{k_2 - k_1\,MA_x} = \int dt$$

where $k_1=G(EA+Ew)$ and $k_2=Mx(tot).Ew.G$.   Integration of this expression yields:

$$-\frac{1}{k_1}\,\ln\left[k_1 - k_2\,MA_x\right] = t + k_3$$

where $k_3=(1/k_1)\ln(k_2-k_1.Mx(tot))$.   Rearrangement of (3) gives:

$$\ln\frac{k_2-k_1 MA_{x_t}}{k_2-k_1 MA_{x_{TOT}}} - k_1\,t$$

This is equivalent to: $MA_{x_t} = \frac{k_2}{k_1}\left[-\frac{k_2}{k_1} - MA_{x_{TOT}}\right]e^{-k_1 t}$

Converting mass concentrations to partial pressures leads to:

$$PA_{x_t} = \left[M_{tot}.E_{tot}\right] + \left[PA_{x_0} - M_{tot}.E_{tot}\right]e^{-G\left[E_A + E_w\right]t}$$

Reverting to effective volumes, and dividing by $PA_x(t=0)$ gives the equation of Figure 2:

$$PA_{x_t} = \left[\frac{V_A}{V_A + \lambda V_w}\right] + \left[1 - \frac{V_A}{V_A + \lambda V_w}\right]e^{-G\left[\frac{V_A + \lambda V_w}{V_A \cdot \lambda V_w}\right]t}$$

2). The running correction for diminishing lung volume

This correction adjusts the observed single-breath traces by performing the following sequence of operations (given simultaneous log-concentration versus time curves for any two soluble gases E and F with fluid/air partition coefficients e and f,:

    (i) reads the slopes E' and F' of the first small time interval
    Dt of the curves

(ii) determines the apparent volume of w, (=Vwl), for that interval, using the equation first developed by Overland et al (1975), i.e.:

$$\frac{V_W}{V_A} = \frac{E'f_b - F'e_b}{F'e_b f_w - E'e_w f_b}$$

where the subscripts b and w refer to blood and water respectively.

(iii) Adjusts the slope of this element of each curve to correct for the diminution in total effective volume of the system VA+Vw, so:

$$S'_{(corr)} = S_{(obsv)} \cdot \left[V_{A_o} - (\dot{V}_E \cdot Dt) + \lambda V_{w_t} \right] / \left[V_{A_o} + V_{w_o} \right]$$

(iv) Calculates the logarithm of the partial pressure that would have existed at the end of the interval if the corrected slope had been followed, so:

$$PA_1 = PA_o - S'_{(corr)} Dt$$

(v) repeats steps (i) - (iv) on the curve elements in each successive time interval, so:

$$PA_n = PA_{n-1} - S'_{(corr)} Dt$$

REFERENCES

ASMUSSEN, E. and M.NIELSEN (1953) The cardiac output in rest and work, determined simultaneously by the acetylene and the dye injection methods. Acta Physiol Scand 27:217-230

BORNSTEIN, A (1910) Eine Methode zur versleichenden Messung des Herzschlagvolumens beim Menschen. Pflugers Arch 132:307-318

BRIGHAM, K.L. (1978) Lung edema due to increased vascular permeability. In: Lung Water and Sclute Exchange, ed.by N.C.Staub New York, Marcel Dekker Inc., pp 235-276.

CANDER, L. and R.E. FORSTER (1959) Determination of pulmonary par-
    enchymal tissue volume and pulmonary capillary blood flow in man.
    J. Appl Physiol 14: 541-551

COTTON, E.K., J.J. COGSWELL and G.J.A. CROPP (1971). Measurement of
    effective pulmonary blood flow in the normal newborn human
    infant.   Pediatrics 47: 520-528

COTTON, E.K. (1976) The measurement of effective pulmonary blood
    flow in the newborn infant using a mass spectrometer
    Crit care Med 4:245-247

DAVY, H. (1800) Researches Chemical and Philosophical, chiefly con-
    cerning Nitrous Oxide, and its Respiration   London
    Johnson

GIL, J. (1978) Lung interstitium, vascular and alveolar membranes
    In Lung Water and Solute Exchange ed. by N.C.Staub New York
    Marcel Dekker Inc. pp 49-73

GROLLMAN, A. (1929a) The determination of the cardiac output of man
    by the use of acetylene. Am J Physiol 88:432-445

GROLLMAN, A. (1929b) The solubility of gases in blood and body fluids
    J. Biol Chem 82: 317-325

HENDERSON, Y. and H.W. HAGGARD (1925) The circulation and its
    measurement. Am. J Physiol 73: 193-253

KROGH, A. and J. LINDHARD (1912) Measurements of the blood flow
    through the lungs of man. Skand Arch Physiol 27: 100-125

LANDAHL,H.D. and R.G.HERMANN (1950) Retention of vapours and gases in
    the human nose and lungs Arch Ind Hyg 1:36-45

MORGAN,M.S., R.FRANK (1977) Uptake of pollutant gases by the respir-
    atory system. In Brain,J.D., Proctor, D.F., Reid, L.M. Ed.
    Respiratory Defence Mechanisms. Marcel Dekker Inc New York
    pp 157-192

OVERLAND,E.S., G.M.OZANNE and J.W.SEVERINGHAUS (1975) A single-
    breath method for determining lung weight and pulmonary blood
    flow from the differential uptake of two soluble gases.
    Physiologist 18: 341

PETERSON,B.T.,M.F. PETRINI, R.W.HYDE AND B.F.SCHREINER(1978) Pul-
    monary tissue volume in dogs during pulmonary edema
    J.Appl Physiol 44: 782-794

PETRINI,M.F., B.T. PETERSON and R.W.HYDE (1978) Lung tissue volume
    and blood flow by rebreathing: theory.   J Appl Physiol 44:782-802

SACKNER,M.A.,D.GREENELTCH, M.S.HEIMAN, S.EPSTEIN and N.ATKINS (1975)
    Diffusing capacity, membrane diffusing capacity, capillary
    blood volume, pulmonary tissue volume and cardiac output
    measured by a rebreathing technique.
    Am Rev Respir Dis 111: 157-165

SUTHERLAND,P.W., T.KATSURA and J.MILIC-EMILI (1968) Previous volume
    history of the lung and regional distribution of gas
    J Appl Physiol 25:566-574

WEST,J.B. (1962) Regional differences in gas exchange in the lung of
    erect man.   J Appl Physiol 17: 893-898

WEST,J.B. (1977) (ed) Regional differences in the lung.   Academic
    Press, New York.

WILLIAMS,S.J., .R.J. PIERCE, N.J.J.DAVIES and D.M. DENISON (1979)
    Methods of studying lobar and segmental function of the lung
    in man.   Br J Dis Chest 73: 97-112

Discussion

QUESTION: Can you explain the difference between the soluble and insoluble gases?

DENISON: I am drawing a graph of the logarithm of the concentration of gas against time. And we will say that at the start of the procedure, when it is just being diluted in the alveolar gas, we will give it a concentration of 1. If we look at the insoluble alveolar gas, concentration is constant and uniform. A soluble gas will show two phenomena. First an almost immediate fall in concentration and then a linear fall, and if we extrapolate to time zero, then this fall must have been due, (or it should be treated as if it were entirely due), to solution in lung water. How much water? Well, you can calculate from simple dilution theory. Suppose now that that was the lung at full size; it would be as if this gas saw an effective volume twice as big as alveolar gas. So we say it sees a volume of water that behaves as if it were 3 litres of gas. How much water would that be? It would depend on the solubility of the gas. The more soluble, the less water. So you would take that additional 3 litres and you divide it by the solubility. And the best paper on this is in the Journal of Applied Physiology, 1959. Although the authors were discussing it for rebreathing, the same principle applies to the single breath. Consider the volume of pulmonary capillary blood compared with lung water and it is very similar, if you wanted to be precise about it you would measure it with a particular soluble gas, CO. And then you can make any precise correction for it.

CUMMING: So the lung water is going to be 450 mls and the volume of blood static, as it were in the lung, capillaries would be 80 or 90 mls, so it would be about 1/5.

DENISON: There is no experimental evidence that these measurements are accurate in healthy lungs.

HORVATH: You seem to have a similar picture to the one we observed with radiokrypton. Was it on gamma camera pictures?

DENISON: Gamma camera.

HORVATH: Gamma camera, two plane gamma camera pictures.

DENISON: No, one plane. Why do you use krypton? Is it because it has a short half-life and it fades, so that when you take a picture on one part of the lung the image disappears and you are ready to take a picture of the next area?

HORVATH: What is the usefulness of the mass spectrometer.

DENISON: The great strength of the mass spectrometer is it can measure many gases simultaneously with exactly the same characteristics. And the importance of the method of using the bronchoscope is that it gives you information in terms that are of interest to the surgeon. Surgeons can't cut out an upper zone with a patchy shadow on the left. What they can cut out is a lobe or a segment. And the beauty of the method is that it tells the surgeon which lobe or segment. I think the main drawback of the method is that it takes time.

CUMMING: If I may offer some encouragement you shouldn't be too worried about a mass spectrometer, because in Eastern Europe they are now making an excellent mass spectrometer, and this is being manufactured by Comecon and you can get one very easily.

LEE: I think I kept up most of the way. If you look at the ether volume of water and compare it with tritiated water, single path methods, what do you get?

DENISON: We haven't done that, but our measurements agree with simultaneous rebreathing procedures, and the rebreathing procedure agree in principle with those measurements that have been made in animals, by lung weight estimation of water and the like. Until you get up to more than about three times normal values. Values of about 400 - 500 ml.

LEE: Could we hear a little bit about distribution of lung water using these techniques?

DENISON: In lateral decubitus, we have preliminary evidence of a gravitational distribution, but we have not done it formally, it is impossible to say anything more than that. There is no doubt that you can detect the differences and similarly, although I have not described them, these are very obvious in diseased lungs. And we have made many studies in patients recovering from open heart surgery and as soon as the lung water becomes a little increased it becomes inaccessible. However, once you have a large amount of water in the lung, it becomes easy to estimate radiographically and we think that the geometric techniques we developed for measuring the displacement volume of the lung and the soluble gas methods are complementary. You use the soluble gas method to look at small quantities of water and you use the radiographic technique for larger quantities. We are able to measure the volumes of lung lobes and segments quite precisely radiographically, and so you can still get information, but it is still too early for us to be more precise.

LOCKHART: May I ask you a very simple technical question? How do you deliver a precisely measured amount of argon. How do you monitor the flow, which is not always very easy to do very precisely?

DENISON: The technique that we use on the whole lung and to make the comparisons is very straightforward. You just have a mixture in which the concentrations of argon, Freon, ether or CO are adjusted so that the electrical signals are equal, or almost equal. If you want to express blood flow, ventilation, or blood flow, lung water, CO transfer per unit of alveolar volume, you don't need to measure the concentration precisely. Then 20 - 50 ml. of the second insoluble gas is delivered down the second lumen of the bronchoscope catheter. If we are breathing a mixture of argon, Freon and ether we inject helium down the catheter into the part under study and look at the dilution of argon to get overventilation, the volume of the structure can be estimated from the dilution of helium. I should have mentioned that all of these techniques are described in a paper in the British Journal of Diseases of the Chest 1973, vol. 80, pages 97 to 112.

LOCKHART: I am sorry, this is not exactly my question. When you measure overall ventilation, using constant injection of argon and you are measuring the dilution factor, you have to know precisely the amount of argon which you inject at the inflow of the mixing box.

How do you get the inflow of argon very precisely?

DENISON: We described that technique in the detail in Respiration Physiology, in January this year. It does not need to be precise, it only needs to be constant. And provided you have a high pressure source, more than 3 atmospheres, you can get sonic flow, that is constant flow, down the long tube, and it's independent of the minor changes in pressure down-stream. And so we have tubes like this going to the intensive care ward to the catheter laboratory and to the bronchoscopy ward, the flow remaining constant day after day. To measure them we go back to Empedocles and just put a syringe in a beaker full of water, put the tube underneath and see how long it takes to displace 20 ml. We use about 100 ml. per minute.

RIEDEL: I have a very stupid but perhaps practical question. Would you recommend the measurement of diffusing capacity as a non-invasive test for the diagnosis of pulmonary hypertension? We found a very poor or perhaps no correlation at all between the PAP and the steady state diffusing capacity in about 60 patients of a very wide range of PAPs.   The second question is about the

reactivity of the pulmonary circulation after diazoxide. Do you
think this is a good drug to use?

DENISON: There are several studies that show reasonable
correlation between CO uptake impairment and pulmonary arterial
pressure in chronic obstructive lung disease. I wouldn't go further
at the moment than to say that if you find this low, measure the
pulmonary arterial pressure, which is the actual method that I gave.
As far as diazoxide is concerned, we were the second group of people
to use it, as a group in Manchester had used it before. We used it
in 9 patients for primary pulmonary hypertension. It has many
disadvantages. It causes diabetes, it causes hirsutism, it causes
systemic hypertension. Yet, at present, it is the only hope that
could be offered to these people. And two of the nine made, and
have maintained, a remarkable recovery. One of the ladies, who was
believed to be very close to death, has since married and is living
an ordinary life. You may see a description of those nine cases
published in the British Heart Journal, which is due to come out
soon. The article points out that the drug is unsatisfactory, and
that there should be a search for the better overall pulmonary
hypotension agent, and we are looking at that now. We'd agree with
you entirely, but it is better than nothing.

TRICOMI: I am a radiologist in Rome. My question is not pertinent
and indeed, impertinent, because I have no qualifications to talk
specifically about your subject. But as a radiologist being used to
reading a chest x-ray through vascularity and being used to
comparing the morphological vascularity of the lung with perfusion
scintigraphy, I was pleased to see that in looking at the radiograph
that you showed, my experience as a radiologist has been confirmed.
My question is this: in your last case of post-surgical failure, do
you have the x-ray after surgery. Can you show us the x-ray of the
case after the operation?

DENISON: I heard the question, I am thinking of an answer. I have
in there a box with around 1000 slides, and it may well be there.
What I will do is this; we will look this evening and if I find it,
I will show you tomorrow. I think if I had your skills, maybe I

wouldn't need to use a mass spectrometer. But then I would have missed a lot of fun. I have shown you gross cases in which many clinicians would have been happy to make a decision without the help of our technique. But we had many examples of more subtle differences in which we are quite happy and our clinicians are quite happy that they would only have made the decision with the help of the technique I have described.

PULMONARY DIFFUSING CAPACITY FOR O_2 AND CO BY REBREATHING TECHNIQUES USING STABLE ISOTOPES

M. Meyer, P. Scheid and J. Piiper

Abteilung Physiologie, Max-Planck-Institut für experimentelle Medizin, D-34 Göttingen, FRG

INTRODUCTION

It is generally held that the alveolar-capillary membrane is not a significant limiting factor to oxygen transport in normal lungs of resting man at sea level. It is also well established that diffusion limitation becomes increasingly important in hypoxia. Therefore, the diffusive conductance or diffusing capacity of the lung (DL) must be finite and is expected to limit maximal O_2 uptake in extreme conditions such as high altitude hypoxia.

The ability of oxygen to penetrate the alveolar-capillary membrane is commonly taken to be 1.23 times that of carbon monoxide which for theoretical and practical reasons is more readily measured. Recent experimental findings (Hyde et al., 1966; Gong et al., 1972a; Cross et al., 1973) have revealed lower DL_{O_2} estimates as compared to the values predicted from DL_{CO} measurements. Thus, in order to assess the importance of diffusion limitation in alveolar-capillary gas transfer of O_2 there is little significance in measurements of CO diffusing capacity unless DL_{CO} can be translated into terms of O_2 diffusing capacity. More information upon the DL_{O_2}/DL_{CO} relation-

167

ship appears therefore desirable from measurements of DL_{O_2} and DL_{CO} both performed under identical physiological conditions.

Moreover, pulmonary diffusing capacity both for O_2 and CO is found to increase at exercise. Whether the increase proceeds to a plateau value which can be considered as the maximal diffusing capacity or increases in proportion to the oxygen uptake is controversial.

Rebreathing methods for measurement of pulmonary blood flow and diffusing capacity have been developed in our laboratory (Adaro et al., 1973, 1976; Teichmann et al., 1974; Cerretelli et al., 1974; Veicsteinas et al., 1976) and applied to man at rest and exercise. The stable isotope ^{18}O has recently been introduced to the rebreathing techniques in order to eliminate some of the theoretical prerequisites and practical problems that were still encountered in the existing methods for measurement of pulmonary O_2 diffusing capacity. The purpose of this communication is, (1) to briefly summarize the rebreathing principle and apparent advantages of using stable isotopic test gases, (2) to describe its application in normal man at rest and exercise, and (3) to evaluate the physiological implications that may be derived from simultaneous measurements of DL_{O_2} and DL_{CO}.

METHODS

Rebreathing principle

The principle of the rebreathing techniques, i.e. breathing in closed system made up by the lungs and the rebreathing bag is shown in Fig. 1. The equilibration kinetics of the different test gases initially contained in the rebreathing bag vary according to their physical properties.

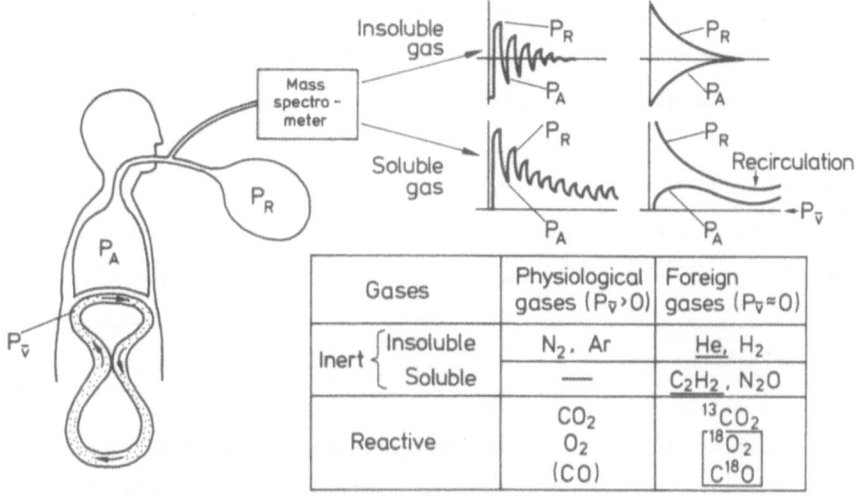

Gases		Physiological gases ($P_{\bar{v}} > 0$)	Foreign gases ($P_{\bar{v}} \approx 0$)
Inert	Insoluble	N_2, Ar	$\underline{He}$, H_2
	Soluble	—	C_2H_2, N_2O
Reactive		CO_2 O_2 (CO)	$^{13}CO_2$ $^{18}\underline{O_2}$ $C^{18}O$

Fig. 1. Principle of the rebreathing technique. The equilibration pattern for the different gases during rebreathing varies according to their physical properties (for detail, see text).

Insoluble gases (e.g. He or H_2) come to an equilibrium depending on the lungs to bag volume ratio as they are not eliminated from the system. The kinetics for attaining equilibrium between bag and lungs is determined by the effective ventilation.

Soluble inert gases (e.g. C_2H_2 or N_2O) are taken up by pulmonary capillary blood, thus, their rate of equilibration is also dependent on pulmonary perfusion. Hence, pulmonary capillary blood flow can be measured from the rate of disappearance of soluble test gases from the rebreathing system. Measurements have to be completed before the onset of recirculation which may be identified by a change in slope of the rebreathing tracing.

The respiratory gases O_2 and CO_2 (and CO) basically behave similarly as soluble gases, the difference is due to their increased

solubility on account of chemical binding in blood. During rebreathing both alveolar and bag partial pressures of these gases approach
their mixed-venous partial pressures that in contrast to foreign
gases ($\bar{Pv}$ = O) are generally not known with high enough accuracy.
It is therefore advantageous to use stable isotopes of these gases
rather than the naturally abundant component as their partial
pressures in mixed-venous blood are practically zero (see below).

Rebreathing lung model

A two compartment lung model comprising an alveolar compartment (V_A) and the rebreathing bag compartment (V_R) appropriately
depicts the situation realized in rebreathing conditions (Fig. 2).
Gas transfer between the alveolar compartment and capillary blood
(flow rate Q) is limited by a diffusion barrier (diffusing capacity, DL). In this system alveolar to capillary gas transfer can
be described in terms of an alveolar-mixed venous blood transfer
conductance, G [transfer rate / alveolar-to-mixed venous partial
pressure difference, $G = M/(P_A - \bar{Pv})$]:

$$G = V_A \cdot \text{ßg} \cdot k \left(1 + \frac{V_R/V_A}{1 - k \cdot V_R/\dot{V}_{eff}}\right) \qquad (1)$$

in which k is the rate constant of exponential approach of P_A
towards its asymptote $\bar{Pv}$:

$$k = -\frac{d[\ln(P_A - \bar{Pv})]}{dt} \qquad (2)$$

$\dot{V}_{eff}$, effective ventilation between the two compartments V_A and V_R;
ßg, capacitance coefficient for gas phase (cf. Piiper et al., 1971).

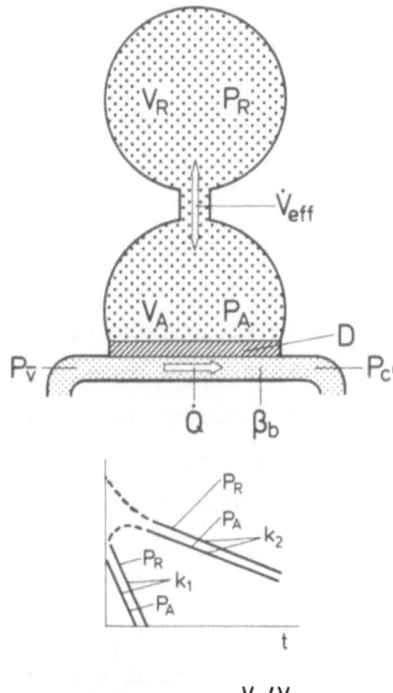

Fig. 2. Model underlying analysis of rebreathing
for determining DL
and $\dot{Q}$. The approach
of P_A and P_R is plotted
on logarithmic ordinate
scale against time.
From the rate constant
of the slow component,
k_2, DL and $\dot{Q}$ are calculated as explained in
the text.

$$G = V_A \beta_g \cdot k \left(1 + \frac{V_R/V_A}{1 - k \cdot V_R/\dot{V}_{eff}}\right)$$

The conductance G differs for the various inert and respiratory gases on account of their respective transfer limitations.

Insoluble gases (e.g. He): $G = O$ (3)

Soluble inert gases (e.g. C_2H_2): $G = \dot{Q} \cdot \beta b$ (4)

Carbon monoxide: $G = DL$ (5)

Respiratory gases (e.g. O_2, CO_2): $G = \dot{Q} \cdot \beta b (1 - e^{-DL/\dot{Q} \cdot \beta b})$ (6)

For <u>insoluble gases</u>, $G = O$, since they are not taken up by the
blood.

For <u>soluble inert gases</u> transfer is exclusively limited by perfusion and G has the meaning of a perfusive conductance, $\dot{Q} \cdot \beta b$ (βb,

capacitance coefficient of gas in blood).

Uptake of <u>carbon monoxide</u> is limited by diffusion alone since
the effective solubility (ßb) for CO is extremely high due to the
high CO affinity of hemoglobin. Hence, G signifies a diffusive conductance or diffusing capacity, DL, of the gas-blood barrier.

Transfer of the <u>respiratory gases</u> O_2 and CO_2, whose effective
solubility in blood (ßb, equal to total solubility or slope of
dissociation curve) is increased by chemical binding, is limited
both by diffusion and perfusion. It is important to notice that the
decisive parameter in eq. (6) determining the characteristics of
alveolar-capillary equilibration is the ratio $DL/\dot{Q} \cdot ßb$, i.e. the
diffusive/perfusive conductance ratio.

The relationships of eqs. (3) - (6) in combination with the
general equation for the conductance G (eq. 1) are used to determine
$\dot{Q}$ and DL. In practice, $\dot{Q}$ and DL are calculated from the equilibration
rate constants (k) and the other parameters of eq. (1), i.e. V_A,
V_R, V_{eff} and ßb that are known or determined in the same rebreathing
procedure.

For soluble inert gases the solution of gas in lung tissue and
pulmonary capillary blood leading to an increased effective alveolar dilution volume, V_A, compared to the alveolar gas volume determined from insoluble gas dilution, has to be taken into accout. The
effective dilution volume is obtained by the extrapolation procedure
introduced by Cander and Forster (1959).

Advantages of using stable isotopes

In principle, DL can be determined from the equilibration kinetics of the naturally abundant isotopes. Indeed, this approach has

been utilized previously in determining pulmonary DL_{O_2} (Cerretelli
et al., 1974; Veicsteinas et al., 1976). The use of stable, naturally occurring but rare isotopes (e.g. $C^{18}O$ and $^{18}O_2$) offers distinct advantages of which two major characteristic features are
considered to be of particular interest.

1. *Mixed venous partial pressure*

The relative natural abundance of ^{18}O is reported to be
0.2039%. Calculations reveal that $^{18}O-^{18}O$ (mass 36) should occur in
air at a fraction of about $8 \cdot 10^{-7}$. Therefore, $^{18}O_2$ can be considered
virtually absent from mixed venous blood as is the case with foreign
inert gases (c.f. Fig. 1). Since mixed venous P_{O_2} constitutes the
asymptote for equilibration of alveolar P_{O_2} small errors in its
value give rise to large errors in determination of DL_{O_2}. In the
experiments by Cerretelli et al. (1974) and Veicsteinas et al. (1976)
mixed venous P_{O_2} for the abundant isotope $^{16}O_2$ was determined either
by a separate rebreathing procedure or by an extrapolation procedure.
However, both techniques appear to yield rough estimates only and
therefore the accuracy that can be achieved in measurements of DL_{O_2}
from rebreathing equilibration kinetics of the abundant isotope
$^{16}O_2$ is very limited.

Similarly, the abundance of $C^{18}O$ should be about 0.2% of $C^{18}O$
and $\bar{Pv}$ for this isotope can be safely neglected. In measurements
of DL_{CO} the asymptote usually termed as ❯ back pressure ❰ corresponds to the P_{CO} in equilibrium with capillary blood. The $\bar{Pv}_{CO}$
may be ❯ 0 in the presence of elevated HbCO concentrations in smo-
kers or arising from multiple DL_{CO} determinations. This factor has
to be taken into account when the normal abundant isotope $C^{16}O$
is used at low concentrations in the DL_{CO} measurements whereas the
$\bar{Pv}$ for the isotope $C^{18}O$ is negligible in most circumstances.

Isotopic CO has to be used for technical reasons since $C^{16}O$ which has a mass number similar to that of N_2 cannot be separated by conventional respiratory mass spectrometers. The stable isotopes ^{13}CO (mass 29) and $^{13}C^{18}O$ (mass 31) have no principal advantages over $C^{18}O$ (mass 30). Most recently, experimental evidence against role of facilitated transport of carbon monoxide in alveolar gas exchange was obtained from simultaneously measuring DL_{CO} with the isotopes $C^{18}O$ and $^{13}C^{18}O$ at various alveolar CO concentrations (Meyer, 1979).

2. *Constant slope of effective dissociation curve*

As outlined above, the effective solubility or capacitance coefficient of blood for any gas species, ßb, is an important parameter for the gas transfer rate by pulmonary blood flow. While ßb is equivalent to physical solubility and thus constant for all inert gases, ßb for the respiratory gases O_2 and CO_2 varies with the slope of the dissociation curve within the range of capillary partial pressures of these gases (ßb = dC/dP).

Analysis of DL_{O_2} (cf. eqs. 1 and 6 solved for DL_{O_2}) assumes constancy of the slope of the O_2 dissociation curve, $ßb_{O_2}$, in the range of capillary PO_2 during rebreathing. This requirement is only approximately met in hypoxia where in the range between 15 and 35 torr the O_2 dissociation curve is close to linear. The changes in ßb are reduced when the PO_2 difference $(P_A-P\bar{v})_{O_2}$ is small, however, a high accuracy with respect to the absolute value of $P\bar{v}$ is required in this case.

A more accurate approach is based on the use of labelled isotopes, e.g. $^{18}O_2$. Under certain conditions the uptake of $^{18}O_2$ occurs in accordance with constant ßb as will be outlined below.

Consider an in vitro equilibration experiment (Fig. 3A) where O_2 is in equilibrium between blood and gas, and thus the total P_{O_2} [P_{O_2} (t)] comprising the oxygen isotopes ^{16}O and ^{18}O as molecular species $^{16}O-^{16}O$ [O_2 (n)] and $^{18}O-^{18}O$ [O_2 (i)] is constant. Assuming that the affinity of hemoglobin is equal for both isotopes the total amount of oxygen molecules (C_{O_2} (t)) represented by the sum of both isotopic species is therefore constant and related to the P_{O_2} (t) on the dissociation curve. If P_{O_2} (i) is varied at constant P_{O_2} (t), O_2 (n) will be replaced by O_2 (i) as both compete for binding at the same hemoglobin molecules. In this case the relationship between O_2 content (C_{O_2}) and partial pressure (P_{O_2}) for both isotopes is identical and equal to that for their sum:

$$\frac{\Delta C_{O_2}(i)}{\Delta P_{O_2}(i)} = \text{ßb}_{O_2}(i) = \frac{\Delta C_{O_2}(n)}{\Delta P_{O_2}(n)} = \text{ßb}_{O_2}(n) = \frac{C_{O_2}(t)}{P_{O_2}(t)} = \text{ßb}_{O_2}(t) \quad (7)$$

Therefore, for the process of isotopic replacement the effective O_2 dissociation curve is a straight line passing through the origin with slope equal to the ratio total O_2 content/total P_{O_2}.

The requirement of constant total O_2 content [C_{O_2} (t)] can be achieved in the lung if there exists equilibrium between lung gas and capillary blood, i.e. under conditions of no net transfer for O_2 and CO_2 (Fig. 3B). Hence, $C\bar{v}_{O_2}$ (t) equals $C_{c'O_2}$ (t) and P_{O_2} (t) is virtually constant along the pulmonary capillary. This situation is met if rebreathing equilibration of $^{18}O_2$ is recorded during equilibrium of the major abundant component ($^{16}O_2$) with $^{18}O_2$ applied at trace concentrations. In lungs equilibrated to mixed venous P_{O_2} the P_{O_2} of the abundant isotopic species $^{16}O_2$ is about 20-40 torr. If about 0.07% of the isoptope $^{18}O_2$ is administered to the rebreathing bag its initial P_{O_2} is about 0.2 torr, rapidly decreasing towards zero (due to natural occurence of $^{18}O_2$ $P\bar{v}$ is less than 10^{-4} torr).

In this situation the $P\bar{v}_{16_{O_2}}$ will nearly exclusively contribute to the $P\bar{v}_{O_2}$ (t) which means that the sum of both isotopes is practically equal to that of the $^{16}O_2$ isotope and stays constant during equilibration of the rare $^{18}O_2$ isotope (concentration ratio $^{18}O_2/^{16}O_2 \approx$ 0.01). Therefore, ßb effective for uptake of $^{18}O_2$ is constant and equal to the $C\bar{v}_{16_{O_2}}/P\bar{v}_{16_{O_2}}$ ratio that can be calculated from $P\bar{v}_{16_{O_2}}$ measured in rebreathing equilibrium and the corresponding $C\bar{v}_{16_{O_2}}$ obtained from a standard dissociation curve.

The condition of constant effective solubility is of extremely valuable advantage validating the use of a linear effective dissociation curve in the range of total partial pressures where the dissociation curve is markedly curvilinear. This approach is not limited to analysis of oxygen equilibration kinetics but may also

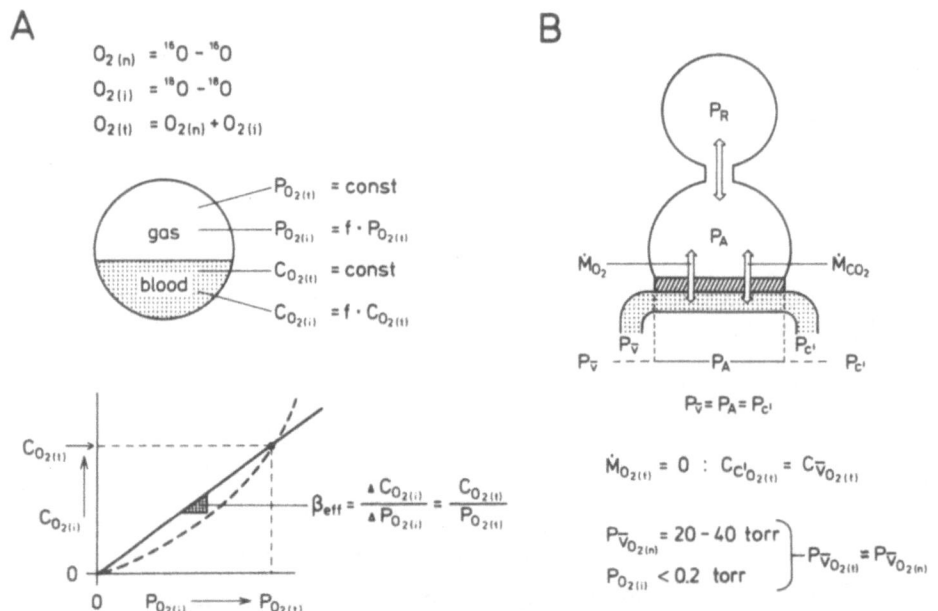

Fig. 3. Model underlying calculation of effective ßb for isotopic O_2 equilibration in equilibrium of the abundant isotopic component. For explanation, see text.

be applied to carbon dioxide as has been demonstrated recently by Piiper, Meyer and Scheid (1979) in measurements of the CO_2 diffusing capacity utilizing the stable isotope $^{13}CO_2$.

Experimental procedures

    The experimental set-up for simultaneous measurement of DL_{O_2} and DL_{CO} is shown in Fig. 4. The subjects were sitting on a bicycle ergometer either resting or pedalling against work loads of 50-125 watts. During a "pre-period" of about 4-5 min the subjects breathed a mixture of 21% O_2 in N_2 to wash out atmospheric Ar from the lung because the isotope ^{36}Ar conflicts with $^{18}O_2$ at the same mass peak. After two rapid priming breaths taken from a spirometer containing an O_2-free hypercapnic mixture (about 8% CO_2 in N_2, to bring alveolar P_{O_2} and P_{CO_2} close to their expected values in mixed venous

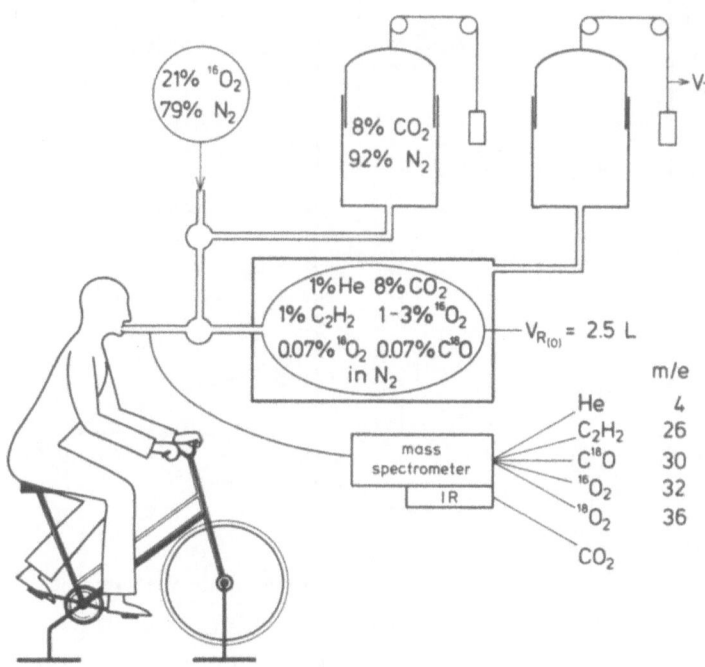

Fig. 4. Schematic set-up for estimation of DL_{O_2} and DL_{CO} in man by rebreathing

blood) the subjects were rebreathing a mixture containing 0.07% $C^{18}O$, 0.07% $^{18}O_2$, 1% He (for measurement of lung volume and effective ventilation), 1% C_2H_2 (for measurement of pulmonary blood flow), 1-3% $^{16}O_2$, and 8% CO_2 in N_2 starting the rebreathing maneuver after a forced expiration. The concentrations of $^{16}O_2$ and CO_2 were adjusted to provide an equilibrium for these gases over the interval between the 5th and 11th breath during rebreathing. Rebreathing frequency was 50/min at a tidal volume of 2.5 L both at rest and exercise.

Fig. 5 shows recordings of the mass spectrometer output for the various gases. Since the mass spectrometer is equipped with 5 channels only (re-designed Varian M3) CO_2 was measured by infra-red absorption. The tracing in Fig. 5 starts with the last breath of the "preperiod" followed by the two priming breaths before the on-

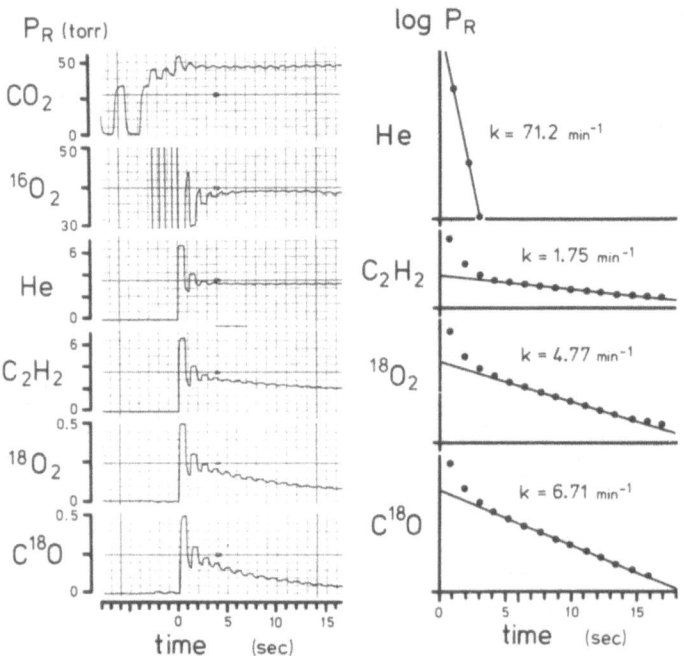

Fig. 5. <u>Left</u>: time course of partial pressures for the various gases during rebreathing. <u>Right</u>: end-inspired partial pressures (P_R) plotted on semilogarithmic scale against time of rebreathing.

set of the rebreathing procedure. While there is initially wide
variation for $^{16}O_2$ between very low and high values the inspired
and expired CO_2 levels are already close to the plateau level in
the following rebreathing period. Plateau levels indicating rebreathing equilibrium were reached for $^{16}O_2$, CO_2, and He within
5 sec while $^{18}O_2$, $C^{18}O$, and C_2H_2 progressively decrease towards zero.

The semilogarithmic plot of end-inspired points against time of
rebreathing is linear for He whereas those for $^{18}O_2$, $C^{18}O$ and C_2H_2
are more complex but allow to identify an apparently linear portion
(exponential equilibration) that extends from the 5th to the 13th
sec after initial mixing and before the onset of recirculation. From
the slopes (k) of the straight parts of these plots V_{eff}, $\dot{Q}$, DL_{CO}
and DL_{O_2} were calculated. The mixed venous values for $^{16}O_2$ and CO_2
were read from the respective rebreathing plateaus and effective ßb
for the isotope $^{18}O_2$ was obtained from conversion of $\bar{Pv}_{16_{O_2}}$ into
content $\bar{Cv}_{16_{O_2}}$ use being made of the algorithms of Thomas (1972).

RESULTS

Average values for DL_{CO} and DL_{O_2} obtained from 6 normal male
subjects (age 20–33 years) are summarized in table 1.

	Rest	Exercise	Exercise/Rest
DL_{O_2}	54	63	1.18
DL_{CO}	47	52	1.11
DL_{O_2}/DL_{CO}	1.14	1.20	

Table 1. Diffusing capacities for $^{18}O_2$ and $C^{18}O$ (in ml STPD·
min^{-1}·torr^{-1}). Overall mean values from 6 healthy
individuals.

In Fig. 6 mean values for $\dot{Q}$, DL_{CO} and DL_{O_2} are plotted against oxygen uptake ($\dot{M}_{O_2}$) at rest and exercise at the various work loads. The following features become apparent.

1. The mean values at rest for DL_{O_2} and DL_{CO} as well as for $\dot{Q}$ are higher when compared to literature data (see Discussion).

2. There is a slight increase in both DL_{O_2} and DL_{CO} on transition from rest to exercise, not exceeding 15% on the average. It appears that the increase of DL_{O_2} and DL_{CO} proceeds to a plateau level as there is little or no further increase at work loads above 75 watts.

3. The ratio DL_{O_2}/DL_{CO} shows a slight tendency to increase with exercise, however, the difference is not statistically significant. The overall mean value for this ratio is 1.18.

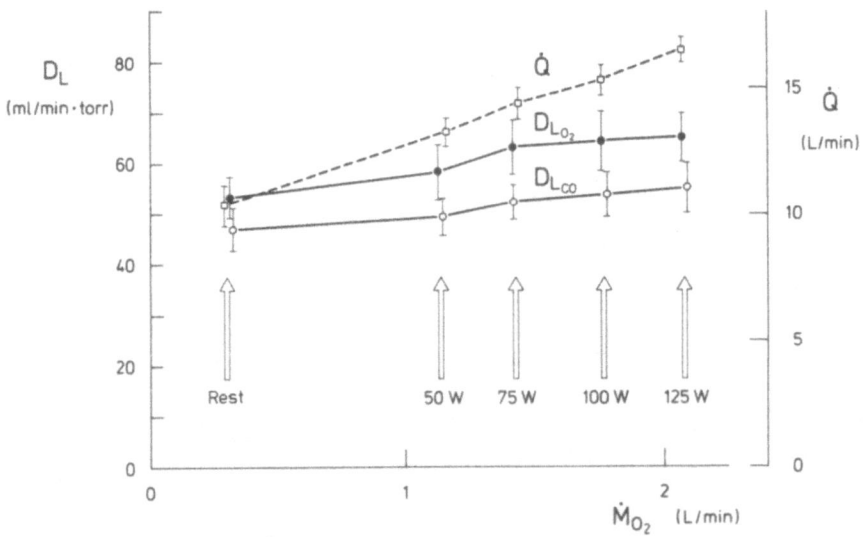

Fig. 6. Cardiac output and diffusing capacities for $^{18}O_2$ and $C^{18}O$ at rest and during various work loads. Overall mean values of 6 healthy males (20-33 years) $\pm$ SD of individual mean values.

DISCUSSION

Pulmonary diffusing capacity at rest

Carbon monoxide

Rebreathing techniques have recently been applied in a limited number of studies for determination of DL_{CO} in normal man (Kruhøffer, 1954; Lewis et al., 1959, 1961; Lawson, 1970; Gong et al., 1972b; Sackner et al., 1975; Adaro et al., 1976; Farney et al., 1977; Rose et al., 1979; Meyer, 1979). The average value from the literature, DL_{CO}= 29 $\pm$ 4 ml·min^{-1}·torr^{-1} is considerably lower than the mean value, DL_{CO} = 47 ml·min^{-1}·torr^{-1}, in the present series. Several factors that mainly reside in differences in experimental conditions may accout for the increased DL_{CO}.

1. In the present study DL_{CO} was determined in transient hypoxic conditions with alveolar P_{O_2} equal to that of mixed venous blood. By contrast, in all other investigations except that of Gong et al. (1972b) the background components of the rebreathing gas mixture was air. In these studies alveolar P_{O_2} is expected to be well above the normal normoxic range at the onset of rebreathing. The increase of DL_{CO} in hypoxia is most probably attributed to the faster rate of association of CO with free hemoglobin, in contrast to the rate at which CO replaces O_2 from HbO_2 in fully saturated red cells.

The alveolar P_{CO_2} was considerably higher in the present study which in turn with alveolar P_{O_2} was equal to mixed venous P_{CO_2}. DL_{CO} by the conventional single-breath technique has been found to increase with increasing alveolar P_{CO_2} (Rankin et al., 1960).

2. The hypothesis of a carrier mediated facilitated transport of carbon monoxide in the lung has recently been invoked by Gurtner

and co-workers (Burns and Gurtner, 1973; Gurtner et al., 1975; Mendoza et al., 1977). The experimental evidence is based on measurements of DL_{CO} at various alveolar CO concentrations. Mendoza et al. (1977) have found an increase of steady-state DL_{CO} in dogs by the order of 30-60% when very low alveolar CO concentrations (about 200-300 ppm) were used in the measurements. These authors have interpreted their results as evidence for the phenomenon of saturation kinetics which is known as a characteristic feature of facilitated transport processes.

In a recent study in which rebreathing DL_{CO} was measured at various CO levels we were unable to substantiate the results by Gurtner and co-workers (Meyer, 1979). It is important to notice that in these measurements low concentrations of the stable isotopes $C^{18}O$ and $^{13}C^{18}O$ in a background of air were used as rebreathing gas mixture. The mean DL_{CO} for both isotopes was 32 ml$\cdot$min$^{-1}\cdot$torr^{-1} which is in close agreement with the average literature value of 29 ml$\cdot$min$^{-1}\cdot$torr^{-1} for similar conditions as mentioned above.

3. Analysis of DL is based on a two compartment rebreathing lung model (c.f. Fig. 2) which takes into account ventilation limitation effects because under experimental conditions the effective ventilation between lungs and rebreathing bag cannot be made high enough to be eliminated in the analysis. With the exception of Adaro et al. (1976) all other authors have analyzed their data on the basis of a more simplified model, in principle by assuming ventilation to be infinite. This leads to an underestimation of DL particularly when the rebreathing ventilation is fairly low as was the case in most other studies cited above.

The discrepancy between our higher DL_{CO} values and those of previous studies may therefore be attributed to a combined effect of factors, notably that of (1) and (3).

Oxygen

Pulmonary diffusing capacity for O_2 has been determined most widely by the steady-state method (Lilienthal et al., 1946). A survey of the literature yields an average DL_{O_2} value of 32 ml· $min^{-1}\cdot torr^{-1}$ which is considerably lower than the mean value, DL_{O_2} = 54 ml·$min^{-1}\cdot torr^{-1}$, obtained in the present study.

There is remarkable agreement between the results of the steady-state method and the breath-holding (single-breath) method introduced by Hyde et al. (1966) for which a mean value of DL_{O_2} = 30 ml·$min^{-1}\cdot torr^{-1}$ is obtained from the literature. It is important to note that the breath-holding technique of Hyde et al. (1966) for determination of DL_{O_2} is similar to ours in as much DL is calculated from the disappearance of isotopic test gases ($^{16}O-^{18}O$, $^{18}O-^{18}O$) from lung gas while the abundant component $^{16}O_2$ is in equilibrium with mixed venous blood. Nontheless, a considerable difference remains with regard to the present results.

Rebreathing DL_{O_2} has been estimated previously by several authors (Micheli and Haab, 1970; Cerretelli et al., 1970, 1974; Piiper et al., 1970; Gong et al., 1972b; Veicsteinas et al., 1976). Except the study of Gong et al. (1972b) DL_{O_2} was calculated from equilibration kinetics of the naturally abundant isotope $^{16}O_2$. The DL_{O_2} values varied from 17 to 47 ml·$min^{-1}\cdot torr^{-1}$, the upper limit of the range being close to the mean value of this study. The difficulties that may be experienced with $^{16}O_2$ as test gas (see above) are expected to account for the large variability and possibly for the discrepancy with regard to the present data.

A major problem in determining DL_{O_2} resides from functional inhomogeneities with respect to unequal distribution of $\dot{V}_A$, DL and $\dot{Q}$. In the steady-state method the ideal-air approach is usually

followed by which all inhomogeneity is attributed to presence of
ventilated but unperfused alveoli, i.e. alveolar dead space ventilation. This approach has been demonstrated to underestimate the
true DL_{O_2} for nearly all $\dot{V}_A/\dot{Q}$ inequalities (Haab et al., 1964;
Chinet et al., 1971; Geiser et al., 1979). Also breath-holding DL_{O_2}
is influenced by unequal distribution of V_A, DL, $\dot{Q}$ and $\dot{V}_A$, however,
the effects of functional inhomogeneities have not been analyzed
systematically.

In the rebreathing technique regional inhomogeneity of alveolar
gas is expected to be reduced by effective mixing. Evidently, the
homogenizing effect is more effective the higher the effective ventilation during rebreathing since with $\dot{V}_{eff}$ all inhomogeneity
must disappear. Therefore, a high $\dot{V}_{eff}$ (fresp = 50/min, V_T = 2.5 L)
was applied in the present study. Model calculations by Scheid et
al. (1973) suggest that, also in the rebreathing technique, unequal
distribution of V_A, $\dot{V}_{eff}$, $\dot{Q}$ and DL result in significant underestimation of DL_{O_2}, particularly when DL is high and $\dot{V}_{eff}$ is only slightly increased. In this analysis the absolute value of $\dot{Q}$ was assumed
to be known rather than calculated from soluble inert gas rebreathing
equilibration kinetics. Preliminary model calculations suggest that
in the presence of regional inhomogeneity $\dot{Q}$ may also be misestimated
in the rebreathing techniques, the direction of error leading to reduced underestimation of DL_{O_2}.

We tend to believe that our high DL_{O_2} values at rest are due to
presence of very high ventilation during rebreathing and/or reduction of inhomogeneities by the rebreathing procedure.

Pulmonary diffusing capacity on exercise

The pulmonary diffusing capacity both for CO and O_2 has been
found to increase as the O_2 requirement increases during physical

exercise. The results in respect of absolute values and relative
changes upon transition from rest to exercise have been highly
variable. In most studies DL_{CO} has been measured by the steady-
state or the single-breath method. The relative increase of DL_{CO}
with increasing exercise level is generally more pronounced in the
steady-state than in the single-breath method but even more pronounced in both methods than found in the present study. There is,
however, reasonable agreement between our values and those by
both steady-state and single-breath techniques at heavy exercise
(O_2 uptake about 2 L/min). It appears that part of the increase in
both methods is due to decreasing inhomogeneity effects as the
discrepancies are most pronounced with the resting values.

Similarly, the discrepancy between our DL_{O_2} values and those
with the steady-state method is most pronounced at rest while there
is reasonable agreement with literature data at heavy exercise.

The following mechanisms may possibly account for an increase
of DL at exercise: (1) Increase of number and/or diameter of pulmonary capillaries, i.e. increase of effective gas exchanging area,
(2) reduction of inhomogeneities ($\dot{V}_A/\dot{Q}$, $DL/\dot{Q}$).

The slight increase of DL_{O_2} and DL_{CO} on transition from rest to
exercise measured with the rebreathing method may well be attributed to a reduction of inhomogeneity by exercise. It is conceivable
that the small increase with no tendency to increase further at
higher work loads represents the maximum of reduced inhomogeneity
that can additionally be gained with exercise in excess of that
already produced by the rebreathing procedure. We therefore neither
can rule out the possibility that the diffusion conditions in our
subjects had changed at all nor can argue in favour of no change
had occurred in heavy exercise.

Relationship of DL_{O_2} and DL_{CO}

The experimental values of the DL_{O_2}/DL_{CO} ratio may be compared to theoretical predictions considering (1) membrane diffusion and (2) diffusion and chemical reaction in red cells as factors determining the rate of alveolar-capillary equilibration. According to Roughton and Forster (1957) the total resistance to alveolar-capillary gas transfer (R_{tot}) can be partitioned into a membrane (R_M) and blood (R_b) resistance (Fig. 7). Both components are incorporated in the well established Roughton-Forster formula for partitioning of lung diffusing capacity DL:

$$\frac{1}{DL} = \frac{1}{DM} \cdot \frac{1}{\Theta \, Q_C} \qquad (8)$$

in which DM is the diffusing capacity of the gas/blood barrier, Θ, the rate of uptake from well stirred plasma of O_2 or CO by red cells (involving both diffusion and chemical reaction) per unit partial pressure difference per unit blood volume, and Q_C capillary blood volume.

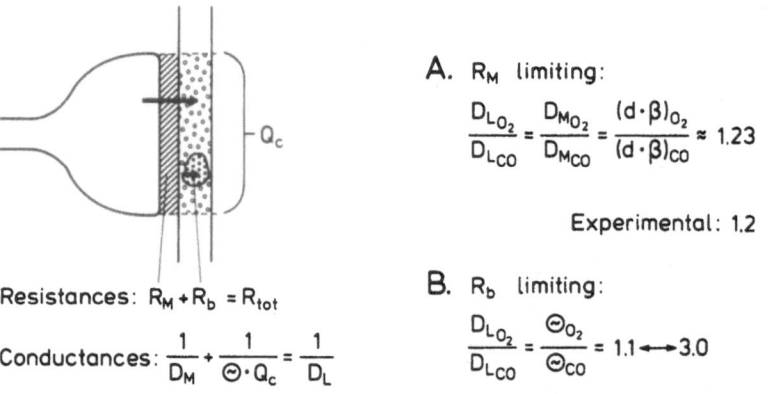

A. R_M limiting:
$$\frac{D_{L_{O_2}}}{D_{L_{CO}}} = \frac{D_{M_{O_2}}}{D_{M_{CO}}} = \frac{(d \cdot \beta)_{O_2}}{(d \cdot \beta)_{CO}} \approx 1.23$$

Experimental: 1.2

B. R_b limiting:
$$\frac{D_{L_{O_2}}}{D_{L_{CO}}} = \frac{\Theta_{O_2}}{\Theta_{CO}} = 1.1 \longleftrightarrow 3.0$$

Resistances: $R_M + R_b = R_{tot}$

Conductances: $\dfrac{1}{D_M} + \dfrac{1}{\Theta \cdot Q_c} = \dfrac{1}{D_L}$

Fig. 7. Schematic representation of the limiting factors in alveolar-capillary transfer of O_2 and CO.

(1) If the total resistance that corresponds to the diffusing capacity DL mainly represents a resistance offered by the alveolar-capillary membrane, the ratio DL_{O_2}/DL_{CO} should be close to the ratio of Krogh's diffusion constants $(d \cdot \beta)$, i.e. about 1.23.

(2) If the rate of uptake of O_2 and CO by red cells constitutes the major limiting factor, the ratio DL_{O_2}/DL_{CO} is expected to be close to the specific conductance ratio, i.e. θ_{O_2}/θ_{CO}. Whereas the θ_{CO} value is usually taken to be 0.9 (in $ml \cdot min^{-1} \cdot torr^{-1} \cdot ml^{-1}$) there is considerable disagreement as to the value of θ_{O_2} which, above 75% saturation, varies between 2.7 (Staub et al., 1962) and 0.9 (Mochizuki, 1966). Thus, the ratio θ_{O_2}/θ_{CO} results to be in the range 1.1 to 3.0.

Simultaneous determinations of DL_{O_2} and DL_{CO} have been performed in a limited number of studies using steady state and single-breath methods. There is a marked disparity as to the DL_{O_2}/DL_{CO} ratio which is found to vary from 0.56 to 1.62. This disparity is even worse considering that 75% of the literature values are below 1.0 which is out of the range that is expected on theoretical grounds.

By contrast, our value is about 1.2 both at rest and exercise. This finding suggests that the uptake of O_2 and CO is mainly limited by a diffusive resistance, chemical reaction rates with hemoglobin being too rapid for a significant uptake-limitation. However, this conclusion is rendered to be at least premature as alternative implications have to be considered.

As discussed already presence of functional inhomogeneity generally leads to underestimation of pulmonary diffusing capacity. The effects of regional inequality as regards to the ratio of DL_{O_2}/DL_{CO} have not been analysed systematically. Preliminary model calculations reveal that in the rebreathing technique the effects of inhomogeneities are more pronounced for DL_{O_2} than for DL_{CO}, resulting in reduced DL_{O_2}/DL_{CO} ratio.

The uncertainties about the Θ values for O_2 and CO constitute a major problem in the analysis of DL_{O_2} and DL_{CO} into their components. In fact, with lowest Θ_{O_2} from the literature (0.9, Mochizuki, 1966; 1.5, Holland et al., 1977) Θ_{O_2}/Θ_{CO} comes close to unity. Similar objections apply to the value of Θ_{CO} which has been measured only in fully oxygenated blood for replacement of O_2 bound to hemoglobin by CO. In hypoxic conditions that prevail in our experimental procedures (and most part of the capillary length in normoxia) Θ_{CO} is expected to increase by an unknown factor as the rate of association of CO with Hb increases in the presence of unsaturated hemoglobin.

Evidently, more accurate data on Θ_{O_2} and Θ_{CO} are required for the analysis of DL_{O_2} and DL_{CO} into their components.

REFERENCES

Adaro, F., Scheid, P., Teichmann, J. and Piiper, J., 1973.
    A rebreathing method for estimating pulmonary D_{O_2}: theory and
    measurements in dog lungs.
    Respir. Physiol. 18: 43-63.
Adaro, F., Meyer, M. and Sikand, R.S., 1976. Rebreathing and single
    breath pulmonary CO diffusing capacity in man at rest and
    exercise studied by $C^{18}O$ isotope.
    Bull. Europ. Physiopath. Resp. 12: 747-756.
Burns, B. and Gurtner, G.H., 1973. A specific carrier for oxygen
    and carbon monoxide in the lung and placenta.
    Drug. Metab. Disp. 1: 374-377.
Cander, L. and Forster, R.E., 1959. Determination of pulmonary
    parenchymal tissue volume and pulmonary capillary flow in
    man. J. Appl. Physiol. 14: 541-551.
Cerretelli, P., Di Prampero, P.E. and Rennie, D.W., 1970.
    Measurement of mixed venous oxygen tension by a modified
    rebreathing procedure. J. Appl. Physiol. 28: 707-711.

Cerretelli, P., Veicsteinas, A., Teichmann, J., Magnussen, H. and Piiper, J., 1974. Estimation by a rebreathing method of pulmonary O_2 diffusing capacity in man. J. Appl. Physiol. 37: 526-532.

Chinet, A., Micheli, J.L. and Haab, P., 1971. Inhomogeneity effects on O_2 and CO pulmonary diffusing capacity estimates by steady-state methods. Theory. Respir. Physiol. 13: 1-22.

Cross, C.E., Gong, H., Kurpershoek, C.J., Gillespie, J.R. and Hyde, R.W., 1973. Alterations in distribution of blood flow to the lung's diffusion surfaces during exercise. J. Clin. Invest. 52: 414-421.

Farney, R.J., Morris, A.H., Gardner, R.M. and Armstrong, J.D., 1977. Rebreathing pulmonary capillary and tissue volume in normals after saline infusion. J. Appl. Physiol. 43: 246-253.

Geiser, J., Chinet, A. and Haab, P., 1979. Pulmonary O_2 diffusing capacity estimates from assumed log-normal $\dot{V}_A/\dot{Q}$ distribution. Respir. Physiol. 37: 31-44.

Gong, H., Kurpershoek, C.J., Meyer, D.B. and Cross, C.E., 1972a. Effects of cardiac output on $^{18}O_2$ lung diffusion in normal resting man. Respir. Physiol. 16: 313-326.

Gong, H., Kurpershoek, C. and Cross, C.E., 1972b. $^{18}O_2$ diffusing capacity measured by a rebreathing method in normal man. Clin. Res. 20: 195.

Gurtner, G., Peavy, H., Summer, W. and Burns, B., 1975. Physiological evidence for the presence of a specific O_2, CO carrier in the lung and placenta. Prog. Resp. Res. 8: 166-176.

Haab, P., Duc, G., Stucki, R. and Piiper, J., 1964. Les échanges gazeux en hypoxie et la capacité de diffusion pour l'oxygène chez le chien narcotisé. Helv. Physiol. Acta 22: 203-227.

Holland, R.A.B., Van Hezewijk, W. and Zubzanda, J., 1977. Velocity of oxygen uptake by partly saturated adult and fetal human red cells. Respir. Physiol. 29: 303-314.

Hyde, R.W., Forster, R.E., Power, G.G., Nairn, J. and Rynes, R., 1966. Measurement of O_2 diffusing capacity of the lungs with a stable O_2 isotope. J. Clin. Invest. 45: 1178-1193.

Kruhøffer, P., 1954. Studies on the lung diffusion coefficient for carbon monoxide in normal human subjects by means of $C^{14}O$. Acta Physiol. Scand. 32: 106-123.

Lawson, W.H., 1970. Rebreathing measurements of pulmonary diffusing capacity for CO during exercise. J. Appl. Physiol. 29: 896-900.

Lewis, B.M., Lin, T.H., Noe, F.E. and Hayford-Welsing, E.J., 1959. The measurement of pulmonary diffusing capacity for carbon monoxide by a rebreathing method. J. Clin. Invest. 38: 2073-2086.

Lewis, B.M., Hayford-Welsing, E.J., Furusho, A., and Reed, L.C., 1961. Effect of uneven ventilation on pulmonary diffusing capacity. J. Appl. Physiol. 16: 679-683.

Lilienthal, J.L., Riley, R.L., Proemmel, D.D. and Franke, R.E., 1946. An experimental analysis in man of the O_2 pressure gradient from alveolar air to arterial blood during rest and exercise at sea level and at altitude. Am. J. Physiol. 147: 199-216.

Mendoza, C., Peavy, H., Burns, B. and Gurtner, G., 1977. Saturation kinetics for steady-state pulmonary CO transfer. J. Appl. Physiol. 43: 880-884.

Meyer, M., 1979. Experimental evidence against role of facilitated transport of carbon monoxide in alveolar gas. Pflügers Arch. 382: Suppl. R17.

Micheli, J.L. and Haab, P., 1970. Estimation de la capacitê de diffusion pulmonaire pour l'oxygêne chez l'homme au repos par la mêthode du rebreathing hypoxique. J. Physiol. (Paris) 62: Suppl. 1, 194-195.

Mochizuki, M., 1966. Study on the oxygenation velocity of the human red cell. Jap. J. Physiol. 16: 635-648.

Piiper, J., Dejours, P., Haab, P. and Rahn, H., 1971. Concepts and basic quantities in gas exchange physiology. Respir. Physiol. 13: 292-304.

Piiper, J., Meyer, M. and Scheid, P., 1979. Alveolar-capillary equilibration kinetics of CO_2 : measurements by rebreathing in man at rest and during exercise. Physiologist 22: 101.

Rankin, J., McNeill, R.S. and Forster, R.E., 1960. Influence of increased alveolar CO_2 tension on pulmonary diffusing capacity for CO in man. J. Appl. Physiol. 15: 543-549.

Rose, G.L., Cassidy, S.S. and Johnson, R.L., 1979. Diffusing capacity at different lung volumes during breath holding and rebreathing. J. Appl. Physiol. 47: 32-37.

Roughton, F.J.W. and Forster, R.E., 1957. Relative importance of diffusion and chemical reaction rates in determining rate of exchange of gases in the human lung, with special reference to true diffusing capacity of pulmonary membrane and volume of blood in the lung capillaries. J. Appl Physiol. 11: 291-302.

Sackner, M.A., Greeneltch, G., Heiman, M.S., Epstein, S. and Atkins, N., 1975. Diffusing capacity, membrane diffusing capacity, capillary blood volume, pulmonary tissue volume, and cardiac output measured by a rebreathing technique. Amer. Rev. Resp. Dis. 111: 157-165.

Scheid, P., Adaro, F., Teichmann, J. and Piiper, J., 1973. Rebreathing and steady state pulmonary D_{O_2} in the dog and in inhomogeneous lung models. Respir. Physiol. 18: 258-272.

Staub, N.C., Bishop, J.M. and Forster, R.E., 1962. Importance of diffusion and chemical reaction rates in O_2 uptake in the lung. J. Appl. Physiol. 17: 21-27.

Teichmann, J., Adaro, F., Veicsteinas, A., Cerretelli, P. and Piiper, J., 1974. Determination of pulmonary blood flow by rebreathing of soluble inert gases. Respiration 31: 296-309.

Thomas, L.J., 1972. Algorithms for selected blood acid-base and blood gas calculations. J. Appl. Physiol. 33: 154-158.

Discussion

LOCKHART: As regards your last slide, it pertains to sea level residents at altitude. Have you made similar calculations or estimates using data from highlanders living at that altitude? Because from what I recall some people have already measured or attempted to measure diffusion of CO by conventional methods in highlanders and found it to be, if anything, higher than in sea level dwellers, suggesting that perfusion is not a limiting factor in highlanders. I wonder whether you would like to speculate on that.

MEYER: Well, unfortunately I haven't been at Mount Everest so I had no possibility to do these measurements, although I would have liked to do it. Now for your question, and it appears that there is obviously some disagreement but the disagreement is mainly due to the fact that it is extremely difficult, and maybe impossible, to calculate diffusing capacities of oxygen from data on CO, because the relationship between oxygen diffusing capacity and carbon monoxide diffusing capacity is not as clear as it is sometimes believed. It is often assumed that the ratio is about 1:2 and you may have realised that from our measurements, that oxygen diffusing capacity was always larger than for CO.   And in fact under all conditions we obtained a ratio of about 1:2 which indicates that the difference between these two gases is mainly due to the differences in their physical characteristics with respect to diffusivity and solubility. And on the other hand, if one accepts the ratio of 1:2 there is more or less no space for limitation of oxygen and/or CO transfer, because it is well known that the rate of reaction for oxygen is much faster than for CO. And coming back to the question I feel that one should be extremely careful to draw conclusions with respect to diffusion limitation or to limiting factors of oxygen transfer from data that have been obtained from carbon monoxide.

THE EFFECTS OF REGIONAL HYPOXIA ON THE

DISTRIBUTION OF PULMONARY BLOOD FLOW

Gordon Cumming

Midhurst Medical Research Institute

Midhurst, West Sussex

When a part of the lung is made hypoxic, the perfusion of that part diminishes and is redirected to the non-hypoxaemic part. Experiments demonstrating this phenomenon have usually been done by cannulating one bronchus, using a Carlens catheter and then ventilating one lung with 21% oxygen and the other with perhaps 10% oxygen measuring the pulmonary blood flow on the hypoxic side using the Fick principle. Whilst such an experiment is rather invasive and the precision of measurement was not high it was sufficient to confirm the hypothesis that alveolar hypoxaemia led to blood diversion.

In order to use a less invasive method in humans, regional hypoxia was induced using a characteristic of the upright lung breathing at residual volume. At full expiration the dependant lobes of the lung receive initially no ventilation, since it goes preferentially to the upper lobes on account of the effective intrapleural pressure being affected by gravity acting upon lung parenchymal density.

It would be possible therefore to produce hypoxaemia of the lower lobes by breathing gas containing the first 21% of its volume as pure oxygen, followed by 79% of its volume as pure Argon, provided that a normal inspirate is taken from residual volume. Under such conditions the first part of the inspirate which is pure oxygen, passes into the upper lobes, whilst the latter part of the inspirate (pure Argon) enters the dependant part of the lungs and there produces local hypoxia. This hypoxia will then produce a fall in arterial oxygen partial pressure. If local hypoxia produces a diversion of blood away from hypoxic areas to well ventilated areas this fall of actual oxygen partial pressure would then restore itself to normal and the rate of such restoration would delineate the time course of vascular adaptation.

Following the time course of arterial desaturation in a non-invasive way is possible by using ear oximetry, especially since the absolute values of the change are not important, but only the fact that such changes occur and that these alter with time.

A special valve was developed which partitioned the resting tidal volume into its two compartments of oxygen and argon and the subject breathed for one minute at F.R.C. whilst measuring end expired oxygen, carbon dioxide and arterial saturation from the ear oximeter. The subject then expired maximally and then continued to breathe with the same frequency and the same tidal volume as before, being careful to return to residual volume on each occasion. Breathing continued in this fashion for 3 minutes after which the subject returned to F.R.C. and continued for a further minute. Since this manouvre involved inspiring a large volume and since the oxygen volume was fixed, the balance was argon and this produced an overall hypoxic mixture in the alveolar. The level of this hypoxia was measurable from the end tidal oxygen concentration and could be correlated with the fall in oxygen saturation observed from the ear oximeter. In this way a direct calibration of saturation change was available.

Normal subjects breathing in this way showed the expected response. At F.R.C. no change was observed in any of the measured variables, but during the first half minute of R.V. breathing a marked arterial desaturation was seen: thereafter, whilst still breathing at R.V. the arterial saturation recovered to its initial level. This behaviour was interpreted as indicating a diversion of pulmonary blood flow away from an area of regional hypoxia.

The next set of experiments were by way of control, in which the same apparatus was used but instead of inspiring oxygen followed by argon, ambient air was inspired in both phases. Thus the subject was breathing air only from residual volume. Perhaps surprisingly this breathing manouvre resulted in an identical fall in arterial saturation, but the subsequent behaviour was different, in that the recovery to normal saturation did not take place, but the desaturation continued for the whole 3 minutes, only reverting to the normal value on resuming the F.R.C. position.

The third set of experiments was arranged so that pure oxygen was inspired first, followed by ambient air so that hyperoxia would be induced in the upper lobes, but no part of the lung would be rendered hypoxic, since the dependant parts would receive ambient air.

The behaviour of the arterial saturation was similar to that seen in the second set of experiments in that saturation did not return to control values during breathing at residual volume, but there was a slight increase of about 10% after the initial fall.

The interpretation of these experimental findings was as follows:- at residual volume ventilation of the dependant parts of the lungs ceases. This does not require that airways closure should occur, although this may happen for a part of the cycle. The alveolar gas in this non-ventilated lung rapidly assumes mixed venous concentration for oxygen and the blood flow through it constitutes a shunt and results in desaturation of the arterial blood. The size of the shunt can be calculated to be about 25% of pulmonary blood flow. This shunt occurs in all the experiments independant of inspired gas and results purely from breathing at residual volume.

Despite the local hypoxia during air breathing in the second and third experiments, no redirection of pulmonary blood flow took place, so that hypoxia equal to mixed venous oxygen saturation was inadequate in these experiments to effect pulmonary vascular adaptation. However, rapid adaptation occurred when pure argon was used. From this it can be concluded that Argon entered the dependant parts of the lung, for it produced vascular adaptation, so that airway closure could not be present throughout the tidal volume taken at residual volume and if present at all, could only be intermittent. Further, since the arterial saturation was restored to normal, argon must have gained access to the whole volume of the lung which was unventilated and producing shunt. Thus ventilation was intermittent in all of the dependant lung.

Perhaps the most important observation in the first experiments was that it was necessary to reduce alveolar gas concentration below mixed venous levels in order to produce a redirection of pulmonary blood flow away from the shunted areas. This behaviour of the pulmonary circulation to local hypoxia is produced under very specific conditions and in no way invalidates other observations made with global hypoxaemia, but does give additional insight into the mechanisms involved.

Discussion

BARER: Have you any evidence that local acute hypoxia differs in different parts of the lung. Have you done your experiments standing on their heads or lying on their side?

CUMMING: It's quite an unusual experiment and it's very easy to do. I'm hoping to have an Australian fellow in September to extend this technique. It gives you a good idea of how to investigate the effects of drugs on hypoxemic shunting with no invasion and very simply. Thank you for your suggestion.

DENISON: I hope that you are not suggesting that the Australian fellow will now need to stand on his head! The question that I wanted to ask you, or to comment, was that in your chappies who went from the coast to Denver, I suspect that their return to Denver would be much too gradual for you to get a real reversal of oxygen flow in any part of the lung. What do you think?

CUMMING: I have no data on this. I'd like to have a look at it. It's just a suggestion. It is difficult to explain the observation by any other hypothesis that is currently being offered. This might equally well not be a valid hypothesis, but it stands for the moment until we can shoot it down by some such methods as you suggest. I don't know how quickly mixed venous blood adapts. Within hours, I would guess. I don't know the mechanism of transportation back to the mountations and so if it took a day it would be very unlikely, if it took an hour it may be possible.

DENISON: Mixed venous adapts, since I've measured it many times, in hypoxia, and it did adapt within minutes.

CUMMING: Within minutes?

DENISON: Yes, and that's why I'd be worried that it would follow very faithfully the re-ascent to Louisville.

ZARDINI: Is it not very difficult starting from residual volume?

CUMMING: Yes, very difficult. Its's painful.

ZARDINI: It is painful and I have some experience in this. Perhaps it happens to you sometimes that when you start to do the Valsalva manoeuvre, and start again to breathe and you couldn't see all the changes that you saw sometimes? When after a full expiration you start to breathe a tidal volume from the residual volume, very often a Valsalva manouvre occurs.

CUMMING: Well, of course, if you do a Valsalva many things happen. Although I say that it is simple to do, it has to be learned. You need several attempts of breathing at residual volume and seeing the needle go up and down, and keeping your glottis open. A very important point.

ZARDINI: What about the difference between argon and nitrogen to extend the regional hypoxia?   The difference between the two gases in diffusing through the smaller airways.

CUMMING: No. Nitrogen has a molecular weight of 28 and Argon of 40, too close to make an important difference.

MECHANISMS OF PULMONARY ARTERIAL HYPERTENSION

Henri Denolin

Professor of Cardio-Pulmonary Physiology, Head of the

Department of Cardiology, University of Brussels

1. INTRODUCTION

Before discussing in a simple way and from the clinical point of view the possible mechanisms of pulmonary arterial hypertension, it may be usefull to remember some of the basic characteristics of the pulmonary circulation.

From the anatomical point of view, we should remember that the pulmonary circulation is a short circuit, that the small arteries have muscular cells in their walls and that there are no valves on the venous side.

From the physiological point of view, we should remember that the pulmonary circulation is a low pressure-low resistance system.

The pressure we measure in the pulmonary artery is an intravascular pressure, relative to atmosphere and different from the transmural pressure, which is the difference in pressure between the inside of the vessel and the pressure in the tissues surrounding the vessels. The driving pressure is the difference in pressure between two points in the circulation. We know also that there are local changes in pressure related to hydrostatic pressure, with difference in perfusion at the different levels; but for the clinician, the pulmonary arterial pressure is measured in the pulmonary trunc or its main branches.

The vascular resistance is generally defined as the drop in pressure between the artery and the end of the vascular system, that is the wedge pressure (representative of the left atrial pressure), devided by flow.

In many books of physiology, it is said that the pulmonary vascular system is highly distensible, but it was demonstrated that this is not the case. Using the method of occlusion of
one of the main branches of the pulmonary artery (P.A.) by a
balloon, Harris and Heath[1] demonstrated that in the normal subject,
lying down, the muscular pulmonary arteries do not distend
greatly in response to a twofold increase in flow.

We will see later this may be true if the immediate
effect of flow increase is considered, but probably not in chronic situations.

Finally, the pressure in the P.A. is related -as in
the systemic circulation- to flow, distensibility of the system,
resistance of the vessels;but also to the pressure in the left
heart, which is passively transmitted to the arterial side.

Normal values of the pressure in the P.A. are
available in the litterature for the lying and the sitting
positions; there are individual differences, or differences
in the series, related probably sometimes to methological
reasons.

2. MECHANISMS OF PULMONARY ARTERIAL HYPERTENSION IN CLINICAL SITUATION

It is classical to devide these mechanisms into
precapillary hypertension, with a normal wedge pressure, and
post capillary hypertension with an increased wedge pressure.
But in many cases several mechanisms are associated.

2.1. Hypertension by increase in flow or hypercinetic hypertension

In _acute_ situations, the most interesting condition
associated by an increase in flow is the begining of physical
exercise. When the cardiac output is increased, the pressure in
the P.A. rises always, in both upright and lying positions.
For some authors, the difference between the arterial and the
wedge pressures is increased more than the flow, and a small
increase in vascular resistance is observed [1]. But others
·consider that, in the lying position, there is a small decrease
in resistance, related to the opening of new channels and/or
to a dilation of the vessels.

The increase in pressure is related to age, and the
answer in old subjects is greatly due to an increase in wedge
pressure : this increase is partly of post capillary origin.

In the sitting position, there is also an increase
in arterial pressure with exercise, with an increase in wedge
pressure[2,3]; in normal middle age subjects, the higher value
of the mean pulmonary arterial pressure is around 30 mm Hg,
for an oxygen consuption of 2 liters/minute[4].

In the sitting position, there is probably some decrease in resistance, related to difference in central blood volume ?
    An other condition associated with a sudden increase
in flow is the occlusion of one of the main pulmonary arteries by
a balloon catheter. The pressure increases in the open artery; the
vascular resistance is probably not decreased[1].
    During graded exercise, the P.A. pressure increase
maximally during the first level of work load; with subsequent
level of exercise, the pressure does not increase substantially.
In prolonged exercise, with a constant cardiac output, the pressure
slowly decrease, by changes in pulmonary resistance or by change
in the left atrial pressure, we don't know.
    In chronic conditions of increased flow, the pressure
in the P.A. may remain completely normal. This is the case after
pneumonectomy, even in the older patients or after many years
in the same patient[5]. An other example of this situation is
represented by some congenital heart diseases, especially in
pretricusped shunts like atrial septal defect, in which a flow of
2 to 3 times of the normal value is associated with a normal
pressure.
    So, if it is true that an acute increase in flow is
associated with an increase in pressure, and only a small or no
change in resistance, there are chronic conditions in which
a large increase in cardiac output is associated with a normal
pressure and a large decrease in vascular resistance.

2.2. Pulmonary hypertension secondary to a passive transmission
of an elevated pressure in the left heart

    An increase of pressure in left ventricle is asso-
ciated with an increase in wedge and in pulmonary arterial
pressures; this is well know from the studies on myocardial
infarction and other ventricular diseases, and the monitoring
of the pressure in the pulmonary circulation is of tremendous
importance in the coronary care unit.
    The problem of mitral stenosis is more interesting
from the point of view of the evolution of pulmonary hypertension. At the begining of the disease, there is only a
passive transmission of the elevated left atrial pressure
to the pulmonary tree. But even at this stage of the disease
their may be a vasoconstriction of the muscular part of the
vessels, probably by a myogenic reaction, as demonstrated by
the hypotensive effect of acetylcholine. In a second stage,
anatomical changes appear in the pulmonary vessels, in response to the sustained passive hypertension : medial hypertrophy of the muscular arteries, internal thikening and
fibrosis [6]; a large gradient between arterial and wedge
pressure appears, with an important increase in valvular resistance.

It is possible also that an increase in interstitial pressure contribute to the elevation of the pressures.

If we consider large series of cases with mitral stenosis, we observe very large differences in the individual arterial pressures, even in patients of the same age, same duration of the disease and same severity of valvular stenosis : the individual reaction to a sustained passive hypertension may be quite different from one patient to another [5].

Finally, in this group of transmission of hypertensive from the post capillary side, we could include the rare cases of venous pulmonary diseases [1.6].

2.3. Anatomical changes in the vascular walls

We have already seen that changes in the structure of the arterial walls of the pulmonary vessels may be secondary to a chronic increase in pressure, as in mitral stenosis. But there are other conditions which are associated with anatomical changes in the vessels. A first example is given by some cases of congenital cardiac defects, especially of the post-tricuspid types (ventricular septal defect, persistent ductus arteriosus) in chich hypertension is present from birth : in these cases, the normal downward trend in the thickness of the media is interrupted, there is a medial hypertrophy and increase in smooth muscle in the vascular wall.

A complete description of the pathological aspects in these diseases is given in the book of WAGENVOORT AND WAGENVOORT[6].

In some cases of congenital heart diseases, of the pre- or post tricuspid type, the same changes appear sometimes later, around 40 years : the pressure in the PA remains normal during the first years of life, and then increases slowly.

In some cases, of primary pulmonary hypertension of unknown etiology, the same pathological changes may be observed without any associated heart defect.

Finally, there are cases of acquired isolated pulmonary hypertension, apparently from toxic origin. In some countries of Europe, a dramatic increase in the number of cases of isolated pulmonary hypertension was observed a few years ago, especially in women, probably related to the use of an anorexigen. But it is important to stress that only 2%o of the users of this drug develop a pulmonary hypertension; this means that an individual sensibility is needed before the drug is able to produce a reaction in the pulmonary vessels.

So, it appears clearly that in many diseases of the heart or in some intoxication, important changes in the anatomy of the pulmonary vascular walls contribute to the development and to the maintainance of hypertension.

2.4. Obstruction of the vessels

        In diseases associated with the obstruction of the
pulmonary vessels, an increase in pressure and resistance may be
observed : thromboembolism, fat embolism, tumor embolism,
parasites (schistosomiasis), etc.
        The mechanism of pulmonary hypertension in thrombo-
embolism remains discussed : simple mechanical occlusion of a
sufficient number of vessels, release of vasoconstrictive
substances (SEROTONIN), or reflex vasoconstriction. From our
own experience in dogs [7] and from some anatomical observations[6]
it appears that the mechanical obstruction of the vessels is
probably the good hypothesis.

2.5. Vasoconstriction or Reactive Hypertension

        The normal pulmonary circulation is probably not
regulated by the nervous system, but in some conditions vasoconstriction may be observed under the influence of local
agents.
        The most important condition in which a constriction
of the muscular arteries is observed in alveolar hypoxia.
        For BERGOVSKY, this vasoconstriction is not related
to changes in the total alveolar pressure, or in blood viscosity,
or in left atrial pressure, or in blood flow, and is apparently
independent of the nervous system [8].
        But for a few observers, as KAZEMI and coworkers[9],
the hypoxie pulmonary vascular response in dogs is considerably
reduced after cervical sympathectomy, and the nervous system
should thus be involved in the development of hypertension.
        But for most of the observers, the situation is the
following :
- the hypertension is related to alveolar hypoxia, and not to
the content or pressure of oxygen in the blood.
- the increase in the pulmonary pressure during hypoxia is
related to an action on the arterial side of the vascular tree.
- the increase in pressure is related to direct action of hypoxia
on the vascular muscle or to the local release of a substance
able to act on the alpha receptors of the small pulmonary vessels
(histamine, angiotensine, cathecolamines, ionic composition of
the vascular smooth muscle, tissue acidose, etc ??).
        Concerning the possible role of prostaglandins in
the anoxic vasoconstriction, the question remains open. For
some authors, it seems unlikely that prostaglandins or their
intermediates are mediators of hypoxie pulmonary vasoconstriction[10].
        Finally, the situation remains confused, as far as
the mechanisms responsible of hypertension in alveolar hypoxie
are concerned [11].

Examples of hypoxie hypertension in man are given by altitude and chronic lung diseases.

In altitude hypoxia, appears again the problem of individual sensibility : not only the hypertensive reactions differ greatly from one animal species to another, but even in man the development of hypertension is strongly different from one subject to another, for the same altitude and the same oxygen pressure in the alveoli.

2.6. Mechanical compression of the vessels

Distribution of blood flow in the lungs is related to transmural pressure. A possible contribution to an elevated pressure could be an increase in intrathoracic or intra-alveolar pressure.

2.7. Transmission from the bronchial circulation

It is considered that in some diseases (bronchiectasis, neoplastie diseases) the development of anatomosis between the bronchial arteries and the pulmonary circulation could be a mechanisms explaining an increase in wedge pressure and pulmonary arterial pressure.

3. CHRONIC OBSTRUCTIVE LUNG DISEASES

In most of the chronic lung diseases of the group of chronic bronchitis and emphysema, several mechanisms are probably involved : changes in vascular walls (thickening, medial hypertrophy, muscularization); loss of capillaries; hypoxic vasoconstriction; increase in alveolar pressure; increase in blood viscosity (polyglobuly).

In opposition with what was sometimes claimed the cardiac output is generally not increased in these cases. The problem of an increase in wedge pressure, and of the participation of the left ventricule in the development of pulmonary hypertension in chronic lung diseases remains unsolved but there are no proofs that the hypothesis of a left heart disease directly related or to associated with the lung disease has to be considered [12]. The great majority of patients have a normal left ventricular function [13-14].

4. CONCLUSION

The regulation of the pressure in the pulmonary circulation is quite different from the regulation of pressure in the systemic circulation and the mechanisms of hypertension are completely different.

Important differences in adaptation between acute and chronic situations are observed (response to an increased blood flow).

Differences in reaction to the same stimulus are observed, not only between species, but also in man (mitral stenosis, congenital heart diseases, hypoxia).

In many clinical conditions, several mechanisms are associated.

REFERENCES

1. P. Harris, and D. Heath. The human pulmonary circulation. Churchill Livingstone Edinburgh. (1977).
2. T. Strandell. Pulmonary blood flow and pressure in old age. Effect of body position, exercise and physical training in Pulmonary Circulation. Progress in Respiratory Research 5. Karger. Basel (1970).
3. S. Degré, A. Decoster, R. Messin and H. Denolin. Normal pulmonary pressure-flow relationship during exercise in the sitting position. Int.Z.Angew.Physiol. 31:53 (1972).
4. V. Stanek, J. Widimsky, S. Degré, and H. Denolin. The lesser circulation during exercise in healthy subjects. in Pulmonary Hypertension. Progress in Respiration Reserach 9. Karger. Basel. (1975).
5. H. Denolin. Contribution à l'étude de la circulation pulmonaire en clinique. Acta Cardiologica. Supplementum X. (1961).
6. C.A. Wagenvoort and N. Wagenvoort. Pathology of Pulmonary Hypertension. J. Wiley and Sons. New-York. (1977).
7. O. Courtoy et N. Salonikides. Hypertension pulmonaire aiguë expérimentale par embolie pulmonaire. Acta Cardiologica. 11:52. (1956).
8. E.H. Bergovsky. Mechanisms underlying vasomotor regulation of regional pulmonary blood flow in normal and disease states. Am.J.Med. 57:378 (1974).
9. H. Kazemi, P.E. Bruecke and E.F. Parsons. Role of the autonomic nervous system in the hypoxic response of the pulmonary vascular bed. Respir. Physiol. 15:245 (1972).
10. D.F. Horrobin. Prostaglandins. Churchill Livingstone. Edinburgh (1978).
11. J.M.B. Hughes. Local control of blood flow and ventilation. IN Regional differences in the lung. Edited by J. West. Academic. New-York. p.419. (1977).
12. H. Denolin. Le ventricule gauche dans les bronchopneumopathies obstructives. Bull.Europ.Physiopath.Resp. 12:407. (1976).

13. R.G. Kachel. Left ventricular function in chronic obstructive
    lung disease. Chest. 74:266 (1978).
14. L.E. Kline, M.H. Crawford, W.J. Mac Donald, H. Schelbert,
    R.A. O'Rourke and K.M. Moser. Noninvasive assessment of left
    ventricular performance in patients with chronic obstructive
    pulmonary disease. Chest. 72:558 (1977).

Discussion

SCHIAVINO: You said that wedge pressure on COLD is always normal even in the case of high PA pressure. I agree with this; we have similar results. What is difficult to explain in these cases of COLD is the frequent presence of pulmonary oedema which is visible on x-ray during acute exacerbations.

DENOLIN: That's a good question but then we go to the regulation of the microcirculation and I hesitate to develop this here because it seems too difficult. But maybe the anatomists have some explanation. We think it is not only in chronic lung disease that we see pulmonary oedema associated with a normal wedge pressure. There are many conditions in which this occurs, probably related to all the factors of pressure, such as changes in the permeability of the walls and things like that.

GUNELLA: I want to ask you your opinion of the pathogenetic aspects of this problem of radiologically visible pulmonary oedema in patients with COLD and who have normal wedge pressure. The first idea was that at the basis of everything there was a preferential redistribution of the flow according to the anatomical situation of the pulmonary arterial meshwork since it is evident that the blood can only circulate where the vessels are patent. We thought that it is possible that where there is an anatomical restriction of the arterial lung bed in these patients, there was a marked increase of pressure in the area where the flow was free, probably associated with an increase of vascular permeability. However, we must still show what actually causes this increase of vascular permeability. We should also ask ourselves if the problem couldn't be considered as lymphatic stasis since these patients often have high pressures in the right ventricle. Showing that in man lymphatic stasis is responsible for this situation of oedema is not very easy and therefore we remain in the field of hypothesis. But the real pathogenetic explanation is, I think, somewhat difficult.

DENOLIN: I have no answer to this question only to say that oedema in the systemic as well as in the pulmonary circulation is related to the pressure in the vessels, to the pressure in the interstitium to the oncotic pressure inside and outside and to the permeability. That is well known but this is not an answer to your question.

WILLIAMS: I would be most grateful for Denolin's thoughts on a case of pulmonary hypertension which we recently had in Liverpool. This was a young girl who was born in the Andes of South America. Her parents were from England and they went to the Andes to undertake some geological research. While there, she was born in the Andes and was presumably exposed to hypoxic pulmonary hypertension. As a child she did not do very well and so her parents decided to return to England. She then had an uneventful childhood. She went to a British university and started to become breathless, particularly on exercise. Subsequently she died, at the age of nineteen, and was thought to have been suffering from pulmonary hypertension. My question is does Denolin think that this young lady was unfortunate enough to have been exposed to two different types of pulmonary hypertension in her lifetime, or does he think that the initial exposure at birth in a Caucasian child had brought about some permanent change in her pulmonary circulation which resulted twenty years later in her apparently dying from primary pulmonary hypertension?

DENOLIN: Well, I have no answer to your question. I have already seen from surgical experience when the cause for hypertension is abolished, say by closure of a heart defect, the pressure in the pulmonary circulation in some cases decreases, sometimes very suddenly, sometimes progressively, and sometimes never. So the individual answer is not only to the causes increasing the pressure, but also, after suppression of the cause the individual answer may be quite different.

DENISON: I would be embarrassed if I missed it in your talk, but could you summarise the changes in pulmonary vascular resistance which occur in benign and malignant systemic hypertension?

DENOLIN: I think this is related to the state of the left ventricle. I don't think that there is a regular association between systemic and pulmonary hypertension. And this is evident because the mechanisms of regulation are completely different. I don't think that those causes able to produce systemic hypertension are able to cause at the same time pulmonary hypertension - this is at least not the rule. So when you go to hypertension you see that the situation in the pulmonary circulation is related to the functional state of the left ventricle.

RIEDEL: I thought that pulmonary hypertension is irreversible in the vast majority of cases, and it has a very bad prognosis. You mentioned many times in your lecture that there is an individual reactivity of pulmonary vessels to various pressure stimuli. So I thought it would be of paramount importance to have clinical means of identifying those patients who are vulnerable. I already asked this question but I didn't get a satisfactory answer. If we had such a clinical procedure and we could identify those patients who might develop pulmonary hypertension at an early stage it would be a break through for managing these patients. So, again, I ask you, or perhaps the audience, if there is any such prospect, and if not I would like to stimulate us all to work on these methods.

DENOLIN: I think that is very important and I suggest to our chairman to remember this topic for a next course in 30 years or something like that.

HORVATH: Allow me a short comment. Denolin has spoken about a parallelism of the mean pulmonary artery pressure with increase in flow during acute exercise. It is interesting to achieve a better resolution of this effect. I remember the early investigation of Donato who measured ventricular output with radiokrypton finding right ventricle cardiac output increase is earlier than the increase of the left. There was a difference in time of about half or one minute. The new possibility with the gamma camera which can measure the ejection fraction at the right ventricle during exercise and the left ventricle.

DENOLIN: The adaptation to long duration exercise could be related to a change in the resistance of the vessels, but could also be related to a change in the compliance of the left ventricle.

CARRATU: I would like to ask you what importance you give to the physiomechanical features in the mechanism of hypertension, since it seems to me that there is a whole area of deformities of the thorax and alterations of the mobility of the thoracic cage expressed in conditions such as kyphosciolosis, pectus excavatum where we have a proponderance of these alterations in the thoracic and diaphragmatic physiomechanics which condition hypertension. To these should be added also those conditions deriving from secondary lung disease. However, the first step is the alteration of the physiomechanics of the lung and chest. Also I would like to take this opportunity to speak about Enson's trial of the balloon - and here we are in agreement that in young patients we don't have hypertension with occlusion of the pulmonary artery. In elderly patients, and we have seen this a number of times before pneumonectomy, we have often found an increase in pressure, not only for 10 to 15 minutes as is seen when the surgeon ties the pulmonary artery in pneumonectomy, but also after a half to three quarters of an hour after the circulation is re-established because we have a substitutive pnenomenon of the vascular area. In elderly patients we constantly have this pressure increase. In many cases of pneumonectomy (and we have written a monograph on this) after 2 or 3 years if the patient was more than 40 there was always an increase in pressure. We explained this because there was a lack of those reserve vascular areas, that distensibility of the vessels which would have allowed the lowering of resistance before a doubling of the flow. Also I would like to ask you with regard to your experience of a lobe perfused in isolation in order to show that in thromboembolism there are no nervous reflexes. I would also like to ask if you recall the very elegant experiment of Nedon and Aviado who with the same methods showed that there was always pulmonary hypertension with the dog's lobe perfused in isolation devoid of nervous connections. Now, how can we explain these two observations, what you obtained and what Nedon and Aviado obtained?

DENOLIN: The fundamental mechanism is one of these seven, whatever
the clinical cause. For the second question, I made years ago a lot
of occlusions, and in fact the changes in pressure are related to
the quality of the non-occluded part of the lung, and of course in
very old patients the increase is a little higher, but not too much.
It depends only on the quality of the remaining lung. And at this
time all our surgeons were anxious to know the results of the
occlusion.

CUMMING: Thank you very much. I think we will have to terminate
the discussion. May I take the chairman's privilege and ask a very
brief Anglo-Saxon question. Although the pressure drop in the
normal circulation is greatest in the capillaries, the capillary
does not figure in your list of the causes of hypertension.

DENOLIN: Yes, they are here.

CUMMING: Direct alveolar compression. Thank you very much.

THE NATURE OF ZONE 4 IN REGIONAL DISTRIBUTION OF PULMONARY BLOOD FLOW

J. Milic-Emili and N.M. Siafakas

Department of Physiology
McGill University
Montreal, Canada

The first measurements of the regional distribution of pulmonary blood flow in man were made using O_2-labelled carbon dioxide.[1] The results in 16 normal upright subjects are shown in Fig.1. The clearance rates were measured during 10-15 seconds breath-holding following an inspiration of one liter of radioactive carbon dioxide from functional residual capacity. If we take the clearance rate of O_2-labelled carbon dioxide as a measure of blood flow per unit lung volume,[2] Fig.1 shows that blood flow increased more or less steadily from the top to the bottom of the upright lung, with very low values at the apex. This general pattern was confirmed by early results with Xenon-133.[3,4] A discrepancy, however, was found between these results and those obtained by West et al[5] on an isolated dog lung preparation.

In the latter preparation, the regional distribution of pulmonary blood flow closely followed a theoretical lung model developed largely by Permutt et al[6] and West et al.[5] This model divides the lung into three zones according to blood flow patterns as determined by the relative magnitude of the alveolar pressure (P_A), pulmonary arterial pressure (P_a), and pulmonary venous pressure (P_v). In zone 1, which was at the apex, $P_A > P_a$ and there is no driving pressure and hence no flow. In zone 2, immediately below zone 1, $P_a > P_A > P_v$; the driving pressure is $P_a - P_A$ and since this increases down the lung, so does flow; the increase in flow being inversely related to P_a. In zone 3, the most dependent zone, $P_a > P_v > P_A$ and the driving pressure is $P_a - P_v$. Despite unvarying driving pressure within zone 3, both P_a and P_v continue to increase downwards. West et al[5] postulated that this rise in intravascular pressures distends resistance vessels, causing the increase in flow which is observed down zone 3. However, the flow increase down zone 3 is less pronounced than in zone 2.

Because of the magnitudes of P_a and P_v, one would expect that the zonal perfusion distribution described above would be demonstrable in normal upright man, but as mentioned above, the early studies of flow distribution in man have shown an approximately linear increase in flow from apex to base (Fig.1).

One reason for this discrepancy between prediction and experimental results is inherent in the radioactive gas techniques used in the early studies which measured flow per unit lung (gas) volume. It has been reported from our laboratory[7] that alveolar volume decreases progressively from apex to base in erect humans and, therefore, one would expect such subjects to show an increase in flow per unit volume down the lung,even if perfusion per alveolus were uniform. Thus, delineation of the perfusion zones in the lung will be best achieved when alveolar volumes are equal down the lung, as probably was the case in West et al's study on isolated dog Lung,[5] since this would have been exposed to a uniform external surface pressure. In the normal human, however, regional pleural pressure is more subatmospheric at the apex than at the base, and as a result the alveoli are not expanded uniformly.[7]

Anthonisen and Milic-Emili[8] used a modified Xenon-133 method to study the regional distribution to perfusion in seated man taking into account the regional differences in lung expansion. Their method gives regional blood flow "per alveolus." The distribution of perfusion per unit lung volume (Q_I) and per alveolus (Q_{alv}) obtained at functional residual capacity (FRC) in three normal seated volunteers at rest is shown in Fig.2. In agreement with previous observations, perfusion per unit lung volume decreased approximately linearly with ascent in the lung. By contrast, the relationship between Q_I alv (the perfusion per alveolus) and vertical distance clearly demonstrates all three zones predicted by West et al.[5] Flow per alveolus appears to be absent in the uppermost part of the lung, defining zone 1. Below this, flow undergoes a rapid and apparently linear increase with further descent in the lung, as expected in zone 2. Increase in flow per centimeter descent (ΔQ_I alv/cm) decreases abruptly below 15 to 20 cm from lung top, the inflection point indicating the upper limit of zone 3. This point defines the level at which $P_A = P_v$, and the Q_I alv = 0 intercept at lung top represents the point at which $P_A = P_a$.

The Q_I alv = 0 intercept should represent the mean P_a and it is of interest to compare this with reported hemodynamic data. Butler and Paley[9] used cardiac catherization in their study of 13 erect normal subjects and found mean P_a to be 6.9 cm H_2O in relation to the angle of Louis. In the subjects of Fig.2

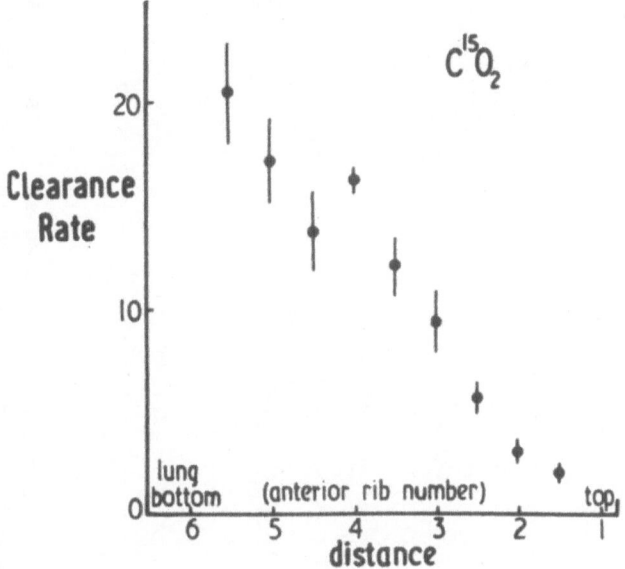

Fig.1.   Clearance rate (percentage per second) of oxygenlabelled
carbon dioxide plotted against counter position (referred
to the anterior ribs in the midclavicular line). Data
from 16 normal volunteers; means and standard errors
(from West[2]).

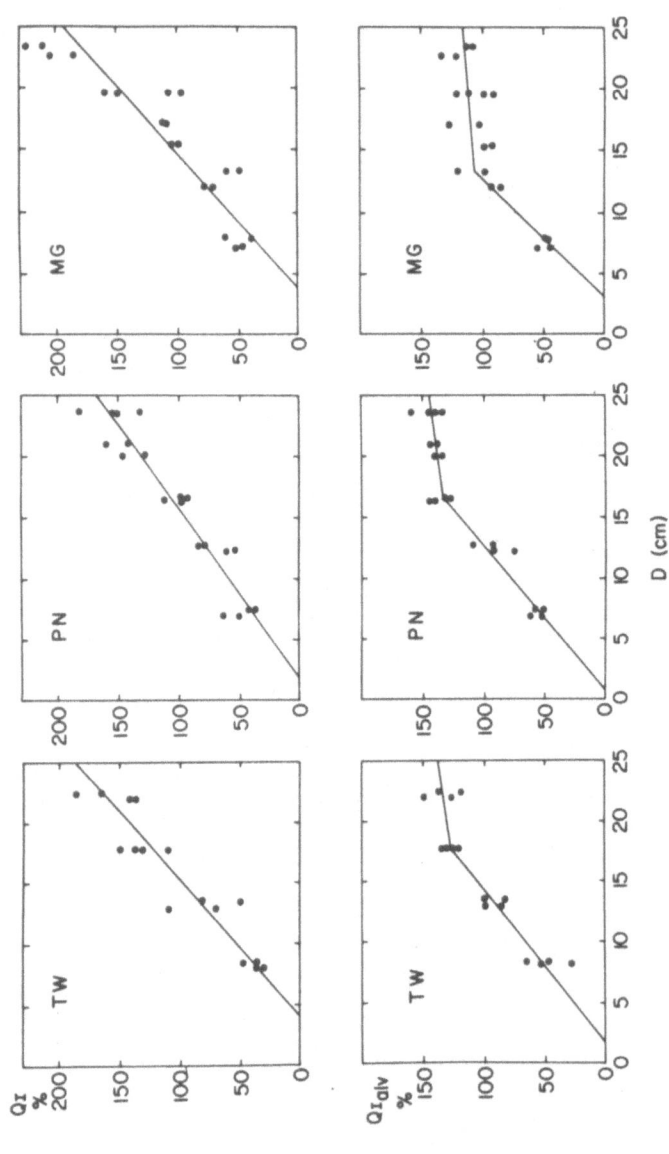

Fig. 2.   Perfusion distribution at FRC in three normal seated subjects at rest.   Above:
perfusion/unit volume (Q_I) as a function of distance (D) down the lung (top = 0 cm).
Below: perfusion per alveolus (Q_I alv) as a function of distance (From Anthonisen
and Milic-Emili[8]).

radiographs showed this reference point to be 10 cm below the top of the lung, so the predicted value for mean P_a would be 7.1 cm H_2O. These data do not necessarily imply that the uppermost 3 cm of the lung in erect humans is entirely unperfused since the intercept Q_I alv = 0 was determined by linear extrapolation. The assumption of a linear relationship between Q_I alv and distance in zone 2 will be valid only if pulmonary capillary flow is nonpulsatile. Pulsatility would cause the relationship to become partly curvilinear, which would result in a higher apical perfusion than would be predicted from a nonpulsatile model with the same mean pressure and flow.

In the subjects of Fig.2, the mean length of zone 2 was about 15 cm, which is somewhat greater than the 11.3 cm H_2O difference between P_a and pulmonary wedge pressure observed by Butler and Paley.[9] However, considering the limitations of both methods, the agreement appears to be reasonably good.

Results of perfusion-distribution studies at residual volume (RV) are presented in Fig.3. Perfusion per unit volume (Q_I) exhibited a zone 2 and 3 behaviour in subjects RW and MG, while a linear decrease in Q_I was observed in subjects RN. Perfusion per alveolus (Q_I alv) at RV was much more even than at FRC, with a trend toward a reduced Q_I alv in the lowermost lung zones. This reduction in basal blood flow at RV was later confirmed by Hughes et al.[10] On the basis of this and other results, a new model of the lungs was introduced by West[2] (Fig.4). A new region (zone 4) was added to the original 3-zone lung diagram, and the basal zone of reduced blood flow was attributed to an increase in vascular resistance of extra-alveolar vessels in this zone.[2,10] This explanation goes as follows. The dependent lung regions, which are subjected to less negative pleural pressure than the upper lung zones, are less expanded and hence interstitial pressure increases. Since the extra-alveolar vessels are pulled open by the tethering action of the tissue surrounding them, a decrease in lung expansion (increased interstitial pressure) will result in narrower vessels. Consequently, at low lung volumes (RV) there is a zone of relatively high vascular resistance in the dependent regions of the lungs (and hence a region of decreased perfusion or zone 4).

While this is an attractive hypothesis, we believe that zone 4 can be explained in an alternate way. In fact, in an attempt to explain the results shown in Fig.3, Anthonisen and Milic-Emili[8] measured in a volunteer the pressure from a catheter wedged 2 cm above the diaphragm during open-glottis RV maneuvers; wedge pressure regularly rose 20-30 mm Hg above control (FRC) values (Fig.5). They were unable to explain the cause of this striking rise in wedge pressure. Similar measurements were later

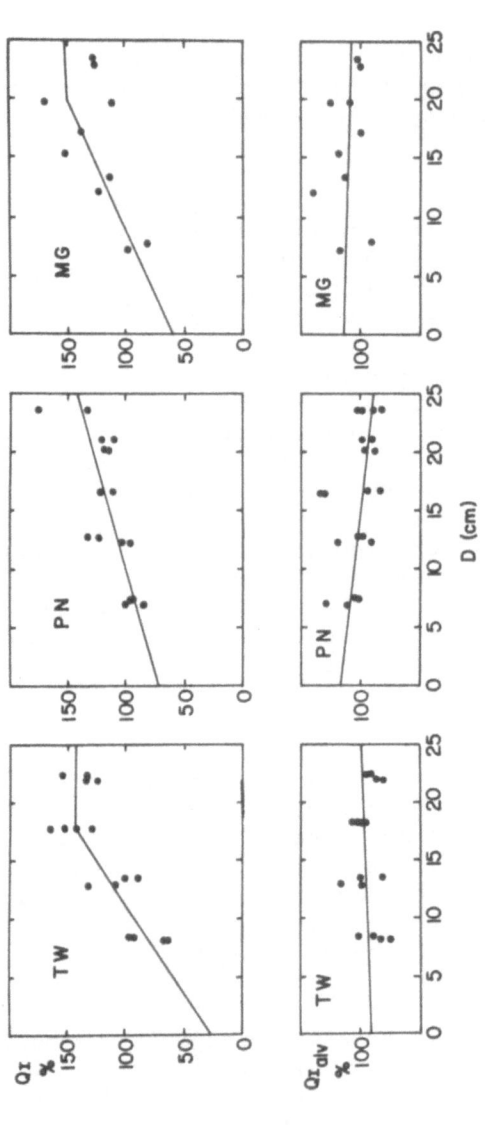

Fig. 3. Perfusion distribution at RV in three subjects. Ordinates and abscissae as in Fig.2. (From Anthonisen and Milic-Emili[8]).

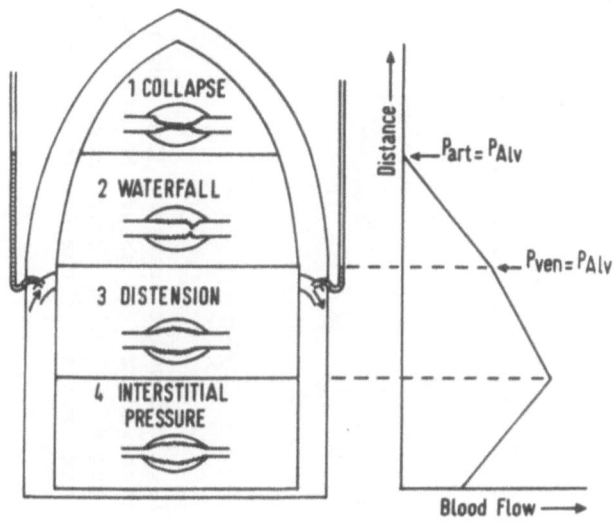

Fig. 4: Modification of the three-zone diagram to include "the effects of increased interstitial pressure in the dependent zone." Because of an increase in the vascular resistance of the extra-alveolar vessels in this zone, blood flow is reduced. (From West[2]).

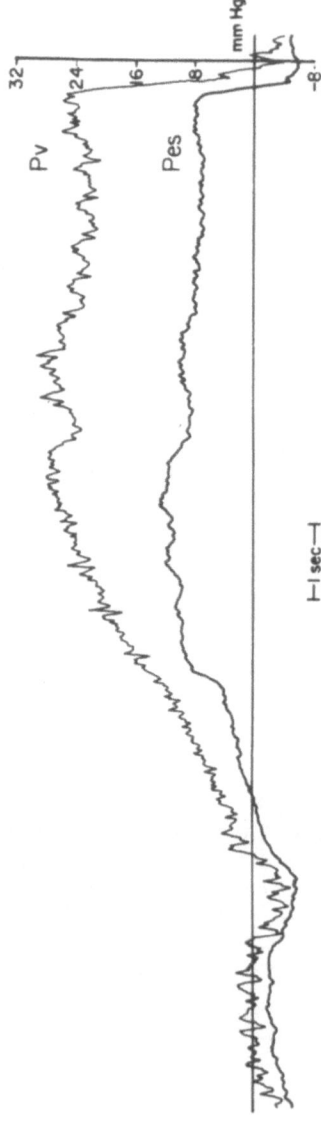

Fig. 5. Tracings of esophageal (P_{es}) and wedge pressure (P_W) during an RV maneuver. P_W
was obtained from a catheter wedged 2 cm above the diaphragm. The reference
level was 5 cm below the angle of Louis. This tracing is representative of six
similar maneuvers in the same subject (From Anthonisen and Milic-Emili[8]).

performed by Arborelius and Lilja.[12] Using a double-lumen catheter,
they confirmed that at RV in erect normal subjects (with glottis
open) the wedge pressure (Pw) measured with a tube wedged close to
the diaphragm increased markedly. More important, in some instances
Pw exceeded systolic Pa by as much as 20 mm Hg. With the catheter
wedged further up from the diaphragm (4th intercostal space) this
was not the case, Pw being invariably lower than systolic Pa. In
addition, Arborelius and Lilja[12] also showed that the changes in
right artrial pressure were similar to those in Pa when exhaling
to RV. They concluded that the high values of Pw observed at RV
in the dependent lung zones (near the diaphragm) were unlikely to
reflect the left artrial pressure for this would imply a reversed
basal pulmonary circulation. They stated that it is more likely
that at RV "the registered Pw was influenced by the intra-alveolar pressure (P_A) where closure occurs at low lung volumes." In
fact in the dependent lung zones, whose airways close as one
exhales towards RV,[7] the intra-alveolar pressure would be expected
to become greater than atmospheric pressure, leading to a decrease
in blood flow. Thus, zone 4 may in fact merely represent a zone 1
($P_A > P_a$) or zone 2 ($P_a > P_A > Pv$) condition located in the lower most
parts of the lungs.

Because of collateral ventilation, one would expect that during a sustained breath-hold at RV the high values of P_A (and hence
P_w) in the dependent lung zones would progressively decrease. This
was indeed found by Arborelius and Lilja[12] whose measurements involved breathholds of up to 20 sec. From the practical standpoint
this means that the duration of breath holding must be taken into
account when regional distribution of blood flow is measured at RV
or in any other conditions where airway closure is present. In
this connection it should be noted that the above phenomenon may
well explain some discrepant results reported by Anthonisen and
Milic-Emili.[8] They measured the regional distribution of gas in
the lungs in two ways, by observing (1) the distribution of inhaled Xenon-133 and (2) the dilution of intravenously injected
Xenon-133 after subsequent inspiration of room air. An example
of data derived by the two techniques is presented in Fig.6 where
regional volume, expressed as percent TLC, is plotted against
overall lung volume, expressed both as percent TLC and percent VC.
Results from three lung regions in one subject are shown, closed ●
indicating data from the inhalation experiment and open circles
those from the perfusion experiment. At overall lung volumes > 20%
VC (ca. 40% TLC) the agreement between the results obtained by the
two methods was good. At RV, regional volumes measured by the two
techniques did not agree completely, the values obtained with Xenon
injection being lower in the dependent lung zones than those
achieved after inhalation of the radioactive gas. At lung top,
the opposite was true. This discrepancy may reflect the fact that
in the inhalation studies no breathhold at RV was involved, whereas a variable breathhold time at RV was inherent in the Xenon

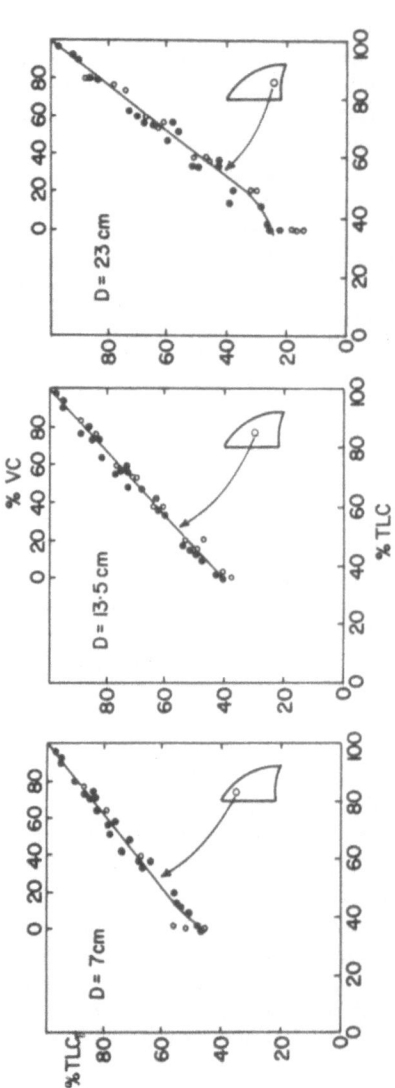

Fig. 6:   Distribution of inspired air. Data obtained 7, 13 and 23 cm below lung top, on
one seated subject. Closed circles indicate results from inhalation of Xe133;
open circles indicate results from dilution of injected Xe133. Ordinate:
regional lung volume, expressed as percent of regional total lung capacity
($\%$ TLC_r). Abscissa: overall lung volume, expressed as percent of overall TLC
or VC (From Anthonisen and Milic-Emili[8]).

injection studies. During breathhold at RV some of the trapped
gas in the dependent lung zones must escape via collateral ventilation, and regional lung volume accordingly decreases in the lower
lung zones.[12]

As pulmonary congestion and edema are known to promote airway
closure[2] and are characterized by the appearance of a distinct
zone 4, [2] the same notions described above should apply in these
pathological conditions. Clearly, future work is required to
provide further information on this point.

REFERENCES

1. J.B. West and C.T. Dollery, Distribution of blood flow and
    ventilation-perfusion ratio in the lung, measured with
    radioactive CO_2, J. Appl. Physiol. 15: 405 (1960).
2. J.B. West(Ed), Regional differences in the lung. Academic
    Press, New York, San Francisco, London, 1977.
3. W.C. Ball,Jr., P.B. Stewart, L.G.S. Newsham, and D.V. Bates,
    Regional pulmonary function studied with Xenon 133,
    J. Clin. Invest. 41: 519 (1962).
4. A.C. Bryan, L.G. Bentivoglio, F. Beerel, H. MacLeish,
    A. Zidulka, and D.V. Bates, Factors affecting regional
    distribution of ventilation and perfusion in the lung,
    J. Appl. Physiol. 19: 395 (1964).
5. J.B. West, C.T. Dollery, and A. Naimark, Distribution of blood
    flow in isolated lung; relation to vascular and alveolar
    pressure, J. Appl. Physiol. 19: 713 (1964).
6. S. Permutt, B. Bromberger-Barnea and H.N. Bane, Alveolar
    pressure, pulmonary venous pressure, and the vascular
    waterfall, Med. Thorac. 19: 239 (1962).
7. J. Milic-Emili, J.A.M. Henderson, M.B. Dolovich, D. Trop, and
    K. Kaneko, Regional distribution of inspired gas in the
    lung, J. Appl. Physiol. 21: 749 (1966).
8. N. R. Anthonisen, and J. Milic-Emili, Distribution of pulmon-
    ary perfusion in erect man, J. Appl. Physiol. 21: 760 (1966).
9. J. Butler, and H.W. Paley, Lung volume and pulmonary circula-
    tion. The effect of sustained changes in lung volume on
    pressure-flow relationships in the human pulmonary circu-
    lation, Med. Thorac. 19: 261 (1962).
10. J.M.B. Hughes, J.B. Glazier, J.E. Maloney, and J.B. West,
    Effect of lung volume on the distribution of pulmonary
    blood flow in man, Resp. Physiol. 4: 58 (1968).
11. M. Arborelius, Jr., and B. Lilja, Haemodynamic changes at
    different lung volumes. Scand. J. Clin. Lab. Invest. 29:
    359 (1972).
12. J. Milic-Emili, and F. Ruf, Effect of expiratory flow rate on
    closing capacity. In: Distribution of Pulmonary Gas Exchange,
    INSERM, 22-24, Sept. 1975, Vol. 51, pp.395-396.

Discussion

CUMMING: Thank you very much Joseph for your stimulating presentation. Just to test that I have got the message, may I put it back to you and check whether I got it correctly. I was particularly interested in whether the CO_2 tension could be explained by mechanical ventilation factors, as you demonstrated quite clearly this would not be applicable. So I must look in some other area for the mechanics of CO_2 retention.

MILIC EMILI: I believe you have understood what Cumming has said and I will take up his question and present you with a classical graph. A lot of you are already familiar with this. Here you have the PCO_2 - this is Howell's graph - arterial blood PCO_2 in mm of mercury. Patients with obstructive disease - a certain lowering of Dmax. There is no change in PCO_2 and then at a certain stage there are subjects that develop hypercapnia while others do not develop it. I talked of these subjects here - non-hypercapnics and hypercapnics. Dmax is an expression of the respiratory occlusion and the PCO_2 is a result of control of respiration. We should recall that Dmax is an expiratory parameter and the measurement of resistance of flow during respiration, but in patients with chronic lung disease or in most patients at rest, the active part of respiration is inspiration. And there is litle relationship between Dmax and inspiratory resistance. Therefore, we cannot take this parameter as an index of the mechanical load of respiration. Perhaps we should put inspiratory resistance or more simply, the inspiratory impedance PO.1 divided by V_T/T_I.

DENISON: Milic, I think in your third slide you showed an impressive series of curves or pressures developed by patients, with PCO_2's that vary from about 40 to 68. And there were really marked differences in the maximum pressures that were developed. But what impressed me equally was that I don't think that I could find a significant difference in their P 0.1 although there are very different breathing patterns. Would you like to comment on that.

MILIC EMILI: Can we have slide number 5? You are saying that there are big differences and here, you see, in this type of representation you are playing the paper very slowly. So when you retrace the spirogram, first of all it is relatively hard to find the beginning of respiration, and therefore it is very easy to have problems with superimposition of the records. If you are interested in the initial portion of the breath you have to play the paper at least 50 mm per second or 100 mm per second. When you record at such speed, you can't put the variables on the same diagram, because it would be a diagram that would be so small, and so long. Of course there is variability, there is a big separation in terms of P

0.1

DENOLIN: I couldn't understand clearly what pulmonary hypertension is doing in this affair.

MILIC EMILI: What I was trying to say is that in pulmonary hypertension you have some well-known changes in blood gases. In general you have a tendency to hyperventilation, and the problem is why do such patients hyperventilate, in the face of an increase in the work of breathing, and in the face of a reduced efficiency of gas exchange in the lungs. Clearly, to do so, they must be making stronger expiratory efforts. Now the question is where do the stimuli come from. You can increase the pulmonary ventilation not only by increasing these efforts, but also by reducing the duration of the expiration. I didn't have time to develop this, but the question is to find out why, in acute pulmonary oedema which is a sequal of pulmonary hypertension, and that there are some patients with a very low oxygen tension, there are the patients who don't develop oedema - we don't know why.

DENOLIN: You have no data on pulmonary pressure, and I think that your discussion is on ventilation in hypercapnia or changes in blood gases. I should not say in pulmonary hypertension, because the relationship between blood gases and pulmonary pressure is, maybe, quite different.

MILIC EMILI: I fully agree.

LOCKART: I wonder whether some of your findings can be explained by a different strength of the respiratory muscles in your patients, that may be due either to a training effect, increase in strength, or to poor nutritional conditions in the patient, which is a loss of muscle. And whether changes in the muscle per se cannot explain the range of P 0.1 that you observed. And also, how does your data here correlate with independent measurement of the strength of these muscles, for instance, maximum inspiratory pressure?

MILIC EMILI: Your point is well taken. What the P 0.1 is measuring is the neuromuscular component of respiratory output or respiratory drive. Can you give me the slide before the last one? You see, that's in French, I prepared it for you! The P 0.1, which is measured here, can be altered, either by changes in the neural drive through the respiratory centres, it can be altered because of problems in the nerve supplying the inspiratory muscles; it can be altered because there are defects in the resultant neuromuscular transmission; because the properties of the muscles have changed, because of nutritional problems as you have said, etc. All we can measure using the P 0.1 is whether the neuromuscular component of ventilation, ventilatory output, has changed or not. Whereas total ventilation is the overall component. We wanted a test which could distinguish between patients who can't breathe, because there are changes in the ventilatory pump and those who won't breathe because the neuromuscular drive is reduced. With the P 0.1 you can distinguish these without any problem. Now you would like to be able to say that's a patient who can't and that's a patient who won't breathe. Either because the neural drive through the respiratory centres is reduced, or because the effectiveness of contraction of the inspiratory muscles has been changed, either because the muscle fibres have changed or the lung volume and so forth. We do not presently have any test which will allow us to distinguish one from the other. Macklem in 1960 introduced the oesophageal electrodes to measure the electrical activity of the diaphragm. This is a technique that one cannot standardise, because the electrical activity that you pick up depends on the anatomy of the patient, the electrode position and so forth. So far, P 0.1 of ventilation is what we can measure. Beyond that we don't have any technique which would allow us, clinically, to know what is going on.

SCHIAVINO: I don't think that there is hypercapnic pulmonary oedema just on the basis of oedema. I think that this depends on the disease or condition existing before the onset of oedema. If these patients have an oedema and suffer from heart disease probably they won't be hypercapnic, because both hyperventilate with rapid shallow breathing, in the case of pulmonary oedema I must consider that the patient is hypocapnic.

MILIC EMILI: I have carried out some work on the problem of hypercapnia and hypocapnia on ventilated patients before and after mitral valve repair. There are changes but unfortunately there are no data wich are helpful. The problem of the clinically controlled ventilation which we find in the literature generally, mechanical respiratory data are not given. One study for example, has been conducted on patients with acute pulmonary oedema, with and without hypercapnia. They were studied after return to the chronic phase and the problem was to see whether ventilatory response to CO_2 in the patients who had developed hypercapnia during the acute episode, whether this was lower than in those subjects whose CO_2 had not increased during the pulmonary oedema episode and they did not find any correlation.

MAN AT HIGH ALTITUDE

David R. Williams

Department of Pathology, University of Liverpool
Duncan Building, Royal Liverpool Hospital
Liverpool L7 8XW

This is an account of the aspects of high altitude medicine and pathology illustrated in the film 'Man at High Altitude', made during two expeditions to the Andes of Central Peru in 1973 and 1975 by Professor Donald Heath and Mr. David Reid Williams.

High altitude studies are important because they explain the nature and components of acclimatization which enable large communities to exist in mountainous areas throughout the world (Heath and Williams, 1977). They have drawn attention to comparatively new disease entities, specific to great elevations, such as acute mountain sickness, high altitude pulmonary oedema, brisket disease and Monge's disease. The significance of such investigations is that they reveal the effects of chronic deprivation of oxygen on the tissues of the body without the added complications of associated disease. As a result there are many clinical and pathological applications of these studies. For example, an understanding of the behaviour of the carotid bodies in cardiopulmonary disease and an appreciation of the nature and clinical significance of splinter haemorrhages.

In this film 'high altitude' is defined as one exceeding 3000 m because at this elevation most people develop unequivocal signs and symptoms associated with the ascent. The most important physical feature of the mountain environment is the progressive fall in barometric pressure that occurs with increasing altitude so that the partial pressure of oxygen in the ambient air falls progressively. Other physical stimuli that have to be faced at high altitude are cold, low humidity, increased solar and ultraviolet radiation, and ionizing radiation.

The highlanders of the Andes and the Tibetan plateau are of Mongoloid stock and their physique is a composite of ethnic background and possibly partial adaptation to high altitude in the form of a full chest. Physical features include erythraemia, cyanosis, beaked fingers, splinter haemorrhages, and a short, light body build. The chest is full but it is not yet established that this is associated with an increased internal surface area of the lung. Vital capacity is increased and this may be due to the influence of a hypoxic environment during childhood. The size of the developing lung in animals in the newborn period is similarly influenced by the partial pressure of oxygen in the ambient air.

Acclimatization is largely achieved by diminishing the pressure gradient of oxygen from ambient air to its site of utilization at the mitochondria. The main factor in reducing this 'oxygen cascade' is hyperventilation, which raises the partial pressure of oxygen in the alveolar spaces. This initial hyperventilation is due to stimulation of peripheral chemoreceptors. Respiratory alkalosis develops. A slow compensatory process to correct this is renal extraction of excess bicarbonate. Sustained hyperventilation is maintained by the stimuli of both hypoxia and heightened sensitivity of the respiratory centres to carbon dioxide. The A - a gradient is diminished in highlanders facilitating diffusion of oxygen across the alveolar-capillary membrane. A factor involved in this may be the fuller chest of the highlander increasing the area of blood-gas interface. Mild pulmonary hypertension may aid a more widespread even perfusion of blood throughout the capillary bed of the lungs.

The transport of oxygen to the tissues is a function of the cardiac output, the quantity of oxygen in the systemic arterial blood, and the affinity of haemoglobin for oxygen, allowing the gas to pass to the tissues. Thus the haemoglobin concentration is of considerable importance. At high altitude there is an increase in the number of erythrocytes, and in the haematocrit. In man the haemoglobin level rises to 20 g/dl and beyond. The number and differential count of the white cells and the number of blood platelets remains normal, thus distinguishing high-altitude polycythaemia from polycythaemia rubra vera. The oxygen-haemoglobin dissociation curve in Quechuas is shifted to the right, maintaining a relatively high PO_2 in the capillaries to aid diffusion of oxygen to the tissues. There is an increase of 2,3-diphosphoglycerate which enters the core of the haemoglobin molecule, stabilizing the deoxy form, and thus releasing oxygen to the tissues. Increased haemoglobin concentration increases blood viscosity which may eventually prove to be deleterious. Animals indigenous to mountains, who are adapted rather than acclimatized to acute hypoxia, do not show the increased levels of haemo-globin for the reasons summarized below. Neither do they show the shift of the oxygen-haemoglobin dissociation curve to the right; it is in fact displaced to the left in adaptation.

The final area in which respiratory acclimatization to high altitude takes place is tissue diffusion. One component is increased capillary density to reduce the distance over which oxygen has to diffuse from blood capillaries to the cells. Another is an increase in the concentration of myoglobin which facilitates diffusion of the gas through the tissues and, less likely, may act as a reserve store of oxygen. There is conflicting evidence as to alterations in mitochondria. Some workers have reported an increase in number of the mitochondria at high altitude but others report no difference in their number or in the surface area of the inner or outer mitochondrial membrane.

The carotid bodies of man and other species of animals, except for animals indigenous to mountain areas, are enlarged at high altitude (Heath and Williams, 1977). The chronic enlargement of the carotid bodies in native highlanders is due to hyperplasia of the chief (Type 1) cells. In cattle this hyperplasia proceeds to histological changes reminiscent of the chemodectoma in a minority of cases. Acute enlargement of the carotid bodies can be induced in laboratory animals in hypobaric chambers, but here the enlargement is due largely to vascular engorgement. Such acute increase in size is readily reversible on removal of the hypoxic stimulus. Similar enlargement of the carotid bodies is found in clinical states associated with chronic hypoxia, such as chronic bronchitis and emphysema. Chemodectomas are commoner in populations living at high altitude. Ultrastructurally there is microvacuolation around the neurosecretory vesicles of the chief cells of the enlarged carotid bodies, but the functional significance of this change is obscure at present. Chief cells of the carotid bodies are APUD cells and they may secrete a poly-peptide hormone, 'glomin'. Increase in size of the chemoreceptors is associated with a blunted ventilatory response to hypoxia. Two factors seem to be of importance in the desensitization to hypoxia, the age of the subject at the time of exposure to the hypoxia and the duration of the exposure. Children who spend only two or three years at high altitude fail to achieve normal sensitivity to hypoxia even after prolonged residence at sea level.

The healthy highlander living at high altitude has a mild degree of pulmonary hypertension which has an organic basis in muscularization of the terminal portions of the pulmonary arterial tree. In infants and children the elevation of pulmonary arterial pressure and the degree of muscularization are greater. The pulmonary hypertension is characteristically reversible. There is only partial immediate reversibility on the inhalation of oxygen which relaxes pulmonary vasoconstriction induced by hypoxia. Long-term reversibility after two years' residence at sea level is complete and is due to loss of muscularization of the pulmonary arterioles. The elevated pulmonary arterial pressure of the highlander represents a persistence of physiological pulmonary hypertension in the fetus. There is considerable variation in individual hyper-reactivity to the hypoxia of high altitude. There is also a genetic factor influencing the development of pulmonary hypertension in cattle at high altitude. The pulmonary hypertension induces right ventricular hypertrophy in highlanders. Similar 'hypoxic hypertensive pulmonary vascular disease' develops in a number of clinical conditions associated with chronic hypoxia, such as chronic bronchitis and emphysema.

The pulmonary trunk of the highlander shows medial hypertrophy in response to the mild pulmonary hypertension. The normal transition of the elastic tissue pattern of the media of the pulmonary trunk from the fetal to the adult pulmonary configuration is delayed and an abnormal pattern of elastica appears. This is the 'persistent' form in which there is a combination of long thick fibres with others which are fragmented. As a result, the pulmonary trunk of the highlander has a histological appearance, chemical composition and extensibility like that of the aorta of sea-level man.

Brisket disease is a vascular form of loss of acclimatization to high altitude which occurs in calves in Utah and Colorado. Its basis is pronounced pulmonary vasoconstriction in susceptible animals, leading to increased pulmonary vascular resistance, right ventricular hypertrophy, and congestive cardiac failure. The latter brings about oedema of the jaws and the region between the forelegs and neck (the 'brisket' of commerce) and hence gives the disease its name. Brisket disease is not a bovine form of Monge's disease which is a respiratory rather than a vascular form of loss of acclimatization. All cattle have a naturally muscular pulmonary vasculature and are thus prone to the condition, although this develops only in a minority which are no doubt genetically susceptible.

Acute mountain sickness has to be distinguished from the features of accommodation such as hyperventilation and tachycardia, which normally develop on acute exposure to high altitude. 'Soroche' is characterized by a wide range of symptoms including nausea and vomiting, anorexia, giddiness, headache and insomnia. It is usually of short duration. The syndrome is thought to have a basis in oliguria and redistribution of blood, leading to oedema of the lungs and brain. Retinal haemorrhages are common and may lead to residual scotomas. Disturbances of sleep are common and periodic breathing may occur at night. Treatment of acute mountain sickness is controversial. Oxygen is not very effective. Diuretics are advocated but this treatment has been criticized as exaggerating the dehydration induced by the low humidity of the mountain environment. Potassium supplements are sometimes advised. Acute mountain sickness can often be prevented by slow ascent and avoidance of over exertion on arrival at high altitude. Psychological aspects are important and reassurance has its place in treatment.

Lowlanders who ascend rapidly to high altitude and then engage in strenuous physical activity and highlanders who return to the mountains after a period of time at sea level may develop acute pulmonary oedema, which may prove fatal. There is associated pulmonary arterial hypertension without pulmonary venous or left atrial hypertension. There appears to be increased vascular resistance in the pulmonary venous capillaries or in the pulmonary venules. Electron microscopy of the lungs of rats exposed to simulated high altitude reveals intracapillary oedema vesicles which could account for capillary obstruction. Increased plasma volume may be a factor in the development of the condition in highlanders returning to the mountains from sea level. Treatment consists of the immediate administration of oxygen and removal to sea level.

After an increased cardiac output on acute exposure to high altitude due to tachycardia, the stroke volume falls so that the cardiac output returns to normal. In the highlander the resting cardiac output is also normal. There is a redistribution of blood flow away from areas of low oxygen extraction such as the skin to increase the oxygen reservoir for the rest of the body. The systemic blood pressure falls on prolonged residence at high altitude in both long-term sojourners and in the native highlanders. Systemic hypertension is said to be improved after prolonged residence at high altitude.

The coronary flow is diminished in native highlanders but coronary arterial disease and myocardial infarction are rare at high altitude. This may be related to the sociological factors in life in under developed mountainous areas.

However, there is increased vascularization of the myocardium. The number of secondary branches of coronary arteries is increased and the vascularization extends down to capillary level. Coronary blood flow is higher in patients with Monge's disease than in healthy highlanders.

Electrocardiographic studies in both European and Sherpa climbers acutely exposed to high altitude show right axis deviation and T-wave inversion in the right precordial leads due to acute right ventricular overload. Lowering of the T wave in the left precordial leads with associated depression of the ST segment is found in European but not Sherpa climbers and is indicative of left ventricular ischaemia consequent upon the hypoxia. In native highlanders during infancy and childhood there is electrocardiographic evidence of right ventricular preponderance. Transitional patterns to left ventricular preponderance are much delayed. In adolescent and adult highlanders electrical evidence of right ventricular preponderance persists, and although it is less evident than in older children the electrocardiographic evidence of left ventricular preponderance characteristic of life at sea level does not develop.

A respiratory form of loss of acclimatization in man occurs in the Andes and is called chronic mountain sickness or 'Monge's disease'. Its clinical picture is composed of haematological, cardiovascular, respiratory and neuropsychic elements. In essence the condition is a hypoventilation syndrome occurring at high altitude. It is characterized by increase in the haemoglobin level, in the degree of arterial oxygen unsaturation, and in an exaggeration of the pulmonary hypertension found in healthy highlanders. Three clinico-pathological variants are seen. The first is 'chronic soroche', in lowlanders who never acclimatize to high altitude. In 'secondary chronic mountain sickness' there is already present in a high altitude dweller a disease capable of producing hypoxic hypertensive pulmonary vascular disease. 'True Monge's disease' is the primary hypoventilation syndrome at high altitude. There is little or no reliable documentation of morbid anatomy of this syndrome. The features described are an exaggeration of those found in healthy highlanders, such as more intense muscularization of the pulmonary arterial tree.

References

Heath, D. and Williams, D.R., "Man at High Altitude",
Churchill Livingstone.   London and Edinburgh (1977).

ULTRASTRUCTURE IN PULMONARY HYPERTENSION

Donald Heath

Department of Pathology, University of Liverpool
Duncan Building, Royal Liverpool Hospital
Liverpool L7 8XW

A very characteristic feature of the human pulmonary vasculature is that it shows progressive intimal proliferation with age. This age-change was studied intensively by Brenner (1935). On histological examination he found it to be ubiquitous and extensive, involving both pulmonary arteries and veins. When one employs standard connective tissue stains such as Van Gieson's reagents, the intimal proliferation appears relatively acellular and gives a tinctorial reaction for collagen suggesting that the process is one of progressive intimal fibrosis. It is of interest to look at the ultrastructure of this age-change intimal proliferation for it represents an integral part of the structure of the normal pulmonary blood vessel which is available to respond to a raised pulmonary arterial pressure.

The cell responsible for the intimal proliferation has features of both the smooth muscle cell and the fibroblast (Smith and Heath, 1980). Thus it has running through its cytoplasm myofibrils, although these form small bundles and do not permeate most of the structure of the cell as in the mature, classical smooth muscle cell. The muscular nature of these cells is also revealed by attachment points on the plasmalemma for these myofilaments, and by focal condensations within the filaments. At the same time the copious dilated endoplasmic reticulum throughout most of the cytoplasm indicates that it is also a fibroblast. The cell is in fact a myofibroblast, the type of connective tissue cell found as an integral part of granulation tissue. It seems very likely that these cells in the walls of pulmonary arteries take their origin in the media and migrate into the intima. One recalls the arguments and controversies of pathologists of a few years back as to whether the cells in the intimal linings of pulmonary blood vessels are muscular or fibrous in

233

nature; in fact they are both at the same time.

What happens to the myofibroblast in the intima depends on the functional conditions obtaining there. Thus in the pulmonary veins the myofibroblasts progressively lose their myofibrils and assume more and more the ultrastructural features of the fibroblast with dilated endoplasmic reticulum. Within the pulmonary veins the intimal age-change becomes progressively less cellular and it largely comprises collagen and elastic fibrils (Smith and Heath, 1980).

In contrast the myofibroblast in the intima of the pulmonary artery is subjected to the stimulus of pulsation. This maintains the population of cells. Hence the interesting point emerges that age-change intimal proliferation is different in pulmonary arteries and pulmonary veins. In veins it is acellular but in arteries it is cellular (Smith and Heath, 1980). Furthermore, in pulmonary arteries the stimulus of pulsation appears to stimulate the development of more myofibrils so that the cells come to resemble fully-fledged muscle cells. Indeed should pulmonary hypertension supervene for any reason the stimulatory effect on the myofibrils increases so that fasciculi of longitudinally-orientated smooth muscle cells develop in the intima. This phenomenon occurs with the raised pulmonary arterial pressure associated with congenital cardiac shunts and with chronic bronchitis and emphysema.

The normal pulmonary artery has a thin media of circularly-orientated smooth muscle fibres while the normal pulmonary arteriole has a wall consisting of only a single elastic lamina. This sparsity of vascular smooth muscle is associated with the normal low level of blood pressure and vascular resistance.

With the development of pulmonary arterial hypertension we can recognise in very general terms four main types of structural change in the pulmonary vasculature, although these will differ in detail in different forms of hypertensive pulmonary vascular disease. The four main components seen on histological examination are:

1. Muscularization and constriction of pulmonary arterioles.

2. Constriction and hypertrophy of media of pulmonary arteries with various forms of intimal proliferation.

3. The development of various types of complex dilatations such as the "plexiform lesion" and

4. Necrotizing arteritis based on fibrinoid necrosis.

When one looks at the ultrastructure of these components of hypertensive pulmonary vascular disease, some rather surprising features emerge which give us a somewhat fresh insight into the nature of the changes in the pulmonary vasculature in pulmonary hypertension.

First, with regard to muscularization of the pulmonary arterioles, electron microscopy reveals that isolated smooth muscle cells are present in the wall of the normal pulmonary arteriole. During the long-term process of muscularization these smooth muscle cells proliferate to form a distinct media which forms internal to the original single elastic lamina. A new elastic lamina then forms internal to the new muscle coat. On electron microscopy the new layer of smooth muscle cells between the original and new elastic laminae can be seen readily (Smith and Heath, 1977). In effect the pulmonary arteriole has now been converted into something akin to a systemic arteriole which can by muscular constriction elevate pulmonary arterial pressure and resistance.

The electron microscopy of collapsed or constricted vascular smooth muscle presents some surprising features which we have considered in detail elsewhere (Smith, Heath and Mooi, 1979). I had always considered in my mind that, when a smooth muscle cell constricts, it merely becomes shorter and thicker. Scanning electron micrographs of constricted smooth muscle fibres show multiple prominences over their surface. These prominences appear to be muscular evaginations which protrude between attachment points for actin and myosin filaments (Smith, Heath and Padula, 1978). The cytoplasm of the evaginations is devoid of myofibrils and organelles and thus appears clear and unlike the cytoplasm of the parent muscle cell. So clear are these evaginations that, unless one is aware of their origin, one may misinterpret them as cysts and not related to muscle. We have studied them in the smooth muscle of pulmonary arteries of rats fed on Crotalaria spectabilis seeds or exposed to simulated high altitude to cause them to develop pulmonary hypertension (Smith and Heath, 1978). Such muscular evaginations protrude into the adventitia in the case of pulmonary arteries and into the intima in the case of pulmonary veins. In the latter situation muscular evaginations are readily induced by hypoxia and unless one is familiar with their nature and origin in electron micrographs they may be misinterpreted as endothelial cysts. Similar clear muscular evaginations may be seen insinuating through the internal elastic lamina in the pulmonary trunk of rats exposed to chronic hypoxia (Smith, Heath and Padula, 1978).

Whereas medial hypertrophy and constriction and muscularization of pulmonary arterioles represent the earliest changes in the pulmonary vasculature in pulmonary hypertension, necrotizing arteritis equals the terminal stage in which pulmonary hypertension is severe and shows an unusually

rapid rise. Histological sections of pulmonary arteries so affected show a
brightly eosinophilic media showing a smudgy staining, the changes stimulating
an acute inflammatory reaction. Electron microscopy reveals that the eosino-
philia is due to infiltration of the media by fibrin which forces its way through
gaps in the internal elastic lamina to enter the media only to be held up once
again at the outer elastic lamina, a state of affairs which has been referred
to in the past as "fibrinous vasculosis" (Heath and Smith, 1978). The infiltration of the media by fibrin is accompanied by death of vascular smooth
muscle cells and the laying down of ground tissue in a manner producing an
appearance of concentric basement membranes (Heath and Smith, 1978). Of
great interest is the fact that such necrotizing arteritis stimulates the appearance of cells with a striking fibrillary cytoplasm. We shall return to their
nature in a moment.

We may now go on to consider the electron microscopy of the plexiform
lesion for this appears to be closely related to the ultrastructure of fibrinoid
necrosis. Plexiform lesions are a characteristic of the variety of hypertensive
pulmonary vascular disease which complicates congenital cardiac shunts such
as ventricular septal defect, primary pulmonary hypertension, and those rare
cases of cirrhosis of the liver or portal vein thrombosis complicated by severe
pulmonary hypertension. The plexiform lesion has two components. The first
is a dilated terminal or side branch of a muscular pulmonary artery which is
one form of dilatation lesion which allows a collateral flow of blood to the
pulmonary capillary network by-passing the occluded terminal portions of the
muscular pulmonary arteries. The second component of the plexiform lesion
is the peculiar proliferation of cells within this dilated sac.

Electron microscopy of the cells which proliferate in the dilated sacs to
form 'plexiform lesions' show that they are of two forms. One might assume
that the cellular proliferation would be due to endothelial cells but in fact
a surprise comes when the cells show themselves to be muscular rather than
endothelial in origin. The cells show myofilaments, focal condensations,
and attachment points and are myofibroblasts (Smith and Heath, 1979). These
cells abound in granulation tissue and give its contractile properties and we
have already seen that they are responsible for age-change intimal proliferation in the human pulmonary vasculature. It is of singular interest to realise
that much of the intimal proliferation in pulmonary hypertension is thus muscular in nature and origin.

The second type of cell which proliferates in the dilated branches of
pulmonary arteries to give rise to the "plexiform lesion" is the fibrillary cell
(Smith and Heath, 1979) identical to that which we found occurring in association with necrotising arteritis. These fibrillary cells are of interest for they
are widespread in the intima and media of the vasculature of the body. They

are what American authors term "vasoformative reserve cells". They seem to be the type cell of the cardiac myxoma and of the so-called "papilliferous tumour of the heart valves". This is of interest since modern opinion accepts that the papillary tumour of the heart is not a neoplasm or hamartoma but is in fact a giant Lambl's excrescence so that it is in fact built up periodically by organization of fibrin. Since fibrillary cells covering the so-called papillary tumour are intimately concerned with the organisation of fibrin it seems likely that they are involved in the same process within the plexiform lesion. This is of considerable significance because, if it is true, it implies that the plexiform lesion, so characteristic of some forms of HPVD, is brought about by organisation of fibrin.

When histological sections are stained with special Stains for fibrin such as picro Mallory or phosphotungstic acid haematoxylin, they reveal in fact that the plexiform lesion is rich in fibrin. Some is extracellular and some is intracellular. Electron microscopy also confirms a close association between fibrillary cells and fibrin (Smith and Heath, 1979). Some fibrin is in fact intracellular. Such appearances lead us to believe that plexiform lesions arise as a result of proliferation of fibrillary cells in response to fibrin. We have already seen that the source of fibrin in the plexiform lesions is fibrinoid necrosis induced by intense spasm of pulmonary arteries. Hence plexiform lesions appear to result from intense contraction of pulmonary arteries and this is the reason why they occur in such different conditions as cirrhosis of the liver and Eisenmenger's complex ; they are the hallmark of intense vasoconstriction in the lung.

References

Brenner, O. (1935)
Pathology of the vessels of the pulmonary circulation.
Arch. Intern. Med., 56, 211.

Heath, D., and Smith, P. (1978)
The electron microscopy of "fibrinoid necrosis" in pulmonary arteries.
Thorax, 33, 579.

Smith, P., and Heath, D. (1977)
Ultrastructure of hypoxic hypertensive pulmonary vascular disease.
J. Path., 121, 93.

Smith, P., and Heath, D. (1978)
Evaginations of vascular smooth muscle cells during the early stages of
Crotalaria pulmonary hypertension.
J. Path., 124, 177.

Smith, P., and Heath, D. (1979)
Electron microscopy of the plexiform lesion.
Thorax, 34, 177.

Smith, P., and Heath, D. (1980)
The ultrastructure of age-associated intimal fibrosis in pulmonary blood
vessels.
J. Path. In Press.

Smith, P., Heath, D., and Mooi, W. (1979)
Observations on some ultrastructural features of normal pulmonary blood
vessels in collapsed and distended lungs.
J. Anat. 128, 85.

Smith, P., Heath, D., and Padula, F. (1978)
Evagination of smooth muscle cells in the hypoxic pulmonary trunk.
Thorax, 33, 31.

Discussion

CUMMING: Thank you very much Donald. Since you have laid down the groundwork for the first question, perhaps we can ask Denolin what is the simple (to use his word) explanation for the pulmonary vasoconstriction seen in disease.

DENOLIN: Thank you very much. The general problem is not only in the pulmonary circulation but also in the muscle. It is the so-called myogenic theory, but I don't know what it is exactly.

HEATH: I think this is a terribly important question and it would be very instructive to me to know if anybody has any idea why occlusion of the portal vein without any evidence of cirrhosis leads in some instances to intense pulmonary vasoconstriction and plexiform lesions in the lung. What is the physiological background.

CUMMING: Gwen, are you able to make a contribution?

BARER: Could you tell us if the smooth muscle in the arterioles is so formed as to encroach on the lumen? Because the vascular resistance of chronically hypoxic rats is greatly increased even when you relieve the hypoxia and maximally dilate them. So there must be some structural cause.

HEATH: Yes, I think it does. I think this is important because when you deal with high altitude for example, if you give these Quechuas oxygen to inhale, there is a certain fall in the level of the pulmonary arterial pressure and resistance, but it doesn't come down to normal levels at once, that may take 18 months. The reason it takes 18 months of course, is what the new muscle that is formed has gradually to resolve. And as a morbid anatomist this is why I always feel a bit uncomfortable with physiologists, because whenever you talk about pulmonary vasoconstriction this element of muscle hyperplasia never seems to come into the argument. I may be wrong, but that's how it seems to me.

CUMMING: If I could clarify the situation about semantics, yesterday I pointed out that pulmonary vasoconstriction and hypoxia mean many things to many people. Specifying what you are talking about in the first place is most important, and you today defined that we are talking about human chronic high altitude hypoxia. But the physiologists may be talking about acute normal pressure in animals. That may be quite different.

HEATH: The point I was trying to make is this, that when you talk about chronic hypoxia in animals, that stage of chronicity begins after about a week. It doesn't take very long for the muscle to grow.

MORPURGO: Do you believe that changes in the structures, in the physical properties of the main pulmonary arteries can play a role in the maintenance of pulmonary arterial hypertension?

HEATH: No, I don't think so. The arteries are of course less distensible but I would have thought that the role of structural changes in the major arteries was much less than in the small peripheral ones. I have always regarded the effects on the larger elastic arteries as the results of pulmonary hypertension in the small ones if we could talk about these Quechuas again. They have this muscularisation out in the periphery of their lungs, and I think that's the thing that makes the level of their pulmonary artery pressure go up on infancy and remain up to a lesser extent in adult life. Now, that increased pressure and resistance in their lungs makes the large arteries in the lung continue to look like the aorta, but that's not what causes further trouble haemodynamically.

SCHIAVINO: I wonder if what you have shown and what is seen at the level of the cell during pulmonary arterial hypertension is also manifest in the same way in interstitial lung disease and in particular in interstitial pneumonitis and whether this fibroblastic proliferation might respond to cortisone or immunodepressants which is our therapy in these cases?

HEATH: Well, vascular disease does of course occur in interstitial fibrosis of the lung. I have examined it at the histological level. There is first a stage of muscularisation followed by a stage of what in the past I have called fibrosis. But I strongly suspect that this is a mixture of muscle and fibrous tissue. With regard to whether that would be susceptible to treatment with steroids, I don't know.

CORRIN: Certain morphological features are indicative of specific causes of pulmonary hypertension. For example, the plexogenic lesion is confined to septal defects, primary pulmonary hypertension is not found in hypoxia. Is this something inherent to the nature of these diseases, or does it merely reflect the severity of the pulmonary hypertension in these particular diseases?

HEATH: I think the fact that certain diseases have a specific pulmonary vascular component is an inherent feature of those diseases in the sense that it is an inherent quality of the underlying mechanism for that particular group. For example I think that intense pulmonary vasoconstriction without the association of pulmonary venous hypertension produces plexogenic pulmonary arteriopathy. I think that once you get a significant pulmonary venous hypertension as well, then you get more plexiform lesions.

So I think that the way I see it is that it's a reflection of basic physiological mechanisms. You have a number of cases of pulmonary veno-occlusive disease. I would suspect that you have never seen plexogenic lesions in those cases.

CORRIN: That's true, but in occasional cases of mitral stenosis, where of course there is venous hypertension, I have seen fibrinoid-necrosis.

HEATH: Oh, yes.

CORRIN: I think you said it is the most severe.

HEATH: That's right, but I bet you have never seen a plexiform lesion.

CORRIN: No.

DENISON: Would you tell us what a morbid anatomist's view if of the function of the longitudinal muscle fibres?

HEATH: Well, I don't know what the function is but let us draw some obvious conclusions. In the bronchial artery of a fetus, you don't find longitudinal muscle in the walls of the bronchial arteries. I think that's true. But after birth it develops, suggesting that it is related in some way to longitudinal stretch.

HEATH: If you get it around emphysematous spaces in the lung pulmonary arteries may also develop a lot of longitudinal muscle. So one might say that in some way it's related to the stimulus of extensive longitudinal stretch. But I wouldn't like to go beyond that.

LOCKART: I wonder whether we could have one of your slides back; the one with a small arteriole embedded inbetween alveoli.
There that's it. Now do you believe, looking at that, that there is such a ting as isolated alveolar hypoxia? After seeing this, it suggests to me that alveolar hypoxia will cause, necessarily, a hypoxia in the vessel which has in its wall acquired smooth muscle.

HEATH: Yes.

LOCKART: And I submit that the reason why physiologists have been studying alveolar hypoxia as the major stimulus for vasoconstriction in the lesser circulation is because it is easy to produce it, either in an isolated lung preparation, or in an intact animal. There is no such thing, looking at this slide as isolated alveolar hypoxia. And it seems to me from a picture like this one, what is important is the gradient of pressure from the alveolar space to the vessel. Whether the fall in pressure somewhere along the gradient is caused by a primary change in the vessel or in the alveolus. It seems to me that they must act about the same, and that alveolar hypoxia, isolated, as a stimulus for vasoconstriction does not exist. Would you agree on that?

CUMMING: May I clarify a semantic point before we go on? You are talking about isolated alveolar hypoxia. Do you mean hypoxia isolate to a single alveolus?

LOCKART: I am usually rather careful about semantics. What Ed Dakowsky published years ago is a rather thorough study of what he called alveolar hypoxia, in an isolated lung preparation, which was caused by breathing the lung with a low oxygen mixture when the mixed venous blood, or so-called mixed venous blood, coming back to the lung was after reoxygenation using an oxygenator, this is supposed to be isolated alveolar hypoxia. As opposed to that, Ed Dakowsky coined the word total hypoxia, which is alveolar hypoxia. I mean breathing the lung with an hypoxic gas mixture plus desaturation of the mixed venous blood, that in his experiments could be controlled using an oxygenated circuit. Now, this suggests to me that when you have alveolar hypoxia you have hypoxia in the vessel at the same time and there is no such thing as isolated alveolar hypoxia.

CUMMING: Do you have a morbid anatomical viewpoint on that Donald?

HEATH: Not really. No.
CUMMING: Can I focus your attention on a small problem. If in that vessel there is a PO_2 of 40, and there is a PO_2 in the neighbouring alveolus of 30, is that a stable situation?, given the dimensions and the characteristics of the cells which form the barrier between the gases.

HEATH: This is a physiological view.

CUMMING: Yes. Would anyone like to answer? Professor Denolin.

DENOLIN: We are now mixing probably the facts and the explanations.

CUMMING: And the hypotheses.

DENOLIN: And the hypotheses. When I say explanation it is always a hypothetical explanation. The fact is that when a normal lung is breathing a low oxygen mixture you see its pressure increased in the pulmonary circulation with no change in cardiac output, and this increase can be reduced, let's say, by acetylcholine, as demonstrated 35 years ago by Cournand.

HEATH: Yes, I'd not disagree with that.

DENOLIN: Yes, that's a fact. Now, what is the explanation? I
don't see why we should refuse the word vasoconstriction because it
means that we have a diminution of the cross section of the vascular
bed. And in such an acute situation it can be only by a decrease in
the calibre of the vessel.

HEATH: Certainly. The point I have made is that the situation
which you describe, I believe to be one which lasts for a very short
time.

DENOLIN: Yes.

HEATH: I think that maybe what you are presenting is something
that becomes associated with hyperplasia of muscle very rapidly.

DENOLIN: But this was observed and can be observed that's a fact.
I don't see why you are so anxious with the word vasoconstriction.

CUMMING: I understand Donald's difficulty. As a pathologist he
sees dead tissue, and as an ultramicroscopist he sees dead tissue
devoid of water, and he finds it difficult to see how this can have
a life of its own to which he can contribute. Had he worked with
Gwen Barer in Sheffield and seen the blood change from one place to
another under a variety of stimuli, he'd take your view that the
only possible way that blood can go from one area of the lung to
another is that the impedence of blood in one area is higher than
that in another. I think I take Donald's point correctly. He said
he would accept this, but be aware that a structural explanation
may be very rapid in onset.

HEATH: That's right.

LEE: I would like to ask Donald why he thinks vasoconstriction is
the cause of the fibrinoid in the plexiform lesion, because any
condition that raises the vascular pressure beyond a certain point
will produce a transudation of fibrin through the endothelial
junction. And so, one should perhaps not close one's mind entirely
to changes in the permeability associated with disorders.

HEATH: Oh, I agree.

LEE: And in this connection it might well be that the plexiform
lesion of cirrhosis is due to circulating vasoactive substances.
And in this connection some authors have shown what appeared to me
very like the plexiform lesion you described in mitral stenosis
associated with very high intravascular pressures.

HEATH: I think that it is an important statement to make, that
plexiform lesions can occur in mitral stenosis, that maximum

publicity should be made of this. But of course my view being that of a morbid anatomist, I'd be more able to conceive it if I could see the evidence.

LEE: You put up a working hypothesis which would enable these lesions to occur in any condition that produced fibrinoid excretions into the interstitium, going to the subintimal, subendothelial areas.

HEATH: Yes, because to have the proliferation in a dilated sac to form the plexiform lesion you must first get the dilated sac, and I think that this is prevented if you have pulmonary venous hypertension. That's my belief.

LEE: Could I ask one other question? In one of your earliest slides you showed fibroblasts becoming muscular and that muscular cell appeared to have a lot of pinocytotic vesicles on it. Can you tell me about their role in that cell?

HEATH: I don't know, but of course its smooth muscle, vascular smooth muscle shows this activity very considerably, it's very typical of smooth muscle cells.

DENISON: I want to return to Lockart's question and to the slide that you put up again. There is good evidence that's been obtained in the optic nerve and the retina of cats, in the cheek pouch of the hamster, and in the lung, that you get considerable gas exchange through vessels of that size. In the cheek pouch of the hamster blood entering small vessels arterioles, would appear to have a PO_2 of 100. By the time the blood got to the far end of the arteriole, before it reaches the capillaries, its PO_2 had already fallen to 25 mm of mercury. And there is no doubt that the vessel we were looking at in that slide that there would be very little difference in the PO_2 inside and outside its wall.

BARER (Robert):   Denison has in fact answered the point that I was going to make as a question. I was going to ask whether there is any evidence that you could get gas exchange in a blood vessel larger than a capillary. Because it seems to me that the lack of agreement does arise from this question of size and degree of organisation of the blood vessel. Now, it is usually said in the textbooks, which are of course very frequently wrong, that the tissues in an artery are not supplied by the blood contained within the artery but that the tissues are supplied with oxygen and metabolites either from external blood vessels or by diffusion from tissue fluid. But obviously when you get down to something of capillary size, this is not necessarily true. The next stage from the capillary would be what some people call either small arteriole or muscular capillary. There is complete gradation between the capillary, consisting purely of endothelium, and an arteriole or even a muscular artery, containing one or several layers of muscle. And I don't want to sound obsessional about this, but let me again emphasise what I said yesterday about this basement membrane. It is characteristic of smooth muscle that it too is surrounded by basement membrane. So in fact you have this material stretching from the deep surface of the endothelium surrounding all the smooth muscle cells individually into the surrounding connective tissue if there is any. Now, oxygen and metabolites could presumably pass out from the blood vessel outwards into this sponge or they could pass in from tissue fluid, blood vessels, connective tissue and so on, to the blood vessel. And I think it is a question of size, distances and degree of organisation, as to which of these processes preponderates. May I make just another point about why portal vein obstruction should cause the presence of fibrinoid. May I ask you, is it known what happens to the production of fibrinogen by the liver, when you obstruct the portal vein?

HEATH: I have no answer.

LOCKART: I just want to come back very briefly to what has been said about gas exchanging vessels. Cardiologists have been using for almost 20 years now platinum tip catheters to look for shunts in the pulmonary circulation. Now, these catheters are about 2 mm in diameter. You just wedge one of these in a distal pulmonary artery and ask the subject to take a breath of pure hydrogen and you get the hydrogen immediately in a 2 mm size of diameter artery. This has been first shown by Jameson in New York, I think, 15 or 16 years ago. I have used this fairly often when I was a cardiologist and also I can tell that using an optical oxygen sensing electrode in Cournand's laboratory in the early 60's, they were able to show changes in oxygen saturation in arteries about that size in diameter that were in phase with breathing. I mean saturation going up with inspiration, down with expiration. And this takes place in arteries about 2 mm in diameter. So again I would like to point out that the concept of alveolar hypoxia as a stimulus to vasoconstriction is very convenient for physiologists, but there is no such thing as isolated alveolar hypoxia. You get it in the alveolus, you have it in the blood. And it may help physiologists thinking, to stop being blind-folded about alveolar hypoxia. Of course it is what happens at altitude, but it is also hypoxia in the blood.

CUMMING: Thank you. May I, as one who worked with Cournand in the 60's when these experiments were being done, perhaps make a point. It is certainly true that a tracer gas appears in a 2 mm artery immediately, as soon as the breath goes down 150 ml you get the hydrogen. But evidence that this can occur gives us no quantitative information about the equilibrium which exists between the alveolar gas and the blood. And it is a complex question the rate of flow of the blood through the vessel, the thickness, and its diffusing capacity, the quantity of oxygen and CO_2 that remains in the alveolus and the accessibility, in terms of distance of the gas to the vessel. And whilst I take Alan's point, that the concept of local alveolar hypoxia has to be looked at again, I think that we shall find that quantitatively there can exist a difference between alveolar gas and the blood in a 2 mm artery.

BAKHLE: You showed us pictures of smooth muscle cells bouching out into endothelial cells, and you said this is what happens when the smooth muscle constricted.

HEATH: That's right.

BAKHLE: Now, how would you ensure that a smooth muscle is still constricted by the time you have a look at it under the microscope.

HEATH: One distends the lung, so that when it fixes in a state of distension in the situation that obtains at the moment of death and in that way the problem of collapse is avoided.

BAKHLE: Is the distension in the blood, in the circulation or in the airways.

HEATH: Through the pulmonary arteries.
BAKHLE: Do you ever see those evaginations in normal lungs which have not been the site of pulmonary hypertension?

HEATH: Yes. If you were to allow the lung to collapse, you could see that. But then of course this is routine for all the causes of vascular pathology that if you allow lung tissue to collapse then you can get very spurious appearances. If you just take a collapsed piece of lung, then blood vessels look thick, naturally.

CUMMING: I wonder if I might extend that question a bit, because I too have some similar problems. Supposing you have an animal and there is within the animal circulation a constricted cell, and then you kill the animal and you remove the lung and you apply a fixative. Now, in good hands you could do that very quickly, perhaps in ten minutes. What happens in a constricted muscle cell in the ten minutes whilst you are doing the preparation, and can you be certain that you are looking at physiology and not artifact? I'm sorry to put it so bluntly Donald, but I'm sure that the audience would wish to do it in that way.

HEATH: Clearly you cannot do these things instantaneously. I must agree with that.

CUMMING: Yes. But do you think this poses a serious problem?

HEATH: I think it poses some problem but what you have got to bear in mind when you get down to this level, under any form of microscope, you are in fact looking at artifact, to some extent, in that when you put a piece of tissue in a fixative, it shrinks. As soon as you prepare it for staining, there is another aspect of shrinkage.

CORRIN: When one biopsies smooth muscle, the artifactual contraction is tremendous, to the detriment of the interpretation of the changes one presumes are present in life. It's usual to allow the muscle to sit on the bench for 15 minutes before immersing it in the fixative which would cause tremendous contraction. And this is enough time for the cell to die and you avoid this tremendous contraction. I think an indicator that your cells are in constriction is the wavy nature of the elastic lamina, and that partly might answer Bakhle's question. I wonder if I can go on to a question of the mechanism by which venous hypertension causes pulmonary arterial hypertension. Denolin suggested this morning that this was a process of passive transmission, and I imagine from this that he envisages the high pressure in the venous system being transmitted backwards to the pulmonary arteries, and we finally have a pressure in the pulmonary arteries higher than normal. So this then is a reversal of the normal pressure gradient whereby the pressure descends from artery through capillary to vein, we have the blood arriving in the pulmonary circulation finding a higher than normal pulmonary arterial pressure, and then the pressure is going up when we reach the capillaries, and I wonder what the consequence is of this hydrostatic force when we consider it against the osmotic forces. I would envisage the patient drowning in his own oedema fluid. There is perhaps a different mechanism where Barer showed these nerves on the pulmonary veins. Could we have a neurogenous vasoconstriction of the arteries, triggered by the venous pressure?

CUMMING: I think I can't let the question stand as it is at the moment, because I think there is in it a misunderstanding. I think that the pressure gradient is continuous from the pulmonary valve to the left atrium. There is no reverse gradient at any point, no one has suggested that. It would be true the patient would drown, but since it does not occur, that eventuality is not very likely. Can we pass on to your question now, about the neurological input which may be responsible. Would anyone offer an opinion on this?

HEATH: Although there has been tremendous discussion over the past few years about the role of the perivascular mast cells in hypoxia, it seems to me that very few people have pointed out that you get just as many mast cells around the pulmonary arteries in mitral stenosis. And I've never understood this. I'm sure that the mechanism that has been postulated for mast cells, that there is a mediator for hypertension and hypoxia is quite different from what people would regard as a mechanism in mitral stenosis.

DENOLIN: A very brief question. Could you, as we have no good anatomical or physiological explanation, suggest another name to replace vasoconstriction?

HEATH: I'm getting the distinct feeling, Chairman, that Denolin doesn't understand my crude methods.

CUMMING: I suggest that you sit down over a glass of vino rosso and sort it out. I hope you have found the discussion enjoyable and perhaps even informative. Thank you.

CARDIO-RESPIRATORY FUNCTION IN SYNDROME OF HYPERSOMNIA
WITH PERIODIC BREATHING

G. Gunella

Institute of Respiratory Patho-Physiology

University of Bologna - 40100 Bologna, Italy

INTRODUCTION

Before beginning the discussion of the topic under consideration, I would like to point out that the study results that will be presented are the result of a close collaboration between the Institute of Neurology of the University of Bologna, headed by prof. E. Lugaresi, and the Institute of Respiratory Patho-Physiology, under my direction, begun ten years ago. In the studies of the "Pickwick syndrome" and of "primary alveolar hypoventilation" have partecipated, on one hand, Lugaresi, Coccagna, Pazzaglia, Ceroni and Mantovani, and, on the other, my collaborators Petrella and Brignani. I would like to thank all of those who contributed to make available the scientific data that will be used in my speech.

The syndromes of respiratory insufficiency arising in the absence of broncho-pulmonary lesions have been grouped under the term "general alveolar hypoventilation" by Fishman et al. (1966).

The most widely known among these are the Pickwickian syndrome and "primary alveolar hypoventilation".

The Pickwickian syndrome consists of extreme obesity, hypersomnia, muscular jerks becoming more accentuated in the course of sleep, cyanosis, periodic breathing, secondary polycythaemia, right heart failure.

According to several investigators, obesity is of
primary importance in the development of the syndrome
since, by increasing the work of breathing, it produces
a chronic alveolar hypoventilation (Auchincloss et al.,
1955; Burwell et al., 1955; Carroll, 1956). On the other
hand, it has been suggested that besides the obesity
there must be a hypoexcitability of the respiratory centre (Sieker et al., 1950). All the other symptoms, including somnolence, have been considered secondary to
the respiratory insufficiency.

"Primary alveolar hypoventilation" (Rodman and
Close, 1959) or "Ondine's curse" (Severinghaus and Mitchell, 1962) is a syndrome of alveolar hypoventilation
clinically similar to the Pickwickian syndrome excepting
the fact that obesity is absent (Lugaresi et al., 1968).
This syndrome is attributed to hypoexcitability of the
respiratory centre, since there are no lesions of the
lungs or of the neuromuscular apparatus of breathing.
In only a few cases anatomical lesions in the respiratory centre were assumed or demonstrated (Naeye, 1961;
Seriff, 1965).

Due to their affinities, Pickwickian syndrome and
primary alveolar hypoventilation may be grouped under
the heading of "hypersomnia with periodic breathing"
(Coccagna et al., 1970). In "Hypersomnia with periodic
breathing" the following basic observations have been
made:
a) the periodic breathing with recurring apnoeas, la-
   sting from 20 to 80 seconds with intercurrent profound respirations, appears at each dozing off and
   persists through sleep (Jung and Kuhlo, 1955; Gastaut
   et al., 1965; Lugaresi et al., 1968; Gunella, 1972);
b) the apnoeas may be central, obstructive or mixed.
   The central apnoeas are characterized by the interruption and simultaneous resumption of mouth and thoracic breathing; the obstructive apnoeas are characterized by the persistence of the thoracic movements
   after the interruption of mouth respiration; the mixed apnoeas are characterized by the initial interruption and subsequent resumption of the thoracic

movements during mouth apnoea (Gastaut et al., 1965;
Gastaut et al., 1966; Gunella, 1972). All these phe-
nomene are shown in the figures n° 1 and 2;

c) the obstructive phenomenon is secondary to the hal-
ting or weakening of central breathing; this is indicated by the variations, in the endoesophageal pressure (Lugaresi et al., 1968; Gunella, 1972) and the
EMG activity of the intercostal muscles (Kuhlo, 1968),
which is less than normal in the initial period of

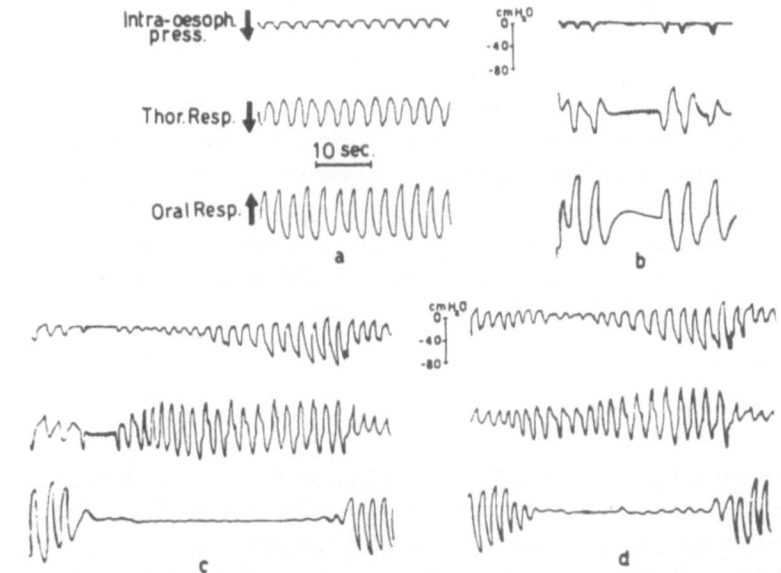

Fig. 1. Simultaneous recording of the endoesophageal
        pressure, thoracic respiratory movements and
        oral respirogram during wakefulness (a) and
        during sleep (b, c, d,) in a typical pickiwi-
        ckian syndrome.
        The arrow indicates the direction of inspira-
        tion. a) Regular breathing during wakefulness.
        b) Central type apnoea. c) Mixed type apnoea.
        d) Obstructive type apnoea.

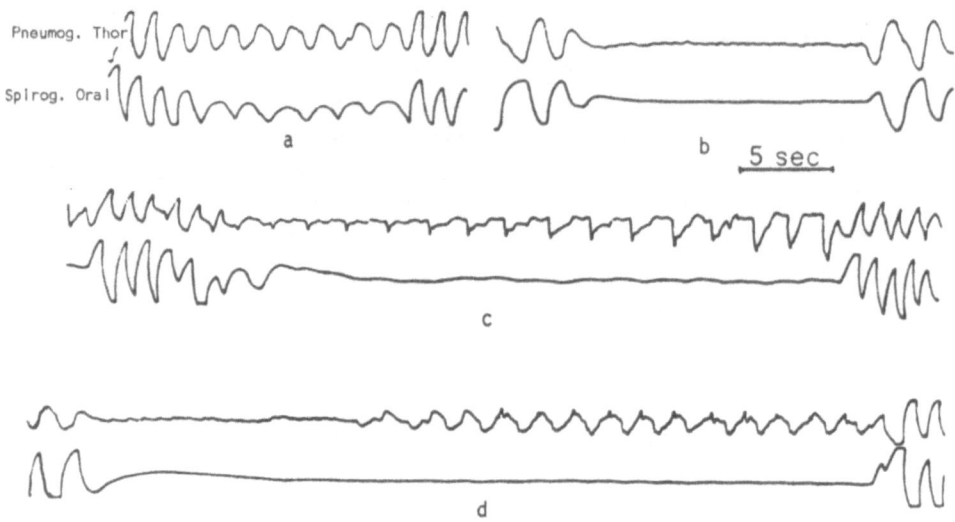

Fig. 2. Simultaneous recording of the thoracic respira-
         tory movements and oral respirogram during wake-
         fulness (a) and during sleep (b, c, d,) in a
         case of primary alveolar hypoventilation.
         a) Simple periodical attenuation of breathing;
         b) Central type apnoea; c) Obstructive type
         apnoea; d) Mixed type apnoea.

   the obstruction. In all likelihood the obstruction of
   the upper respiratory tract is due to a decrease in
   tone of the pharingeal muscles which causes the obstruction of the pharynx by means of a valve-like
   mechanism (Gastaut et al., 1965; Coccagna et al.,
   1968; Schwartz and Escande, 1968; Gunella, 1972);
d) daytime drowsiness is not due to hypercapnia as hypothesized by several authors (Auchincloss and Gilbert,
   1959; Drachman and Gumnit, 1962): in fact in both
   Pickwickian syndrome and in primary alveolar hypoventilation the $PaCO_2$ measured during waking may be normal (Gastaut et al., 1965; Lugaresi et al., 1968;
   Gunella, 1972);

e) the periods of sleep are much longer than in normal
   subjects. In spite of this fact, the sleep is pertur-
   bed by frequent and prolonged nocturnal wakings and
   by a reduction in the phase of deep slow sleep. The
   phases of paradoxical sleep are little shorter than
   those of normal subjects. In both the Pickwickian patients and in the subjects with primary alveolar hypoventilation, periods of respiratory arrest are seen
   during all the phases of sleep (Lugaresi et al., 1968;
   Gunella, 1972.

   This behaviour of the sleeping-waking rhythm and of
the respiratory rhythm, which is associated with a picture of normal, or almost normal, arterial blood gases
during wakefulness, suggests that there may be a basic
abnormality of the central nervous system. In the case
of "primary alveolar hypoventilation", this abnormality
would involve the centres which control the sleeping-
waking rhythm and respiratory rhythm. In the "Pickwickian syndrome" there is, in addition, an abnormality
of the appetite centres leading to pathological hunger
which is responsible for the obesity. However, this obesity plays a purely accessory role in the genesis of the
respiratory disorders.

   Right heart hypertrophy and congestive heart failure are considered the usual complications in "hypersomnia with periodic breathing". On the other hand it has
been established that for long periods of time this syndrome may be characterized exclusively by hypersomnia
and the presence of apnoeas during sleep, without the
evidence during waking hours cf cardiac or respiratory
involvement. These facts suggest that the apnoeic periods,
occurring regularly during sleep over a period of years,
may be responsible for the development of a pulmonary
arterial hypertension and of a "cor pulmonale".

   To verify this hypothesis we carried out a systematic study of the pulmonary and systemic circulatory si-
stem during spontaneous sleep in patients with "hypersomnia with periodic breathing" (HPB).

MATERIALS AND METHODS

   We studied a group of seven patients six of whom

were obese and one was affected by primary alveolar hypoventilation. All the subjects complained of diurnal
and nocturnal hypersomnia and suffered from periodic respiration with apnoeas which occurred regularly throughout the sleep period. While awake, the patients were
given spirographic examinations and measurements of
airway resistance concomitantly, arterial gas analyses
were made. All the patients underwent one or more poly-
graphic recordings of an entire diurnal and nocturnal
cycle of spontaneous sleep.

These involved simultaneous recordings of EEG, horizontal oculogram, EMG of the mylohyoid muscle, EKG,
cardiotachogram, thoracic respiratory movements, oral
or nasal respirogram (by means of small thermoelectric
couples placed in front of the mouth or in one nostril)
or intrathoracic pressure (through an endoesophageal
catheter equipped with a terminal balloon), pulmonary
and sistemic arterial pressure. In order to develop statistically relevant data we took into account only the
values of the pulmonary and systemic arterial pressures
and heart rate recorded at the end of each apnoea, during periods in which ventilation was being resumed.
The blood samples for arterial gas analysis were taken
as ventilation was being restored and during the following apnoea. The sleep stages were classified according
to the criteria suggested by Dement and Kleitman (1957).

RESULTS

During wakefulness the patients had moderate restrictive ventilatory insufficiency. The gas analysis
values showed moderate arterial hypoxemia (mean PaO_2
values = 72,6 mmHg), moderate arterial hypercapnia
(mean $PaCO_2$ values = 48,7 mmHg), moderate respiratory
acidosis (mean pHa values = 7,35 units). In four of the
seven patients the pulmonary arterial pressure was
within normal limits; in the other three cases the
values were above normal. The mean value of Pap, in
these seven patients was 29,5 mmHg. With the onset of
periodic breathing during sleep, the pulmonary arterial
pressure rose rapidly in all cases. The highest pressure values occurred at the resumption of pulmonary ventilation; during the obstructive phase of the apnoeas,

the pressure showed marked oscillations in relation with the variations of the intrathoracic pressure (Fig. 3).

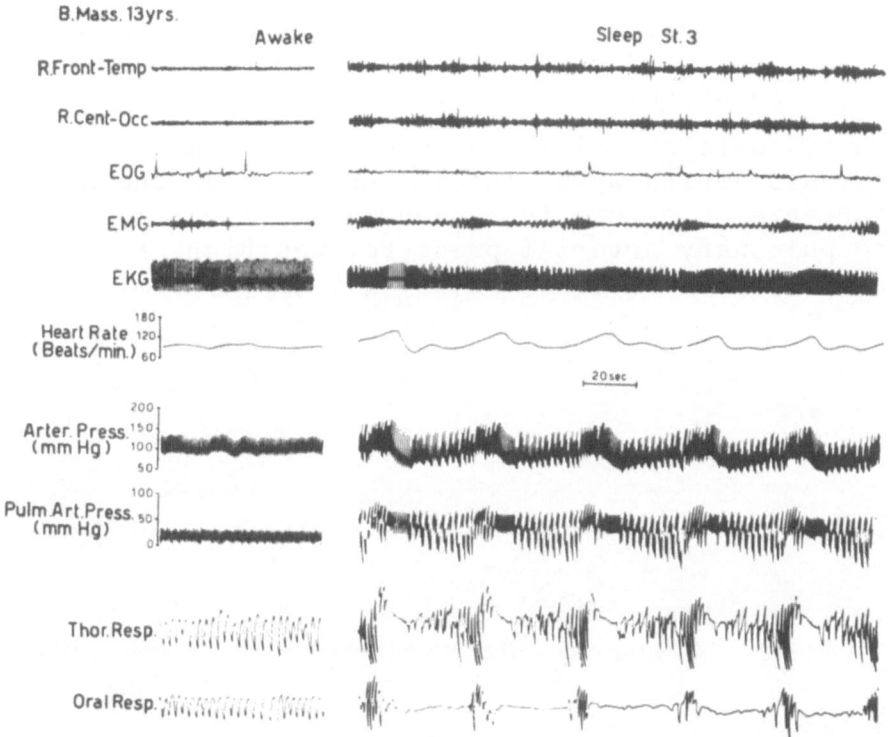

Fig. 3. Simultaneous recording of EEG (first two chan-
        nels), horizontal electrooculogram (EOG), elec-
        tromyogram of mylohyoid muscle (EMG), electro-
        cardiogram (EKG), heart rate, systemic arterial
        pressure, pulmonary arterial pressure, thoracic
        respiratory movements and oral respirogram in a
        case of "primary alveolar hypoventilation".
        During wakefulness the pulmonary arterial pres-
        sure is within normal limits; during stage 3
        sleep a series of mixed type apnoeas occurs.
        The highest pulmonary pressure values are obtai-
        ned at the resumption of ventilation. During the
        obstructive phase of apnoea pulmonary arterial
        pressure undergoes marked oscillations. Syste-
        mic arterial pressure and heart rate increase
        during sleep, the highest values occurring at
        the end of the apnoea.

The pulmonary arterial pressure increased progressively in slow sleep from stage 1 to stages 3-4 in all cases; the highest values occurred during REM sleep (Fig., 4, 5, 6). Often, at the moment of transition from a slow sleep to a REM stage, the pulmonary arterial pressure also rose sharply (Fig. 5).

The systemic arterial pressure was increased in four patients during wakefulness. During sleep the systemic arterial pressure increased in all the cases and, likewise pulmonary arterial pressure, was highest at the end of each apnoea (Fig. 3, 4, 5). The systemic ar-

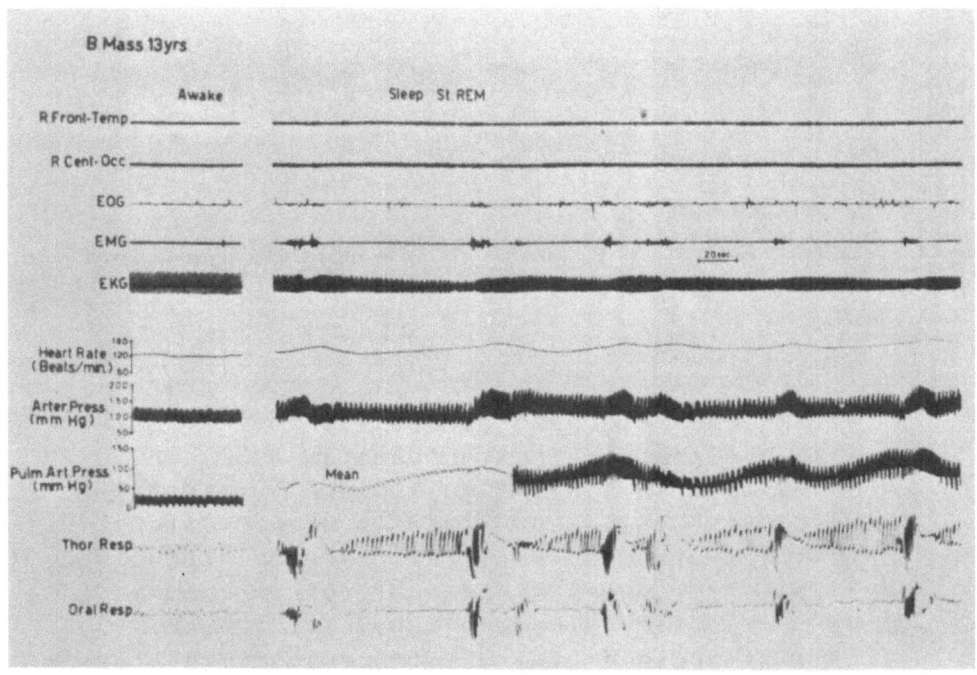

Fig. 4. Same subject as figure 3. During a phase of REM sleep the maximum pulmonary arterial pressure reaches 150 mmHg at the end of apnoeas; the mean Pap 90-100 mmHg. Note the enormous increase of the pulse pressure. The systemic arterial pressure increase substantially to reach systolic pressure values of 200 mmHg (sec. Fig. 3 for legend).

terial pressure rose progressively in the successive
slow sleep stages and underwent an additional increase
in the REM stage.

Changes in heart rate paralleled those in systemic
arterial pressure values (Fig. 7).

During sleep all patients developed severe arterial
hypoxemia, severe arterial hypercapnia and severe respiratory acidosis, all of which increased significantly
from wakefulness to slow sleep and from the latter to
REM sleep (Fig. 8).

These results demonstrate that in all cases of "hypersomnia with periodic breathing" a severe pulmonary
hypertension develops during sleep and this is closely
related to the degree of alveolar hypoventilation; the
severity of these changes is totally independent of the
cardio-respiratory conditions present during wakefulness.
On the other hand, during the course of the night, pul-

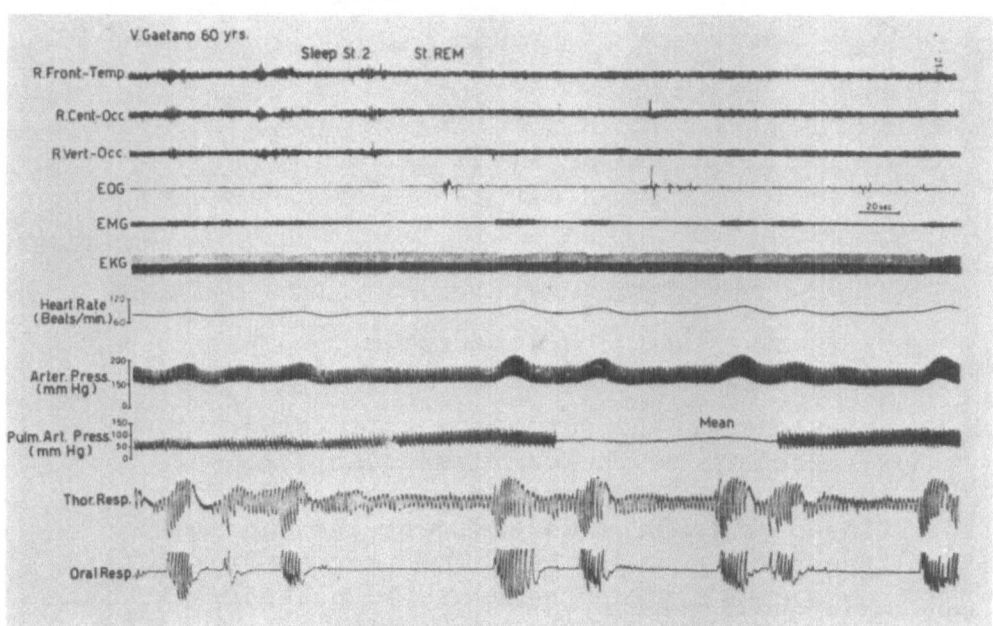

Fig. 5. Pickwickian syndrome: obstructive type apnoeas.
        In passing from a slow sleep stage (stage 2) to
        a REM sleep stage the pulmonary and systemic ar-
        terial pressure rise. sharply (legend as Fig. 3).

monary arterial pressure and arterial gas analysis values
undergo marked oscillations which can be significantly
correlated with the different sleep stages. This last
correlation can be explained by the different times that
the patients spent in apnoea in the various sleep stages.

If we remember that the periods of sleep are much
longer than in normal subjects (the patients with HPB
can sleep 16 or more hours a day), it can be understood
that constant state of pulmonary arterial hypertension
during sleep can, over a period of years, lead to the
development of cor pulmonale. Moreover it must be stressed that the hemodynamic changes during sleep involve

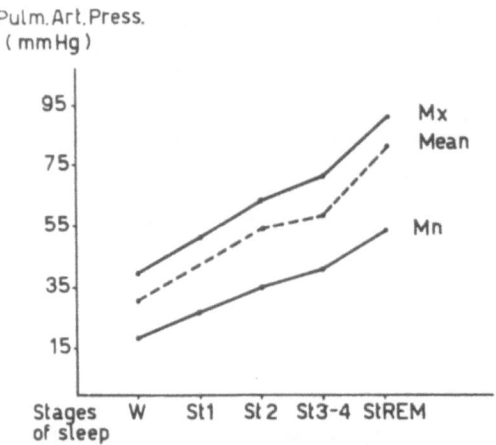

Fig. 6. Behaviour of the pulmonary arterial pressure
        with regard to the various sleep stages.
        The increase in pressure is progressive and
        linear going from wakefulness through sleep
        stages 1,2,3,4 and REM. The increase in pressu-
        re is greater for the systolic pressure so that
        there is also a progressive rise in the pulse
        pressure. The values represent the mean of the
        values of all subjects examined.

not only the pulmonary arterial system but, also, the systemic circulatory system.

    In fact, systemic arterial pressure and, to a lesser degree, heart rate increase significantly during sleep. This explains why systemic arterial hypertension, signs of left ventricular overload and hypertrophy and general enlargement of the cardiac area are found in "hypersomnia with periodic breathing".

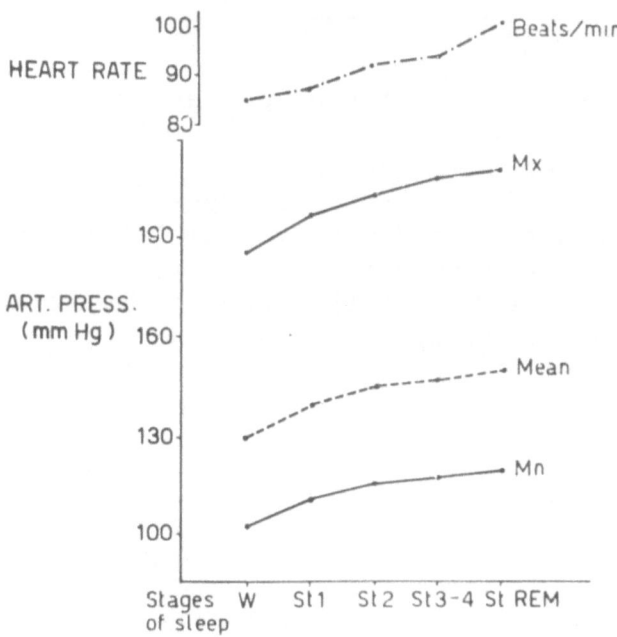

Fig. 7. Behaviour of the systemic arterial pressure and the heart rate in the various stages of sleep. The pressure values increase progressively from wakefulness through stages 1,2,3,4 and undergo a further rise in REM sleep, with a progressive increase in the pulse pressure. The heart rate increase significantly only between deep slow sleep and REM sleep.

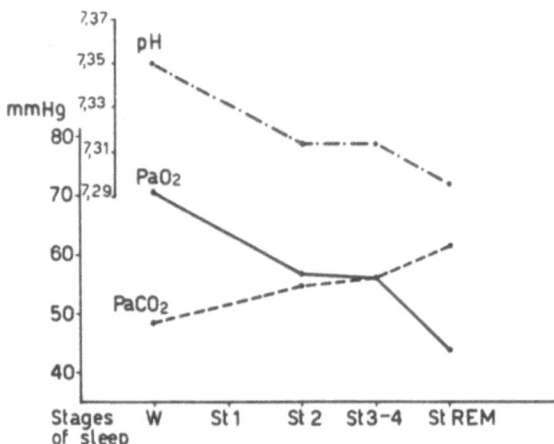

Fig. 8. Behaviour of the arterial gas analysis values
        in different sleep stages.
        During sleep severe respiratory acidosis, arte-
        rial hypoxemia and arterial hypercapnia develop
        and increase significantly from wakefulness to
        slow sleep and from the latter to REM sleep.
        The values represent the mean of the values of
        all subjects examined.

REFERENCES

Auchincloss J.H. jr., Cooke E., Renzetti A.D., 1955,
    Clinical and physiological aspects of a case of
    obesity, polycithemia and alveolar hypoventilation,
    J. Clin. Invest., 34:1537.
Auchincloss J.H. jr., Gilbert R., 1959, La sindrome
    cardiorespiratoria da obesità: quadro clinico e
    fisiopatologico, Progr. Cardiovasc. Dis., 2:215.
Burwell C.S., Robin E.D., Whaley R.D., Bickelmann A.G.,
    1956, Extreme obesity associated with alveolar hy-
    poventilation a Pickwickian syndrome, Am. J. Med.,

21:811.

Carroll D., 1956, A peculiar type of cardiopulmonary fai-
    lure associated with obesity, Am. J. Med., 21:819.

Coccagna G., Mantovani M., Ceroni G., Pazzaglia P.,
    Petrella A., Lugaresi E., 1970, Sindromi ipersomni-
    che-ipoventilatorie. Considerazioni sui rapporti fi-
    siopatologici e nosografici tra sindrome di Pick-
    wick, ipoventilazione alveolare primario e narco-
    lessia a sonno lento, Min. Med., 61:1073.

Dement W., Kleitman N., 1957, Cyclic variations in EEG
    during sleep and their relation to eye movements,
    body motility and dreaming, Electroenceph. Clin.
    Neurophysiol., 9:673.

Drachman D.B., Gumnit R.J., 1962, Periodic alteration
    of consciousness in the Pickwickian syndrome,
    Arch. Neurol., 6:471.

Fishman A.P., Goldring R.M., Turino G.M., 1966, General
    alvéolar hypoventilation: a syndrome of respirato-
    ry and cardiac failure in patients with normal
    lungs, Q. J. Med., 35:261.

Gastaut H., Duron B., Papy J.J., Tassinari C.A., Waltre-
    gny A., 1966, Etude polygraphique comparative du
    cycle nycthémerique chez les narcoleptiques, les
    Pickwickiens, les obèses et les insuffisants re-
    spiratoires, Rev. Neurol., 115:456.

Gastaut H., Tassinari C.A., Duron B., 1965, Etude poly-
    graphique des manifestations épisodiques (hypniques
    et respiratoires) diurnes et nocturnes, du syndrome
    de Pickwick, Rev. Neurol., 112:568.

Gunella G., 1972, Evolution des conceptions pathogeni-
    ques sur le syndrome de Pickwick, Bull. Physio-
    path. Resp., 8:981.

Gunella G., 1972, Interprétation pathogenique des trou-
    bles du sommeil et de la respiration dans le syn-
    drome de Pickwick et dans l'hypoventilation alvéo-
    laire primaire, Bull. Physio-path. Resp., 8:1257.

Jung R., Kuhlo W., 1965, Neurophysiological studies of
    abnormal night sleep and the Pickwickian syndrome.
    In "Sleep mechanisms", Akert K., Bally C., Schadé
    J.P., Eds, Progress in Brain Research, vol. 18,
    Elsevier, Amsterdam.

Lugaresi E., Coccagna G., Ceroni G., Petrella A., Manto-

vani M., 1968, La "maledizione d'Ondine": il disturbo del respiro e del sonno nell'ipoventilazione al-
veolare primaria, Sistema nervoso, 20:27.

Lugaresi E., Coccagna G., Petrella A., Ceroni G., Pazzaglia P., 1968, Il disturbo del sonno e del respiro
nella sindrome Pickwickiana, Sistema Nervoso, 20:38.

Naeye R.L., 1961, Alveolar hypoventilation and cor pulmonale secondary to damage to the respiratory center, Am. J. Card., 8:416.

Rodman T., Close H.P., 1959, The primary hypoventilation
syndrome, Am. J. Med., 26:808.

Schwartz B.A., Escande J.P., 1968, Respiration hypnique
Pickwickienne. In "The abnormalities of sleep in
man", Gaggi A. Ed. Bologna.

Seriff N.S., 1965, Alveolar hypoventilation with normal
lungs: the syndrome of primary or central alveolar
hypoventilation, Ann. N.Y. Acad. Sci., 121:691.

Sieker H.O., Estes E.H. jr., Kelser G.A., Mc Intosh H.D.,
1955, A cardiopulmonary syndrome asscciated with
extreme obesity, J. Clin. Invest., 34:916.

Sieker H.O., Heyman A., Birchfield R.I., 1960, The effects of natural sleep and hypersomnolent states
on respiratory function, Ann. Int. Med., 52:500

Discussion

DENOLIN: What are the limits of changes in blood gases during sleep in normal subjects?

CUMMING: The PO_2 in normal subjects shows a progressive fall with age. And the value of 80 would not be abnormal in a person of 65, such as the case we have seen. But the values which Gunella did show were very much lower than this. They were 40 and 50. So I think we can accept this as a significant deviation. Though the point is well taken that there is a large variability in oxygen tension particularly.

? SPEAKER: The pulmonary circulatory phenomena connected with the data of the gas analysis which we have in the situations of hypoxia at high altitude; these brief episodes of hypoxia or anoxia cause a considerable increase in pulmonary arterial pressure which are the same as found in subjects exposed to low values of partial oxygen pressure - individuals in a decompression chamber for example. I would like to ask what relationship is there between these phenomena and hypoxic phenomena proper? It would seem that these conditions are due not to a primary nervous factor but is a consequency of a peripheral factor which, by occluding the upper airways triggers off a whole series of respiratory problems. Therefore, I think that the cause should be sought in those factors which cause this occlusion of the upper airways rather than trying to find out the reason for the respiratory effects. Perhaps the two aspects are linked to each other. It is not the increase in pulmonary arterial pressure or of systemic pressure that we should identify, but the cause of this increase. It is not the cause for the altered values of the gas analysis but rather the cause of the obstruction of the upper airways which in turn triggers off all those episodes which have been so well and correctly described.

GUNELLA: First of all both in Pickwickins as well as in primary alveolar hypoventilation purely central apnea does exist where there is no peripheral mechanism at work. Probably these patients during sleep undergo a vast series of alterations at the cerebral and cortical levels. At a certain point there is a generalised disappearance of muscle tone. We detect this at the level of the mylohyoideus and we have done so in order to assess the peripheral type of apnea. But we see this lack of tone also at the level of the tracheal bifurcation which is certainly not involved in peripheral type apnea. The disappearance of tone at the mylohyoideus in a person lying down makes the tongue fall back. If this happens in the nasopharynx the upper airways are completely obstructed. What is the pathogenesis? It is evident that during these apneic periods during sleep, arterial PO_2 falls, arterial PCO_2

rises. This fall in PO_2 and rise in PCO_2 are the result of repeated apneic episodes. During the nocturnal cycles we have recorded something like 400 apneic episodes in a Pickwickian. Therefore, it can be supposed that a considerable fall in PO_2 and an increase in PCO_2 can cause the onset of pulmonary arterial hypertension. However, a role is also played by the large ventilatory oscillations observed in pulmonary arterial pressure. What is not so easy to explain is the onset of a state of systemic hypertension in these subjects. However, the point of departure is a primary damage - we should have anatomo-pathologic data in order to see what happens at the cerebral level - unfortunately the data in the literature are scant. The starting point is the hypofunction during sleep of the respiratory centres which is associated with true hypersomnia due to primary damage to the regulating control centres, everything follows on from there. The important thing for us doctors and I understand that the physiologist sees things from a particular viewpoint but doctors, who have to treat these patients know that the important thing is that we simply must record the flow at the mouth and the movement of the thoracic cage to be able to say whether our patients are central, peripheral or mixed type apneics. Then we can ask ourselves whether tracheotomy is necessary or not. As we know that during the whole cycle there is an enormous prevalence of peripheral or mixed type apnea, in practice, tracheotomy is always indicated. We are interested in treating people and preventing the preventable.

HEATH: It is interesting, Mr. Chairman, that so far in the discussion this morning, we haven't mentioned Monge's disease, the hyperventilation syndrome of high altitude. It's interesting with regard to what are the normal falls in arterial oxygen saturation in the normal person and the progressive fall in arterial oxygen saturation with age. The Peruvian school would regard Monge's disease or the hyperventilation of high altitude as merely an expression of ageing at altitude. These people are totally normal, they are just getting older at high altitude. I'd be interested in your comments on that and its relation to what you have been discussing this morning.

GUNELLA: I have no comment to make on the alterations that take place at high altitude. This is not something that interests me in particular.

LOCKART: I would like to know whether this Pickwickian syndrome or hypoventilation in adults relates to the sudden death syndrome in babies, which looks exactly the same with respect fo the presence of obstructive, central or mixed forms of apnoea. Secondly, I would like to know whether any family studies have been done in cases like those you've shown? I suggest it might be interesting to look at the way relatives of your patients sleep, and whether they do not have some other forms of apnoea.

GUNELLA: We have not carried out any studies on the familial nature of the condition. Besides, the baby was an only child, nor have we carried out studies with Pickwickians. I am not aware that data exists in the literature on this. As to your first question regarding the sudden death syndrome in babies, we cannot exclude that there is, at birth, a situation of primary alveolar hypoventilation. What I would say is that there are anatomo-pathological studies, not in the Pickwickian but of the few cases described of primary alveolar hypoventilation. In 2 cases only, there were findings of encephalitic processes but in the other cases there was no trace of cerebral lesion.

CUMMING: I'd like to draw the attention of the meeting to the fact that although the Pickwickian syndrome is very uncommon, there is another syndrome which has almost similar manifestations and which is very common indeed. Sackner in the United States has estimated that there are 5 million sufferers from this disease. This is the disease of snoring, during which in Phase 4 the REM sleep the genioglossus muscle relaxes and completely occludes the trachea. This causes systemic hypertension and pulmonary hypertension and the great problem is in patients under treatment for systemic hypertension. Enormous rises of blood pressure occur during the night. And this is a difficult clinical problem.

DENISON: Two points. Firstly there is a superb review of respiration during sleep in normal subjects by Elliot Phillipson in the current or last annual Review of Physiology, and he has a vast amount of data in all stages of sleep. Like Cerretelli, I believe that the primary defect, having seen your data for the first time, is certainly up here or in the control of these muscles. Everything else could be regarded as secondary. But I was surprised by the extent of pulmonary hypertension. Is it possible that the changes in gas tension that were observed were sufficient to explain the very large rises in pulmonary hypertension. And you, sir, commented that you didn't understand systemic hypertension. I think if someone strangled me when I was asleep my blood pressure would rise too. I don't find that too surprising. But the pulmonary hypertension seems alarming.

GUNELLA: Now as regards the origin of systemic arterial hypertension, we should realise that in a normal subject who is about to be strangled during his sleep and who therefore wakes up, is afraid, and has a hypertensive episode is one thhing, but is completely different in these patients. They continue sleeping but in fits and starts. If they wake up they do so for a very short period and immediately drop off to sleep again. They are not aware of what is happening to them. As to the genesis of pulmonary arterial hypertension, I am sure that the fall of PO_2 and the rise in PCO_2 - given the values that we have recorded - is not sufficient to justify the enormous increase of pressure on the pulmonary artery. Probably there are other mechanisms to be sought. Cumming referred to snoring. In fact snoring can be considered a bland form of primary alveolar hypoventilation.

GEDDES: Can I ask two questions? First, in the patients you successfully treated with tracheostomy, was there any subsequent diminution in their weight? And secondly, have you any experience with the use of progestogens in either form of hyperventilation?

GUNELLA: I have no experience with progesterone. What was the other question.

CUMMING: Loss of weight.

GUNELLA: Loss of weight in our opinion is of importance. It is very difficult for a Pickwickian to lose 20 or 30 kilos; they eat continuously until they fall asleep, even if these patients take large quantities of anorexic and amphetamine drugs. Therefore, it is difficult to get these patients to follow a strict diet which would allow them to shed 20 or 30 kilos. However, our data and those of the literature show that weight loss improves the restrictive volumetric deficiency; it can slightly improve the behaviour of arterial gas analysis during waking periods but it does not cause the disappearance of apnea during sleep nor the hypersomnia of these patients. Therefore, this is another reason which leads us to believe that here we have primary damage to the respiratory centres. In fact, it is sufficient to consider what happens in all other forms of respiratory coma - those working in intensive care wards know this - no patient in a respiratory coma has respiratory disturbances like these patients even if they have 120 mm of PCO_2. You see a respiratory periodicity similar to Cheyne-Stokes breathing in the period immediately preceeding death.

CUMMING: I wonder if I might ask Geddes in order that the audience shall know what you are talking about, to say a few words about the use of progesterones in alveolar hyperventilation.

GEDDES: I'm not really prepared to describe this, I've just read reports presented I think at the American Thoracic Association recently, where progesterone has been used in these patients with success in a high proportion of a small number, both in improving the number of periods of apnoea and all the secondary phenomena afterwards, and also resulting in a loss of weight following the use of progesterones. And so it may be that there

DIAGNOSIS OF CHRONIC COR PULMONALE BY NON-INVASIVE METHODS.

Henri Denolin

University of Brussels

1. DEFINITION OF CHRONIC COR PULMONALE (CCP)

A definition of CCP was given in a WHO report in 1961[1]: "Hypertrophy of the right ventricle resulting from diseases affecting the function and/or the structure of the lung, except when these pulmonary alterations are the result of diseases that primarly affect the left side of the heart or of congenital heart disease". Several other definitions were proposed [2,3,4], but the WHO definition seems to remain the best : CCP is a disease of the right ventricle and not only a pulmonary hypertension.

The <u>incidence</u> of the disease is difficult to appreciate for the following reasons: the clinical diagnosis of CCP is difficult (see below); the definitions are different from one author to another; the autopsy criteria of right ventricular hypertrophy are different; the recruitment of the cases is related to many conditions such as climatic or socio-economic conditions, vocational activity, etc, which influence the frequency of the pulmonary diseases leading to the cardiac complication.

The etiologies are numerous[1], but the most important causes are chronic obstructive lung diseases (70 to 90%), thoracic diseases, and chronic thrombo-embolism. In chronic obstructive lung diseases (COLD), the mechanisms of pulmonary hypertension leading to CCP are apparently numerous : vasoconstriction associated to alveolar hypoventilation, increase in resistance of the airways with compression of capillaries, destruction of parenchyma and reduction of the vessels, increase in blood viscosity and, for some authors, abnormalities in the function of the left ventricle.

2. DIAGNOSIS

A critical description of most of the diagnostic
methods of CCP is given in the proceedings of the meeting on Cor
Pulmonale Chronicum held in München in 1976 [5].

The invasive methods (pulmonary artery catheterization) allow us to measure the pressure in the pulmonary artery
but an increase of the latter is not always a proof of right
ventricular hypertrophy; only if the end diastolic pressure in the
right ventricle is increased, an abnormal function of the right
myocardium could be suspected.

Many non invasive methods were proposed to
evaluate the right ventricular shape, thickness or function.

2.1. Electrocardiography

Many papers in the litterature are devoted to
the electrocardiographic diagnosis of right ventricular hypertrophy, and many criteria were proposed, based on changes in
P waves, R waves, QRS axe, T waves, conduction abnormalities,
etc. In all the serie, the number of false negative and false
positive cases remains very high, and this is related to many
causes, including the position of the heart in the thorax.

The simple criteria proposed by WHO in 1961[1],
remain probably the best : alteration in the ratio R/S in the
left chest leads, with R/S less than 1 in V5; predominant S wave
in standard lead 1, presence of an incomplete right bundle
branch block with QRS less than 0.12 second.

In a study of BERNARD and all[6], the normal
limits of the Ecg were established on 452 subjects, aged 46 to
65 years; then, based on a comparison of pulmonary arterial
pressure with the Ecg in 274 cases of chronic lung diseases,
the following criteria were selected for the diagnosis of
pulmonary hypertension : negative T wave from V1 to V3; electrical axe over 90°; (R + S)/100 lower than 50 in V5; P wave
higher than 2 mm in lead 2; 100 P/(R + S) higher than 20 in
lead 2; 100 R/(R + Q) higher than 50 in AVR; 100 R/(R + S)
higher than 50 in V1. When 2 of these criteria are positive,
pulmonary hypertension is probable, with 3 positive criteria,
the pulmonary hypertension is highly probable.

Changes in the configuration of the ECG are
probably of greater interest than a single record; this is
the principle of dynamic electrocardiography [7,8].

2.2. Vectocardiography

For some authors, the vectocardiogram provide an indirect method of detecting hemodynamic abnormalities in patients with COLD [9].

But, it is generaly agreed that this method is of little valve in the evaluation of right ventricular hypertrophy, at least in COLD [10].

2.3. Mecanography

Right ventricular hypertrophy can be appreciated by an apexcardiogram in many heart diseases, at least with a significant degre of pulmonary hypertension. In COLD, the registration of the tracing is very difficult or completely impossible. New possibilities are now proposed with the Kinetocardiogram, but more research are needed to evaluate the value of this method [11].

2.4. Echocardiography

The patterns of pulmonary valve echo motion may provide informations concerning pressure and flow characteristics in the pulmonary artery. But the correlation between echocardiographic study of the pulmonary valve and the pulmonary arterial pressure remain debated, at least in COLD where the examination is difficult and the increase in pressure in small [12,13]. For the same reason, evaluation of the right ventricular will thickness is difficult.

2.5. Radiography

Three parameters are recommanded to identify pulmonary hypertension on plain chest radiographes : prominence of the pulmonary arc segment; transhilar distance, defined as the distance between right and left main arteries; diameter of the descending branch of the right pulmonary artery or lower lobar artery. In fact, it was demonstrated that the values read by different observers on the same document were considerably different, especially because of the difficulties to define the point where the measurements should be made.

Better results could probably be obtained with tomography or xerotomography of the lungs, but this should be demonstrated in large series of cases.

The value of measurement of right ventricular volume by single plane on biplane angiography in the diagnosis of CCP should also be evaluated.

2.6. Isotopic methods

The right ventricular chamber is not visualized on a resting thallium-201 scan in normal subjects and its presence suggests pressure and/or volume overload of the chamber [14]; the value of this method should be evaluated in large series of COLD.

On the other side, quantitative radionuclide angiocardiography demonstrate an abnormaly low right ventricular ejection fraction in patient with COLD [15].

So, the approach of the right ventricle by isotopic methods with measurement of the thickness of the walls or evaluation of the function appears very promising, but the few data already published require confirmation.

2.7. Lung function tests

Correlations between lung function tests and pulmonary pressure are very poor. It was suggested that a decrease in the normal difference between lying and standing diffusion capacity could be a proof of pulmonary hypertension, [16], but the validity of this method in COLD was not demonstrated.

3. CONCLUSION.

We have no good non invasive method for the evaluation of right ventricular hypertrophy, or even of pulmonary hypertension, in chronic lung diseases before the failure of the right heart.

In only a small number of cases is the diagnosis of CPC possible, when one or two signs are clearly present.

This means that the expression "chronic cor Pulmonale" should probably disappear from the jargon of the clinician; it could be used only by the pathologists, if they agree on the criteria for right ventricular hypertrophy [17].

Even pulmonary hypertension, the cause of CCP, remain difficult to evaluate by non invasive methods. The only think we can do actually is to measure the pulmonary artery pressure and, when it is elevated, to suspect a right ventricular hypertrophy. A hope is represented by the development of nuclear technique. Otherwise, the natural history, the prevention or the treatment of the so called chronic cor pulmonale will remain very difficult.

.REFERENCES

1. Chronic Cor Pulmonale. WHO technical reports series. n° 213.
    Geneva (1961).

2. R.K. BHARGAVA. Cor Pulmonale : Pulmonary Heart Disease. Futura
    Publishing, New York (1973).

3. D. BURCKART. Zur Diagnostik der Chronischen Cor Pulmonale.
    Hans Hubert Bern. (1972).

4. I. SZAM. Cor Pulmonale Chronicum. Akademiai Kiado. Budapest
    (1975).

5. Cor Pulmonale Chronicum, an European Congress. Edited by
    S. DAUM, München (1977).

6. R. BERNARD, and H. DENOLIN. Le diagnostic électrocardiographi-
    que du coeur pulmonaire chronique : état actuel de la question.
    Acta Cardiologica: 3,295 (1967).

7. M.M. KILCOYNE., A.L. DÁVIS and M.I. FERRER. A dynamic electro-
    cardiographic concept useful in the diagnosis of Cor Pulmonale.
    Circulation, 42:903 (1970).

8. E. WEITZENBLUM, A. LOISEAU., C. HIRTH, R. MIRHOM and J.
    RASAHOLINJANAHARY. Course of pulmonary hemodynamics in
    patients with chronic obstructive pulmonary disease.
    Chest, 75:656 (1979).

9. J.R. WILSON, U.G. MASON, R.C. BAHLER, E.H. CHESTER, J.J. PICKEN
    and G.L. BAUM. Vectocardiographic detection of early hemo-
    dynamic abnormalities in chronic destructive pulmonary disease.
    Chest, 76,160 (1979).

10. T. MOCCETTI, M. LUGANO and M. MORPURGO. The contribution of
    vectocardiography to the diagnosis of chronic cor pulmonale.
    Cor Pulmonale Chronicum. Ed. S. DAUM. München (1977).

11. W.H. BANCROFT, and E.E. EDDLEMAN. Methods and physical
    characteristics of the kinetocardiographic and apexocardiogra-
    phic systems for recording low-frequency precordial motion.
    Am.Heart J. 73,756 (1967).

12. A.E. WEYMAN. Pulmonary valve echo motion in clinical practice.
    Am.J.Med. 62,843 (1977).

13. H. ACQUATELLA, N.B. SCHILLER, D.N. SHARPE and K. CHATTERJEE.
    Lack of correlation between echocardiographic pulmonary valve
    morphology and simultaneous pulmonary arterial pressure.
    Am.J.Cardiol. 43:946 (1979).

14. F. KHAJA; M. ALAM; S. GOLDSTEIN, D.T. ANBE and D.S. MARKS.
    Diagnostic value of visualization of the right ventricle
    using thallium-201 myocardial imaging.

15. H.J. BERGER, R.A. MATTHAY, J. LOKE, R.C. MARSHALL, A. GOTTSCHALK
    and B.L. ZARET. Assessment of cardiac performance with quan-
    titative radionuclide angiocardiography : right ventricle
    ejection fraction with reference to findings in chronic
    obstructive pulmonary disease. Am.J.Cardiol. 41:897 (1978).

16. P. JEBAVY, J. WIDIMSKY, J. HURYCK and V. STANEK.
    Relationship between orthostatic changes of pulmonary diffusing
    capacity and haemodynamics of lesser circulation. Respiration,
    28:101, (1971).

17. H. DENOLIN. Le coeur pulmonaire chronique : ce diagnostic
    est-il à maintenir en clinique ? Acta Cardiologica, 34:1 (1979).

Discussion

TRICOMI: I speak with 30 years of experience in a specialised hospital where we see an enormous number of diseases which can lead to pulmonary arterial hypertension to cor pulmonale and COLD. As a radiologist who has also an interest in xerography, I think that the criterion linked to vascularity must not so much be related to the measuring of the pulmonary trunk or intermediary tract but rather to a proportional assessment between the artery of the hilum and those periphery. In other words, as if we upturned West's parameters and instead of reading them vertically, 1,2,3 we should read them horizontally. Radiology can only give what can be objectively shown, naturally we must not make the same mistake as was seen in legal medicine when the radiologist was asked to assess the damage caused by silicosis. But there is no doubt that the objective reading of pulmonary vascularity perhaps also associated with perfusional scintigraphy are able to show the alterations that take place in COLD. Secondly as regards the evaluation of hypertrophy of the right ventricle is concerned some merit should be attributed to the classical oblique projections in x-rays since the anterior convexity behind the sternum of an enlarged heart must have significance.

HORVATH: We have found the oximetric method very useful for screening. It is useful to make this with combined Valsalva manoeuvre.

RIEDEL: It takes us about ten minutes to measure the PAP with a floating catheter, and the procedure is invasive in the sense that we use a needle as big as for drawing a blood sample. So, it takes far more time to have an echocardiogram or a diffusing capacity besides the results being very inconclusive. Criteria of any method constitute sensitivity and specificity and authors were trying to improve specificity, which was the major drawback of ECG and x-rays, that the specificity was very low. There was a very interesting study in Czechoslovakia in 1953, directed on the eradication of syphilis. It was done by screening of the whole 40 million people by the very simple Wasserman reaction. This is a very unspecific but very sensitive method. Several thousand people were identified as being positive and Treponema immobilisation test was applied to them. This study or survey resulted in complete identification of all syphilitic patients in Czechoslovakia and their subsequent treatment, and there was no case of syphilis in Czechoslovakia by 1965 which is one of the very few remarkable and outstanding results of Czechoslovakia in medicine. I think we have same possibility with practical identification of pulmonary hypertension. Perhaps we might look at the ECG and x-rays and find signs which are very sensitive, but signs which would just suggest that it may be pulmonary hypertension, and then use these ten minutes with the floating catheter to either prove or disprove that. And I think that something could be done in that respect.

CUMMING: Thank you very much. Now, ladies and gentlemen, we have a familiar problem, since we had two presenters this morning we have used rather more time in the initial presentation, and the session should now come to an end. There is however considerable pressure from you to ask questions. So I return to my question to you, whose session it is; do you wish to prolong the session for a further ten minutes or not? Those who wish to continue please signify. No, I think that no's have it. I think that the majority of the people do not wish the session to continue, and therefore since that is what is advertised, that is what we must do. Now, before you go, at the end of the session it is hoped that all the members of the course will assemble on the steps outside so that we may have a photograph taken of all participants.

LECTURER: ZARDINI

Discussion

GUNELLA: As regards emboli of the pulmonary artery I would recall
your attention briefly to the danger posed for a whole series of
patients. You mentioned this briefly - I would like to go into this
in more detail. The frequency and the dangerous nature of
thrombo-embolism in chronic lung disease and in those with chronic
respiratory failure. My experience which includes some 1200
emphysematous patients with hypoxemia and severe hypercapnia
suggests that in 28% of these patients there is the onset of
pulmonary thrombus. These are all patients with arterial PCO_2
higher than 60 mm of mercury. There are anatomo-pathological
studies of French authors Bignon and Parian who show that in chronic
lung disease and respiratory failure there is not so much embolus
but rather arterial thrombosis. The danger of such thromboses lies
in the fact that they are unforeseeable and it is not possible to
diagnose them rapidly and with certainty. Rapid dignosis is of
paramount importance because these patients die after a very short
interval - either there is sudden cardiac arrest or ventricular
fibrillation with subsequent cardiac arrest, or they go into severe
shock and death ensues. Arterial gas analysis data do not help to
diagnose in these cases because they are already hypoxemic and
hypercapnic. At best we observe a worsening of the hypoxemia. Now
in practical terms, what I want to say is that it is useless to try
and diagnose pulmonary thrombosis and thrombo-embolus in chronic
respiratory patients. Therapy is difficult because the patient is
always in a very serious condition anyway. All the cases we have
managed have died despite the fact that we used urokinase.
Therefore the best way of approaching these patients is by
prevention of these thrombotic episodes. We have for years carried
out preventative measures when PCO_2 exceeds 60 mm of mercury, using
Calciparin as is commonly done in France. For us, the prevention of
lung thrombosis in chronic lung patients with Calciparin has proved
very effective.

ZARDINI: I am in agreement with you as regards prevention but I
wonder how many of these patients you can administer Calciparin to.
These are patients who often not only manifest pulmonary oedema but
suffer perhaps hypertension and therefore anticoagulant treatment is
dangerous. They have ulcers too perhaps and other diseases and
therefore I would think twice about what preventive treatment to
give. I agree with you that there is the diagnostic problem of
pulmonary oedema and local thrombosis in chronic obstructive lung
patients. I agree, but I ask myself, in how many cases have you
been able to carry out this treatment with Calciparin? I have
thought of doing this and never have because almost always there
were considerable attendant risk factors.

275

GUNELLA: We administer Calciparin to all patients referred to us who have more than 60 mm of mercury of CO_2.

ZARDINI: How long do you continue this?

GUNELLA: Until therapy gives an improvement in the respiratory failure and then we continue Calciparin treatment at home according to the patient's hematocrit values. High blood viscosity is a factor which encourages thrombosis in these patients.

CUMMING: Thank you.

TRICOMI: A radiograph must be carried out in these conditions where possible because the x-ray must be exact.   Since scintigraphy is a very sensitive though highly non-specific technique, comparison with a chest x-ray is all the more important since the chest x-ray may be "negative". If the x-ray of a young patient with no history of COLD is negative and the scintigraph is positive, for me the standard chest x-ray, together with the scintigraph has helped to corroborate the diagnostic value of perfusion scintigraphy.   There is another point: let us radiologists and those who avail themselves of our services, try to forget the expression "hyperdiaphania" - increase of transparency. Often it is simply a technical error. Hyperdiaphania is of significance in that particular x-ray where pulmonary vascularity is readily visible. Beyond that it is of little significance.

CUMMING: Thank you. Would you like to comment on that, Zardini?

MORPURGO: Quite rightly Zardini has said two or three times that we doctors must consider the possible diagnosis of pulmonary embolus. Do we really take into consideration pulmonary oedema? I think not and I will explain why. Out of a total 13,300 autopsies we have identified 538 cases of pulmonary oedema. In pulmonary oedema with embolisation of at least a segmentary branch or its equivalent, patients are divided into three classes: internal medicine; post-operative forms and isolated phlebopathies. During the periods 1940 - 1966 and 1966 - 1974 two large Milanese hospitals with the same teams with the same qualifications followed the same criteria of diagnosis. Correct diagnoses were as follows: 1st group, internal medicine; 10.8% of cases in the first period; 18% in the second, statistically significant. In the post-operative group: 31% exact diagnoses in the first period; 28% exact diagnoses in the second, not statistically significant. Third group - and here are very few cases of isolated phlebopathy: 18% exact diagnoses in the first period; 28% in the second - exact diagnoses at autopsy - not statistically significant.

CUMMING: Thank you. I think there are one or two questions which we have left unanswered. Are the 13,000 case autopsies or live patients?

MORPUGO: Autopsies.

CUMMING: And what were the criteria by which you made the diagnosis?

MORPURGO: The criteria of pulmonary embolisation is embolisation of at least one segmental pulmonary artery or its equivalent.

CUMMING: This means occlusion, visible occlusion of a pulmonary artery branch.

MORPURGO: Yes, with confirmation at autopsy.

CUMMING: Zardini, any comment on that?

ZARDINI: I agree.

SCHIAVINO: I am interested in the reduction of compliance during pulmonary embolus also seen in some cases of primary pulmonary hypertension. If you attribute this reduction of compliance to the oedema it is more difficult to know what to incriminate in the case of primary pulmonary hypertension. A correlation has been drawn between pulmonary arterial hypertension and the ventilatory picture.

ZARDINI: Explaining the clinical data is more difficult. From 1975 we have studied pulmonary hypertension on isolated dog lungs. We studied the pressure volume curves - input, output volume at the various degrees of pulmonary arterial pressure. Starting with values of 10 cm. and up to 60, 70, 80, 90 cm. of water we have never seen significant variations in compliance. Another thing that came out in Milic Emili's paper yesterday, we have never seen in experiments on isolated dog lung variation in the distribution of ventilation in the various degrees of pulmonary arterial pressure. This is all documented in a series of experiments and appeared in the Journal of Applied Physiology in 1966. I took my statistical data and asked myself how many of these data could I transfer to the clinic. I have never seen experimental surveys. You say that you have seen these clinically? I don't know how to explain this. I know that in pulmonary oedema it is very easy to have a histological and radiological investigation of the perivascular oedema. This is something which might suffice to explain to me the alteration in the lung's mechanics. In pulmonary hypertension I have some difficulty in considering interstitial oedema. On the other hand, I find it very difficult to believe that this element of lung resistance can cause an alteration in the mechanics of the lung. It might be attributable to a change in the distensibility of the pulmonary vascular bed or perhaps in pulmonary hypertension there is a variation in the pulmonary volume at the maximum degree of expansion - I don't know. One thing is certain and that is that the two conditions are very difficult and here I would add - since the evidence is scant - and I would be pleased to hear if anyone else subscribes to one of the interpretations given to the experimental work being the instability of the small airways in interstitial oedema of the lung. Especially those bronchioles which trap the air and being without cartilaginous musculature, this causes instability of the small airways.

LEE: I would like to ask a question to Zardini, relating to his experimental work and its application clinically. In his microembolisation experiments, he showed a lot of peripheral oedema. Now, that would suggest that if there is a state of affairs clinically where you have multiple peripheral emboli leading to pulmonary hypertension, you would expect to have evidence of oedema that one could pick up perhaps on a radiograph, as opposed to the opposite, where there is a block of a main blood vessel, so that the periphery is not affected. Is that your experience?

ZARDINI: I can't make any interpretation on the clinical experience of this. You can give much better interpretation of this, I think.

LOCKART: Before starting a potentially harmful treatment, maybe life-saving, but with a lot of undesirable side effects in a patient with pulmonary emboli one should perform pulmonary angiography. I will never, or almost never, make a decision either on surgery or fibrinolytic treatment in a life-threatening potential pulmonary emboli without one. If you think there is life-threatening emboli why don't you go straight away to angiogram and forget all the rest?

ZARDINI: I agree with you. It would be useful for the patients to have the angiogram if we suspect pulmonary embolism. But there are some situations that are not so severe and these cases can do it quite easily. Where I can I do the perfusion scintigraphy, when I can I try to relate the perfusion defect to the gas analysis and other clinical data.

CUMMING: Clearly we have a very complex situation in pulmonary embolus, when the problem is initial diagnosis, and when diagnosis has been made, the next problem is that of therapeutics, and although we have had some indications of therapeutic nihilism, I think that we must do our best to find new methods of treatment that may avert side effects or, as Gunella says, methods of prevention. That's the end of our session this morning, but instead of having an aperitivo before lunch today, you are getting an intellectual aperitivo because it is my pleasure to introduce my friend and colleague Antonio Zichichi to address us.

INTERACTION BETWEEN VENTILATION AND CIRCULATION IN BRONCHIAL ASTHMA AND PULMONARY EMPHYSEMA

P. Even, H. Sors, D. Safran, P. Reynaud

Department of lung diseases - Laennec Hospital
42, rue de Sèvres - 75007 Paris - France

That the heart works as a pump in the respiratory pump and can be influenced by ventilatory events was recognized as early as the eighteen century by Valsalva and Morgani. However in normal conditions the ventilatory effects on the functionning of the cardiac pump are slight and negligible, but in extreme situations, such as Valsalva or Muller maneuvers, the ventilatory forces may overcome the circulatory forces. Similarly, bronchial asthma attacks, chronic upper airway obstruction in children and sleep apnea syndrome resemble Muller maneuver (MM) during inspiration and, otherwise, bronchial asthma and emphysema resemble Valsalva maneuver (VM) during expiration, giving rise in the most severe cases to a kind of cardiac tamponade, reducing the venous return and limiting the circulatory adaptation to exercise.

I - PULSE PRESSURE - INTRA, EXTRA AND TRANS-MURAL PRESSURES.

To make clear the relation between respiration and circulation we have to remind of a few definitions. The arterial pulse pressures (PP) are the differences between systolic and diastolic pressures. The PP depends on the stroke volume (SV), the heart rate, the compliance of elastic arteries and the resistances of muscular arteries. The last three factors being constant, the PP reflects the cardiac output (CO). Now, if we consider the pressures in each side of a vessel wall, the internal pressure measured during catheterization and referred to barometric pressure (P_B) is denominated intramural pressure (imP). The pressure outside the vessel, also referred to P_B, is denominated extramural or surrounding, pressure (emP). The difference between intra and extramural pressures is the transmural pressure (tmP), also termed net, effective or distending pressure and the imP is the total pressure, i.e. the sum of tmP and emP. The pressures which distend the

279

vessels are the tmP, the pressures which preload and afterload
the ventricles are also the tmP and the pressure which makes the
blood flow , overcoming the frictional losses through the vascular
bed, is the difference between the input and output total or imP.

Because the heart and the large thoracic vessels are submitted
to a similar emP, different of the emP surrounding the lung capillaries and the extrathoracic arteries, the pressures afterloading
the right and left ventricles are the tmP of pulmonary artery (PA)
and thoracic aorta (TA). In other words, the mechanical energy
that the heart has to produce to overcome the pulmonary or systemic
arterial impedances, is related to the emP and not to the imP.
Similarly, if a pump in a valley (the thorax) has to fill a reservoir on a hill, (the peripheral systemic arteries) the pressure
that the pump has to develop must be measured by reference to the
level of the pump and not to the level of the hill. So, the lower
the valley, the higher the energy needed to fill the reservoir and
the lower (i.e. the more negative) the intrathoracic pressure, the
higher the cardiac afterload.

The emP of the small alveolar vessels (AV), i.e. lung capillaries and pre and post-capillary vessels, is the alveolar pressure
(P_{AL}), whereas the emP of the heart and large extraalveolar vessels
(EAV), i.e. pulmonary arteries and pulmonary veins (PA and PV) are
the pericardial pressure, near equal to the pleural pressure (P_{PL})
and the pulmonary interstitial pressure, very near the P_{PL}, although
still more negative specially at high lung volume.Therefore the
lung capillaries and the PA are submitted to different emP and this
difference is maximal at TLC, owing to the simultaneous increase
in transpulmonary pressure. During the respiratory cycle, the P_{AL}
oscillates around the P_B with a nul mean value, whereas the P_{PL}
is permanently negative during quiet breathing, and becomes only
positive at expiration during strenuous exercise, its mean value
remaining negative in all circumstances.

Accordingly, the pulmonary arterial resistances are increased
by 2 differents ways at high lung volume. At first, the emP of the
large EAV is very negative, whereas the emP of the AV remains
around 0, so that the lung capillaries are relatively compressed
by the P_{AL}, so opposing an increased resistance to the pulmonary
blood flow. Then the lung inflation increases the volume and the
storage capacity of the large EAV, but stretches and narrows the
AV, so raising again the pulmonary vascular resistances (Howell
et al., 1961),and extending the zone I and II of West and reducing
the zone III.

II - VALSALVA MANEUVER.

The Valsalva maneuver (VM) is a forced expiratory effort
against a closed glottis at TLC. Because of the contraction of the
abdominal expiratory muscles and the associated tension of the
diaphragm, the P_{PL} and, even more, the abdominal pressure (P_{ABD}),
raise to 40-80 mmHg. Accordingly, the venous return to the

abdominothoracic cavity, and then to the right heart, is extremely
reduced. By contrast with the imP of the right heart and of thoracic vessels which augment by approximatively the increase in P_{PL},
the tmP of the right atria (RA) and right ventricle (RV) drop and
the heart size shrinks. As a consequence of the reduction in RV
preload, the right ventricular stroke volume (RVSV) falls down
and the PA pulse pressure (PAPP) wanes. Otherwise, the pulmonary
circulation introduces a phase-lag between right and left ventricles, so as the left ventricular stroke volume (LVSV) and the
systemic arterial pulse pressure (SAPP) are maintained at the
beginning of the VM, during 2 to 3 systoles, at the expense of the
pulmonary blood volume, which is squeezed out of the lungs.
Simultaneously, the intramural systemic arterial pressure (imSAP)
rises by the amount of the increase in P_{PL}, which is transmitted
throughout the systemic arterial tree. However, afterwards, the
pulmonary venous return declines, the tmP of PV, left atria (LA)
and LV are reduced, the LVSV falls down, the SAPP fades and the
intramural systemic artery systolic pressure (imSASP) wanes at
such a degree that syncope may result (Sharpey-Schafer, 1962).
Simultaneously, the carotid body baroreceptors are stimulated and
the systemic arterial resistances increase by a sympathetic reflex,
so reducing the fall of SASP and explaining the overshoot of the
SASP at the end of the VM.

III - MULLER MANEUVER.
        The Muller maneuver (MM) is exactly the reverse of the VM.
However the cardiac performance is yet reduced, although by a
number of different ways, only recently clarified. When a subject
inspires forcefully against a closed glottis at residual volume
(ResV) or FRC, both P_{PL} and P_{AL} decrease to - 50 to - 90 mmHg
(Crowden and Harris, 1929 ; Sharpey-Schafer, 1962) and P_{ABD} rises
because of the diaphragmatic contraction, so that the transdia-
phragmatic pressure may reach 100 mmHg or more.
        As a first consequence, all the imP of the cardiac cavities
and thoracic vessels subside. Simultaneously the imP of the
abdominal veins raises, the imP gradient between inferior vena
cava (IVC) and RA enlarges, the venous return increases, the
effective tmP of the RA and RV rises sharply about to 25 mmHg,
preloading the RV, so as the RVSV raises, as do the PAPP. However,
this large initial increase in venous return is transient and
followed after a few seconds by a return to a level only slightly
elevated, probably because of the collaps of the IVC at its
thoracic entrance (Wexler et al. 1968).
        Because of the increase in venous return the blood is trans-
ferred from peripheral veins towards the thorax and all the tmP
of the right heart cavities and pulmonary circulation are very
enlarged resulting : a) in an increase in pulmonary blood volume,
pooled in large EA vessels and b) in a filtration through the
lung capillaries, producing an interstitial pulmonary edema.

Accordingly, the MM produces radiological changes opposite to those
of VM : enlargement of the heart size, increased density of the lung
roots and marked engorgement of the pulmonary vessels (Crowden
and Harris, 1929).

However, in spite of the increase in venous return and RVSV
observed during the MM, the LVSV and the SAPP decrease ,as they do,
at a lesser degree, during normal or sustained inspiration (Lauson
et al. 1946) and during loaded inspiration. For years, this fall
is conventionally ascribed to a blood pooling in the lungs and
hence to a decreased pulmonary venous return (Lauson et al. 1946).
However, the decrease in P_{PL} elicits a rise in LA and LV tmP,
inconsistent with a decrease in pulmonary venous return (Robotham
et al. 1978 ; Summer et al. 1979). In fact, it has been recently
demonstrated that the inspiratory decrease in LVSV results mainly
from 2 other factors, the increase in LV afterload and the enlargement of the right heart, compressing the LV.

The increase in LV afterload derives from the negativity of
its surrounding pressure, so that the LV has to yield an extra
mechanical work to pump the blood from the thoracic negative emP
compartment into the positive or barometric extrathoracic emP
compartments. The lower the P_{PL}, the larger the gradient from intra
to extrathoracic vessels which has to be overcome, so that the LV
performance may be altered, giving rise to a decrease of the LVSV
inducing an increase of the LV endsystolic volume (LVESV) (Robotham
et al. 1978, 1979 ; Summer et al. 1979).

The second main factor explaining the inspiratory reduction
of the LVSV is the ventricular interference. Because of the tight
anatomic relation between the cardiac chambers enclosed in an quasi
inextensible pericardial sac, it is well established that the
filling of one ventricle affect the volume, the compliance and the
performance of the other (Elzinga et al. 1974 ; Fowler, 1978 ;
Santamore et al. 1976). Therefore, the inspiratory increase in
venous return and RV volume induces a bulging of the septum towards
the LV and a competition for space in the pericardium between both
ventricles, resulting in an increase in LV filling with only a
minor increase in LA and end-diastolic LV volumes(LVEDV)(Summer
et al. 1979), suggesting a decrease in LV compliance, possibly
responsible for a shortage in subendocardial flow (Robotham et al.
1978) and ,accordingly, for a reduction in myocardial contractility.

In experimental situations of right heart by-pass at constant
pulmonary arterial inflow, the ventricular interdependence is
suppressed and the inspiratory LVSV is still decreased, but without
any changes in LA tmP (Robotham et al. 1979). Therefore, the increase in tm LA and tm LVDP during inspiration results mainly from the
ventricular interference and from the increase in right ventricular
output, but hardly from the reduction of the LV ejection. By
contrast, the inspiratory reduction in LVSV results both from the
increase in LV afterload and from the ventricular interference
(Robotham et al. 1979 ; Summer et al. 1979).

IV - NORMAL BREATHING.

The circulatory system is so sensitive to the respiratory events that even during quiet inspiration the PAPP raises by 20% and the SAPP declines by 10%, reflecting an increase of 18-33% of the RVSV and a reduction of 7-12% of the LVSV. Therefore, only minor changes in ventilatory conditions may induce important alterations in cardiac function.

V - PULSUS PARADOXUS.

As recently reviewed (Fowler, 1978), the pulsus paradoxus is only an accentuation of the normal inspiratory weakening of the arterial pulse, but it is termed paradoxical because it contrast with normal heart sounds. In pericardial tamponade, it results from the competition of the ventricles for space in presence of a normal venous return in a fully distended and inexpandable pericardial sac. In chronic obstructive lung diseases and bronchial asthma, it results : a) from an increased inspiratory venous return in a normal pericardium, impeding the LV performance ; b) from an increased tmTA pressure, afterloading the LV during inspiration ; c) from the direct transmission to the systemic arteries of the changes in P_{PL} ; d) from the phase-lag between right and left heart, the expiratory reduction in venous return and RVSV inducing an inspiratory decrease in pulmonary venous return and LVSV.

VI - BRONCHIAL ASTHMA.

That the circulatory function is usually compromized in severe asthma attacks (AA) is suggested by : a) the high frequency of cardiac abnormalities : sinus tachycardia (120-200), marked pulsus paradoxus, systemic hypotension, increase in radiological cardiac size, ECG alterations (right axis deviation, P pulmonale, right bundle, branch block, T wave inversion, right ventricular strain, supra ventricular dysrythmias, ectopic ventricular beats (Ambiavagar et al. 1967 ; Gunstone, 1971) and, in the most severe cases, acute cor pulmonale ; b) the occurence of sudden and unexpected deaths in hospital or home which appears to be due, sometimes to severe hypoxaemia and acidosis, but otherwise to an unexplained acute cor pulmonale without asphyxia.

However, and surprisingly, the scarce hemodynamical data collected in AA (less than 30 cases) are at quite variance with these observations, showing nearly normal right heart pressures even in severe attacks with acute cor pulmonale, the PAMP being 23 ± 8 mmHg, usually $<$ to 25 mmHg and rarely $>$ to 35 mmHg (Ambiavagar et al. 1967 ; Gunstone, 1971 ; Helander et al. 1962). Necropsic evidences also are against any anatomical cardiac or pulmonary vessels abnormalities (Gunstone, 1971). Recently, new facts and ideas were developped by Permutt (1971) which tend to reconcile these discrepant observations in demonstrating a true pulmonary hypertension in AA and proposing enlighting concepts to explain it.

Standard teaching is that asthma is characterized by a paro-
xystic attack of a wheezing expiratory dyspnea, due to a widespread
airways narrowing, interesting small and/or medium sized bronchi
and giving rise to an increase in airways resistances, with a
severe reduction in $FEV_{0.1}$. Because of the higher expiratory
airways resistances and since the patients complain of a great
difficulty in emptying their lungs, it has been assumed that they
have large positive expiratory and mean P_{PL}, able to limit the RV
filling and to compress the lung capillaries, so inducing an
increase of the RV afterload, explaining the acute cor pulmonale
observed in the most severe cases. These traditional notions
remain today largely widespread, in spite of the common clinical
observation that patients complain that inspiration is, in fact,
more difficult than expiration (Woolcock and Read, 1966), with a
feeling of uncomfortable thoracic distension, confirmed by the
clinical evidence of lung overinflation with an inspiratory
depression of intercostal spaces, all observations suggestive of
a very negative intrathoracic pressure.

In fact, modern physiological studies underline that mild
or moderate asthma is characterized by a narrowing of large non-
cartilageneous airways, inducing a marked decrease of the specific
airways conductance (SGaw) and of the slope of the maximum expiratory flow-volume (MEFV) curve, a moderate decrease in $FEV_{0.1}$ and
$FEV_{0.1}/VC$ ratio and only mild modifications of VC, Res.V and FRC,
with no change in TLC and moderate swings of P_{PL}. By contrast,
the major change which occurs in severe asthma, is the closure of
the subsegmental airways resulting in a large increase in Res.V
and FRC, a shift in MEFV curve without change in its slope, a
severe and nearly parallel reduction of VC and $FEV_{0.1}$ without
important decrease in $FEV_{0.1}/VC$ ratio. In such a situation, the
only way to maintain open a part of the airways, is to increase
lung volume and transpulmonary pressure. The higher the bronchial
tone closing the distal airways, the higher the lung volume must
be to reopen these airways and maintain the ventilation and gas
exchange. So, severe AA are usually characterized by an enormous
increase in lung volumes, the Res.V being multiplied by a factor
of 3, sometimes 4 (Woolcock and Read, 1966) and in one case
7 (Mac Fadden and Ingram, 1976), so approaching the predicted TLC,
the FRC reaching twice the normal value and the TLC itself being
increased by 10 to 100%, in mean by 35% (Mac Fadden and Ingram,
1976 ; Woolcock and Read, 1966). Because at such high volume,
the airways are either closed or nearly fully open, the SGaw are
hardly affected (Permutt, 1971). As the level of the tidal
volume increases above the normal FRC towards TLC along the
exponential pressure-volume curve of the lung (Finucane and
Colebatch, 1969 ; Mac Fadden, 1976), the pulmonary compliance
diminishes progressively, so that the elastic inspiratory work
reaches 5-12 times its normal value, so explaining the increase
in oxygen uptake and the severe asthmatic dyspnea which appears

to be related rather to lung overdistension than to frictional energy losses produced by airways obstruction (Permutt, 1971 ; Woolcock and Read, 1966).

In spite of all these evidences suggesting the development of extremely negative intrathoracic pressures during AA, the traditional notions of expiratory difficulties of asthmatic patients were so inveterate that large positive P_{PL} have consistently been assumed. Accordingly, all authors, measuring the oesophageal pressure ($P_{Œ}$) in asthma were quite surprised in observing exactly the opposite (Permutt, 1971 ; Stalcup and Mellins, 1977) i.e. a peak expiratory P_{PL} (PEP_{PL}) hardly positive, but a very negative peak inspiratory P_{PL} (PIP_{PL}) with large swings in P_{PL} (ΔP_{PL}) and a markedly negative mean P_{PL} (MP_{PL}), (Table I) decreasing by 2 cm H_2O for each 10% decrease in VC (Stalcup and Mellins, 1977). Because such large P_{PL} oscillations were observed in mild or moderate AA, it might be predicted that more negative mean and PIP_{PL} could be recorded in severe asthma or in status asthmaticus, as longer as the patient is able to maintain a normal alveolar ventilation.

Because of these large changes in P_{PL}, the ventilation in asthma is tantamount to the performance of a series of MM and VM in rapidly alternating sequence over a long period (Ambiavagar et al. 1967), which have tremendous hemodynamic consequences probably explaining the major part of the cardiovascular disturbances observed in severe AA, as Permutt has very ingeniously hypothetisized (1971). As in MM, the negative P_{PL} observed in AA account for an augmentation in RA, RV, PA, PV and TA tmP and volumes, the LVSV being lessened by the same factors that it is in MM.

Table I.
Pleural pressures in asthma attacks (cmH$_2$O)

	Permutt 1971	Even 1972	Stalcup 1977
	5	7	8
PIP_{PL}	− 22 + 3	− 34 + 8	− 28 + 14
PEP_{PL}	+ 4 + 1	+ 7 + 3	− 2 + 2
ΔP_{PL}	26	41 + 15	26
MP_{PL}	− 10	− 11 + 4	− 16 + 6

However, asthma differs from MM by 2 facts : a) the lung volume is extremely inflated ; b) the mean P_{AL} is nearly equal to P_B and largely positive if referred to P_{PL}. So the alveolar vessels (AV) are stretched and reduced in diameter by the lung volume distension (Howell et al. 1961) and they are submitted to a much higher emP than PA and RV, so that the tmP of lung capillaries is not enlarged. Two important consequences derive from these differences.

At first, there is no important fluid filtration through the lung capillaries and in fact AA is not associated to a clinical evidence of pulmonary edema, even though a small degree of interstitial edema was sometimes present on chest X-Ray, probably owing to the transiently negative P_{AL} (Stalcup and Mellins, 1977) and to some fluid filtration through the smallest extraalveolar vessels (EAV) the tmP of which is increased.

The second difference with MM is that, by comparison to PA and RV entrapped in a very negative compartment, the lung capillaries are in some way lifted up by the P_{AL} in a barometric compartment. To perfuse such relatively compressed AV with an imP sufficient to overcome their frictional resistances, the RV, which is mechanically disadvantaged by its negative surrounding pressure, has to develop a high tmPAP, much higher than in MM for a same degree of negative P_{PL}. Therefore, the tmPAP measures the afterload of the RV exactly as the tmTAP measures the afterload of the LV. So, the relative compression of the lung capillaries by the barometric P_{AL} could be the main raison of the pulmonary hypertension and of the <u>acute cor pulmonale observed in asthma</u>. Therefore, if we want appreciate the magnitude of this pulmonary hypertension, we have to measure the tmPAP and not the imPAP as usually done (Permutt, 1971). Finally, the most important difference between AA and MM is that in AA both ventricles are afterloaded, the LV by the extrathoracic surrounding pressure, positive relatively to P_{PL}, and opposing the blood ejection towards the systemic arterial bed, the RV by the P_{AL} also positive relatively to P_{PL}, and opposing the RV ejection through the alveolar vessels. So, both ventricles are like in a well and both ventricular pumps have to lift up the blood over the top of the alveolar and extrathoracic barriers, a supplementory task more easily accomplished by the forceful LV than by the less vigourous RV, so resulting in a rather acute cor pulmonale than a pulmonary edema. A situation similar to AA could also be observed in severe upper airway obstruction in children and in sleep apnea syndrome.

We have studied 7 patients during AA of moderate severity (Table II) confirming the data published by Permutt (1971) about 2 similar cases. Marked pulmonary hypertension with tmPAMP so high that 50 mmHg have been observed, even in moderate attacks, suggesting that a number of sudden unexpected deaths in asthma could be due to the development of severe RV strain.

Table II.
Asthma attacks. (7 cases ; Even, 1972)

MP_{PL} (mmHg)	$- 8 \pm 3$	imPAMP	26 ± 6
PIP_{PL} -	$- 25 \pm 6$	tm PAMP	34 ± 8
PEP_{PL} -	5 ± 2	PCP (im = tm)	8 ± 2
ΔP_{PL} -	30 ± 10	CI $(1.min^{-1}/m^2)$	3.3 ± 0.4
PaO_2 -	76 ± 9	$\dot{V}O_2/m^2$ $(ml.min^{-1})$	164 ± 15
$PaCO_2$ -	39 ± 6	PAR (tm)	7.8 ± 1.2
$\dot{V}E/m^2$ $(1.min^{-1})$	8.2 ± 2.5	(PAMP - PCP) tm	26 ± 7
Cd (ml/cmH_2O)	65 ± 8	SASP (E - I)*	37 ± 13
$R_{aw}I$ $(cmH_2O\ 1^{-1}.s^{-1})$	18 ± 4	SAPP (I/E)	0.6 ± 0.2
$R_{aw}E$ -	24 ± 6	PAPP (I/E)	1.5 ± 0.4

* Pulsus paradoxus.

However the hemodynamic situation in asthma is certainly more complex that this oversimplified view suggests. At first, the P_{AL} is probably heterogenous, nul in mean in the ventilated regions but positive or negative in the regions beyond closed airways. Owing to the mechanical coupling of lung units and in the absence of an important collateral ventilation, very negative pressures, markedly inferior to P_{PL}, could be developped at inspiration around, and chiefly in, the unexpanded closed airways regions, whose transpulmonary pressure would be reduced. At expiration, positive P_{AL} pressures could be generated in these obstructed zones and finally the P_{AL} averaged on the respiratory cycle remains unknown. If the major part of the lung was beyond closed airways during AA, the difference between mean P_{AL} and P_{PL} would be reduced and the Permutt model of pulmonary hypertension, developped above, would be invalidated. That it is not the cases is suggested by the absence of any shunt in AA, the hypoxaemia of which being entirely due to the presence of very low $\dot{V}A/\dot{Q}$ zones.

The tremendous decrease in P_{PL} is probably not the only cause of pulmonary hypertension or circulatory failure in AA. Probably, severe hypoxaemia, hypercapnia, acidosis and stretching of the pericardium at high thoracic volume (Robotham et al. 1979) are also contributory in a few cases. In addition, some patients develop a very positive expiratory pressure which, similarly to a Valsalva maneuver, reduces the expiratory venous return, so that

Table III.
Pleural pressures in chronic obstructive lung diseases.
(Potter et al. 1971 ; Even, 1979)

	Quiet breathing	Exercise $(\dot{V}_E : 25 - 80 \ 1.mn^{-1})$
ΔP_{PL}	5 to 25	25 to 75
PIP_{PL}	$- 5, - 20$	$- 15, - 32$
PEP_{PL}	$- 5, + 6$	$+ 7 , + 48$
MP_{PL}	$- 2, - 6$	$- 12, + 6$

the RVSV, the PAPP and potentially the cardiac output are extremely diminished during the major part of the respiratory cycle. As
a consequence, the O_2 arteriovenous difference can be extremely
and even dangereously enlarged because of the increase in oxygen
uptake due to the augmented ventilatory work. Finally, if the
majority of the patients develop a very negative P_{PL} and pulmonary hypertension during severe AA, after hours, respiratory muscle
fatigue appears, ventilation and overinflation of the lung decrease
and the extreme negativity of P_{PL} and its hemodynamical consequences
disappear, exactly at the time when hypoxaemia, hypercapnia and
acidosis arise, subtituting humoral to mechanical factors to
maintain acute cor pulmonale.

VII - PULMONARY EMPHYSEMA.
    In patients with severe chronic obstructive lung diseases the
peak expiratory P_{PL} (PEP_{PL}) is frequently positive during quiet
breathing and highly positive during exercise,whereas the mean
P_{PL} (MP_{PL}) is also often slightly positive at exercise (Table III).
Such P_{PL} changes could impede the venous return and impose a
limitation to the cardiovascular adjustments to exercise (Potter
et al. 1971).
    We have studied 3 groups of patients (Table IV) by catheteri-
zation, pulmonary angiography, ventilation and $P_{Œ}$ measurements
(when $P_{Œ}$ were not available, the line joining the values of the
diastolic PAP were taken as an image of the changes in P_{PL}) :
Group I : 10 patients with diffuse emphysema and unilateral giant
bullae (UGBE) compressing the lung parenchyma and shifting the
heart towards the controlateral side ; group II : 30 patients with
advanced panlobular emphysema (PLE) (pink puffers) ; group III :
30 patients with chronic bronchitis and/or centrilobular emphysema
(CB), (Blue bloaters). All patients were markedly short of breath
at exercise.

Table IV
Significantly different criteria in diffuse emphysema with
unilateral giant bullae (UGBE), panlobular emphysema (PLE) and
chronic bronchitis (CB) with identical $FEV_{0.1}$ (0,8 $\pm$ 0,3 1)
and $FEV_{0.1}/VC$ (35 $\pm$ 8%) (abbreviations in text).

	10 UGBE	30 PLE	30 CB
Chronic Cor pulmonale	0	3	16
TLC (% pred.)			
. He dilut.	88 $\pm$ 12	116 $\pm$ 14	94 $\pm$ 7
. Radiological	128 $\pm$ 11	139 $\pm$ 13	103 $\pm$ 8
PaO_2 (mmHg)	76 $\pm$ 8	73 $\pm$ 8	57 $\pm$ 8
$PaCO_2$ (-)	41 $\pm$ 3	40 $\pm$ 3	51 $\pm$ 6
Hematocrit	47 $\pm$ 4	46 $\pm$ 4	55 $\pm$ 7
PAMP (mmHg)	21 $\pm$ 2	23 $\pm$ 4	34 $\pm$ 5
CI ($1.min^{-1}.m^{-2}$)	2.4 $\pm$ 0.3	2.6 $\pm$ 0.3	3.4 $\pm$ 0.4
ΔP_{PL} (mmHg) (quiet breathing)	23 $\pm$ 3	18 $\pm$ 3	13 $\pm$ 3
max PAPP/min PAPP	1.5 - 5.0	1.3 - 4.0	1.0 - 1.5

Patients of group III were hypoxaemic, hypercapnic and polycythaemic, with cardiomegaly and pulmonary hypertension, but normal
cardiac index (CI) at rest and exercise. In spite of the clinical
severity of their disease the patients of groups I and II had near
normal PaO_2 and $PaCO_2$ at rest and hardly abnormal at exercise ;
they had neither polycythaemia or pulmonary hypertension ; their
cardiac size was normal or frequently markedly diminished and
CI was reduced at rest and severely impaired at exercise (Table V).
A similar difference between pink puffers and blue bloaters was
observed by Filley et al. (1968) and by Jones (1966) and a much
lower anaerobic threshold at exercise was noticed in pink puffers
by Marcus et al. (1970).
    In all patients of group II and in a number of patients of
group I, the PAP records elicited the following characteristic
features, which were never observed in group III :
a)large swings in P_{PL} and PAP $>$ 15 mmHg (Table IV).

Table V
Cardiac output at rest (R) and exercise (E) in chronic
bronchitis (CB), panlobular emphysema (PLE) and diffuse
emphysema with unilateral giant bullae (UGBE).

	10 CB		7 PLE		4 UGBE	
	R	E	R	E'	E	E
CI $(1.mn^{-1}.m^{-2})$	3.8	6.4	2.8	4.8	2.5	3.6
	0.7	2.5	0.4	0.6	0.2	0.3
VO_2/m^2 $(ml.mn^{-1})$	166	518	139	476	128	394
	38	110	22	96	19	72
$\Delta CO/ \Delta \dot{V}O_2$ (ml/100ml)	733		553		421	
	270		78		61	

b) absence of any pulmonary hypertension (im PAMP < 24 mmHg).
c) extreme and progressive narrowing of PAPP during expiration
coming sometimes to a nearly complete vanishing, after 3 or 4
systoles, at the end of expiration. The maximum PAPP at the end
of inspiration or at the beginning of expiration (Max. PAPP) being
1.5 to 5.0 times the minimum PAPP (Min. PAPP) (Table IV).
d) inverse relationship between the individual values of the PAPP
(taken as an image of the RVSV) of successive systoles and the
values of the P_{PL} (or the diastolic PAP taken as an image of the
P_{PL}) measured during the RA and RV filling period immediately
preceding each systole. So, the higher the P_{PL} (or the diastolic
PAP), the lower the PAPP, with a slope of $- 0.8 \pm 0.2$ mmHg/mmHg
(against $- 0,20 \pm 0,08$ in group III).

   All these abnormalities were markedly accentuated by hyperventilation at respiratory frequency 15-30, by exercise and by non
maximal forced expiration and apnea at lung volume inferior to
FRC and the CI was simultaneously decreased by 24 to 120%. On the
contrary, during slow hyperventilation at respiratory frequency
5 - 10 or during apnea at lung volume superior to FRC, PAPP and
CI increased dramatically, returning to normal or supernormal
values.

   By analogy with the VM, we hypothesized that venous return
was reduced during expiration, as a consequence of the elevation
of intrathoracic pressure and/or the displacement of the RA and
thoracic IVC by unventilated and rather uncompressible bullae.
Venous return and ventricular filling were reestablished during
inspiration, allowing for an unic normal systolic ejection at the
beginning of the next expiration. In 4 cases, cineangiography in
IVC clearly supported this hypothesis. Similar observations were
made by Nakhjavan et al. (1966) in 9/15 cases but the reverse
was demonstrated in the 6 others patients. In 8 cases, the surgical
removal of bullae (group I) or of highly distended and destroyed
emphysematous parts of the lung (group II) completely normalized

the cardiac size, the PAP records and the CI at rest and exercise, drastically improving the dyspnea and the clinical condition, without any important change in respiratory function data.

We concluded that in UGBE and in some PLE a kind of expiratory emphysematous cardiac tamponade occurs, severely limiting the cardiac adaptation to exercise. We suggest that is the reason why the surgical removal of such bullae improves the patients without changing significantly neither the spirometric data or the arterial blood gas. Finally, and paradoxically, in chronic bronchitis with cor pulmonale, the disability is not "cardiac" but rather "pulmonary", due to small airways lesions, altering the distribution of the local $\dot{V}A/\dot{Q}$ and severely impeding the gas exchange, whereas in severe emphysema (with large bullae or not) without cor pulmonale, the disability, traditionally considered as "pulmonary" and due to the reduction of the gas exchange surface area, could be mainly "cardiac" due to a mechanical circulatory failure induced by the large changes in pleural pressure. The questions which have now to be solved concerns the proportion of the patients with PLE suffering of this syndrome and the identification of reliable criteria to decide surgical treatment. Extreme overinflation, very small size of the heart, blockpnea, malaise or syncope at exercise, discrepancy between respiratory function tests and severity of the dyspnea, absence of hypoxaemia, hypercapnia, polycythaemia and chronic cor pulmonale, presence of specific abnormalities of the PAP records and abnormal adjustments of cardiac output to exercise are among these criteria.

REFERENCES

Ambiavagar, M., Sherwood-Jones, E., Roberts, D.V. 1967. Intermittent positive pressure ventilation in severe asthma. Anæsthesia 22 : 134.

Crowden, G.P., Harris, H.A. 1929. The effect of obstructed respiration on heart and lungs. Brit Med J. 1 : 440.

Elzinga, G., Van Grondelle., Westerhof, N. and Van Den Bos. 1974. Ventricular interference. Am J Physiol. 226 : 941.

Filley, G.F., Beckwitt, H.J., Reeves, J.T. and Mitchell, R.S. 1968. Chronic obstructive bronchopulmonary disease. II. Oxygen transport in two clinical types. Am J Med. 44 : 26.

Finucane, K.E. and Colebatch, H.J.H. 1969. Elastic behavior of the lung in patients with airway obstruction. J Appl Physiol. 26 : 330.

Fowler, N.O. 1978. Physiology of cardiac tamponade and pulsus paradoxus. I. Mechanisms of pulsus paradoxus in cardiac tamponade. Modern Concepts Cardiovasc Dis. 67 : 109.

Gunstone, R.F. 1971. Right heart pressures in bronchial asthma. Thorax. 26 : 39.

Helander, E., Lindell, S.E., Söderholm, B. and Westling, H. 1962. Observations on the pulmonary circulation during induced bronchial asthma. Acta Allergol. 17 : 112.

Howell, J.B.L., Permutt, S., Proctor, D.F. and Riley, R.L. 1961. Effect of inflation of the lung on different parts of pulmonary vascular bed. J Appl Physiol. 16 : 71.

Jones, N.L. 1966. Pulmonary gas exchange during exercise in patients with chronic airway obstruction. Clin Sci. 31 : 39.

Lauson, H.D., Bloomfield, R.A. and Cournand, A. 1946. The influence of the respiration on the circulation in man. Am J Med. 1 : 315.

Mac Fadden, E.R. 1976. Respiratory mechanics in asthma, in Bronchial Asthma. E.B. Weiss and M.S. Segal, Ed. Little Brown publ. Boston, p. 259.

Mac Fadden, E.R. and Ingram, R.H. 1976. Spirometry lung volumes and distribution of ventilation in asthma, in Bronchial Asthma. E.B. Weiss and M.S. Segal, Ed. Little Brown publ. Boston, p. 279.

Marcus, J.H., Mc Lean, R.L., Duffell, G.M. and Ingram, R.H. 1970. Exercise performance in relation to the pathophysiologic type of chronic obstructive pulmonary disease. Am J Med. 49 : 14.

Nakhjavan, F.K., Palmer, W.H. and Mc Gregor, M. 1966. Influence of respiration on venous return in pulmonary emphysema. Circulation. 33 : 8.

Permutt, S. 1971. Some physiological aspects of asthma. Ciba Found. Symp. Identification of Asthma. Churchill (Livingstone) London. p. 63.

Potter, W.A., Olafsson, S. and Hyatt, R.E. 1971. Ventilatory mechanics and expiratory flow limitation during exercise in patients with obstructive lung disease. J Clin Invest. 50 : 910.

Robotham, J.L., Lixfeld, W., Holland, L., Mac Gregor, D., Bryan, C. and Rabson, J. 1978. Effects of respiration on cardiac performance. J Appl Physiol. 44 : 703.

Robotham, J.L. and Mitzner, W. 1979. A model of the effects of respiration on left ventricular performance. J Appl Physiol. 46 : 411.

Santamore, W.P., Lynch, P.R., Meier, G., Heckman, J. and Bove, A.A. 1976. Myocardial interaction between the ventricles. J Appl Physiol. 41 : 362.

Sharpey-Schafer, E.P. 1962. Effect of respiratory acts on the circulation, in : Handbook of physiology. Section 2 : Circulation. III. American Physiological Society, publ. Washington.

Stalcup, S.A. and Mellins, R.B. 1977. Mechanical forces producing pulmonary edema in acute asthma. N Engl J Med. 297 : 592.

Summer, W.R., Permutt. S, Sagawa. K., Shoukas. A.A., Bromberger-Barnea, B. 1979. Effects of spontaneous respiration on canine left ventricular function. Circul. Res. 45 : 719.

Wexler, L., Bergel, D.H., Gabe, I.T., Makin, G.S. and Mills, C.J. 1968. Velocity of blood flow in normal human venæ cavæ. Circulation Res. 23 : 349.

Woolcock, A.J. and Read, J. 1966. Lung volumes in exacerbations of asthma. Am J Med. 41 : 259.

Discussion

BARER: I think this is probably very naive and I didn't understand, but are your pulmonary artery pressures in asthmatic attacks really raised relative to atmospheric pressure, or just to the pleural pressure?

EVEN: I think if you want to assess the stress applied to the right ventricle one must measure pulmonary artery pressure by reference to the pressure around the right heart that is to the pleural pressure.

BARER: That's quite right, but which pleural pressure.

EVEN: A difficult problem. What are you measuring when you are measuring pleural pressure? The first question is that the heart is surrounded by the pericardium and there are many workers who have demonstrated that changes of pericardial pressure are very similar to changes in pleural pressure except in very rare circumstances for example, continuous pressure breathing ventilation or something like that. The pleural pressure is a good reflection of pericardial pressure in the majority of the cases. Regarding your second point, to know what part of the pleural pressure is lost through the thoracic wall I cannot answer that question.

BARER: Which was your method?

EVEN: We have measured during asthma attacks, with the technique of Milic Emili in the supine position with the limitations of such a measurement when the weight of the heart exerts some action on the oesophageal balloon. I agree.

LOCKART: Do changes in posture affect the haemodynamic values in your subjects? Have you tried to do similar measurements in seated patients compared to what you've done lying?

EVEN: No never.

LOCKART: May I ask a second question? I've been told by my clinician friends that when these patients are taught respiratory manoeuvres they are taught to breathe very slowly, to have a very long expiration, and a very deep one. From your data I understand this may harm them rather than improve them. Have you tried this in your patients so that they perform similar type of breathing manoeuvres, such as those that they learn when they are trained so that you could see what is happening with a very deep and long expiration?

EVEN: You talk about emphysematous patients or asthmatic patients?

LOCKART: Emphysema.

EVEN: We have no measurements in other positions but fortuitiously, we have successive measurements at very different respiratory frequency. When the respiration is very slow there is no large increase in expiratory pulmonary artery diastolic pressure, suggesting that when pleural pressure is not too high, the pulse pressure in the pulmonary artery is maintained. But it is difficult to obtain that result, because a very small change in pleural pressure of perhaps 2 or 3 mm will suddenly change the pulse pressure. We have many records where the pulse pressure is normal, and with a very small increase in diastolic pressure the pulse pressure is squashed.

GUNELLA: On what basis and with what criteria do you diagnose panlobular emphysema and centrilobular emphysema.

EVEN: You ask about the selected criteria to classify centrilobular or panlobular emphysema. I use general criteria including clinical x-rays, blood gas analysis and so on. It is difficult to give you the list of all the criteria adopted, but schematically, the patients with history of chronic bronchitis with dyspnoea, fat patients with disorders of blood gas, moderate lung distention, but sometimes distention of an upper lobe, the existence of polycythemia and chronic cor pulmonale are in favour of the diagnosis of centrilobular emphysema or chronic bronchitis. It's very difficult, in vivo, to distinguish between severe chronic bronchitis and centrilobular emphysema, except by the procedure I have described. And we have classified the panlobular emphysema as the thin man (the pink puffer type) with an enormous overdistention predominating in the lower lobes, without increased bronchial markings on x-ray without sputum and so on. In any case, we have rejected the difficult cases where the symptoms were difficult to analyse and to classify.

GUNELLA: We have a series of 150 cases of chronic bronchitic patients, post-bronchitic pulmonary emphysematous cases. We could therefore consider them centrilobular as you say. In these patients at rest the arterial blood gas is normal and cardiac index is normal; pressure in the pulmonary artery is also normal as well as wedge pressure. In a standard exercise of 40 watts for 15 minutes there is no change in arterial gas analysis. We have an increase of about 30% of cardiac output compared to values at rest. This means that the cardiac output goes from an average of 3 litres per square m. to 4 litres. In 70% of emphysematous patients and 10% of bronchitic patients pressure in the pulmonary artery increases on average 30 mml of mercury and wedge pressure remains normal. I would like to know if you have an explanation. I think that among other things there may be an anatomical restriction of the pulmonary arterial bed but I would like to know whether you have any other explanation.

EVEN: I am not sure I have understood the question. You have studied many patients, in two groups: chronic bronchitis and emphysema. And in your emphysema group arterial blood gas was nearly normal. And you have studied at rest and on exercise, and you have observed either an improvement in artery blood gas or no change.

GUNELLA: No, no change.

EVEN: No change? I agree. And a normal increase in cardiac output, without a significant increase in driving pressure of pulmonary circulation. I am not sure that the question concerns the problem I have discussed. You speak about the shape of the pressure flow in the pulmonary circulation in chronic obstructive lung disease, and the cornerstone of your question, I think, is why the flow increases and driving pressure increases minimally. I think the explanation lies in recruitment when you increase a litre of the pulmonary artery flow you recruit new vessels formerly closed or partially closed, probably by the existence of zone I, zone II or zone IV of West distributed in the lungs where there is regional vasoconstriction in hypoventilated areas or localised increase in alveolar pressure squashing the capillaries in zone IV where the airways are totally obstructed and so on. In patients with severe panlobular emphysema and with that very special decrease in pulse pressure during expiration, have you considered a surgical solution? It is a practical but difficult problem to solve, I think.

THE ROLE OF THE PULMONARY VENOUS SYSTEM IN REGULATION OF

LUNG CAPILLARY BLOOD FLOW AND TISSUE EXCHANGE

Grant de J. Lee

Cardiac Department, John Radcliffe Hospital

Oxford, England

The prime function of the lungs is to accomplish efficient gas exchange between the blood flow through the pulmonary capillaries and the air ventilating their relating alveoli. Normally this process occurs over an enormous cardiac output range from 5 litres per minute at rest to perhaps thirty litres per minute in extreme exercise. Yet the lung capillary blood volume probably never exceeds 200 millilitres (Roughton & Forster 1957) and blood flow is accomplished in such a manner that the intra-vascular pressures within the capillaries rarely exceed the plasma osmotic filtration pressure, so that the Starling relation between the vascular and extra vascular compartments of the lungs is maintained and pulmonary oedema is avoided.

Dr.Gwenda Barer (1979) in her masterly review of the active control of the pulmonary circulation, has given a wide ranging detailed account of the physiological mechanisms responsible for regulating vascular haemodynamics to maintain homeostasis in the lung capillary circulation for optimal gas exchange.

In disease of the lungs, adaptive mechanisms must operate which re-distribute both blood flow and gas delivery away from diseased areas to the more normal parts of the lung. Again, in heart disease, particularly those conditions leading to increased impedence to venous outflow from the lungs into the left side of the heart, mechanisms must develop which partially protect the lung capillaries from experiencing the high vascular pressures present in the pulmonary venous system as a consequence of left heart disease. These mechanisms must exist to preserve the alveolar capillary system as a gas exchanging area rather than converting it to a plasma filtration system, manifest clinically

by pulmonary oedema. The activity of the lung lymphatic system
in draining the extra vascular spaces of the lung must also assist
in preserving the gaseous environment of the alveoli.

Because the peripheral resistance of the pulmonary arterial system
is low the pulsatile ejection of blood flow from the right ventricle
still remains pulsatile as it is propelled through the lung
capillaries (Lee and Du Bois 1955). Du Bois and his colleagues
(Menkes et al., 1970) also showed that this pulsatility was
achieved by recruitment of lung capillary systems dynamically in
the same way as West and his colleagues (1964) had shown to be
the case in the steady state in the isolated lung. These hydrostatic relationships are plainly dependent on the fact that the
alveolar capillary systems act as parallel resistors stacked
vertically upon one another in the erect posture, and indicate
how vascular pressure adjustments as well as zonal distribution
of flow can be achieved under real life conditions of pulsatile
blood flow. Thus at peak capillary flow rate the pulmonary arterial
pressure will momentarily exceed the alveolar gas pressures in all
areas of the lung so that all lung capillary systems will open to
accomodate blood flow. During diastole alveolar capillary systems
in the upper zones of the lung will cease to conduct blood flow as
the pulmonary arterial pressure within them falls below alveolar
gas pressure. This very simple physical relationship I believe
to be the most fundamental factor in regulating blood flow for
gas exchange through the lung capillaries and maintaining pressure
optimal to avoid excessive water transfer across the membrane.
It is the final common pathway in regulation whether or not changes
in pre-capillary or post-capillary impedence are affected passively
by such factors as alterations in lung mechanics during respiration,
changes in left atrial pressure, or changes in venous return resulting
from attenuations in systemic circulation. It is also the final
common pathway for homeostatic regulation in attenuation of
impedence due to active factors such as vaso active amines,
reflexes or vaso constriction due to alterations in arterial
oxygen tension, CO_2 tension and pH. The pattern of blood flow
in the capillaries is thus a function of the driving pressure
generated in the right ventricle modified by the transmission
characteristics of the pulmonary arterial bed, taking place both
physiologically and pathologically. Reuben and his colleagues
(1970) have shown that a reciprocal relationship exists between
pulmonary arterial resistance on the one hand and pulmonary
arterial compliance on the other hand. This relationship
implies that as the pulmonary arterial resistance increases, the
compliance of the arterial bed falls so that the product of
resistance and compliance remains constant. It is this
relationship which acts to preserve unchanged inflow pulsatility
to the capillaries, for an increase in pulmonary arterial
resistance alone would attenuate capillary pulsation. (Reuben
et al 1970; Reuben 1971).

The role of the pulmonary venous system in the regulation of
capillary blood flow is much less clear. Under normal conditions
the shape of the lung capillary flow pulse, measured by nitrous
oxide uptake in a body plethysmograph, resembles the profile of
the pulmonary artery pressure curve though somewhat delayed from
it in time (Karatzas & Lee 1969). Blood flow through the lung
capillaries seems largely uninfluenced by pressure events in the
left atrium in spite of the fact that there are no valves in the
pulmonary veins to prevent back pressure effects from reaching
the capillaries. This implies that episodic events due to left
atrial contraction must be damped out before reaching the capillaries
by virtue of some physical property of the pulmonary venous system.
Gillespie and his colleagues (1967) tried to study this assumption
in man by examining a situation in which isolated episodic, but
predictable changes in left atrial pressure occurred. They
examined the effects of left atrial cannon waves on capillary
blood flow in patients with congenital heart block, who have
normal left atrial pressures. They compared these with the same
effects on capillary blood flow pulsatility in patients with
acquired heart block and left ventricular failure in whom high
left atrial pressures were found. The patients with congenital
heart block had normal capillary flow pulsatility while in
patients with elevated left atrial pressures marked attenuation
of capillary blood flow pulsatility took place. This suggested
that in the normals the pulmonary veins were highly compliant
while in conditions of high venous pressure this compliance had
been eliminated. However, direct measurements of the distensibility
of the large extra-parenchymal pulmonary veins in man revealed
that they were virtually inextensible under all conditions(Banks
et al (1978). We have therefore undertaken studies to investigate
the nature of the de-coupling mechanisms which prevent left atrial
pressure events from attenuating lung capillary blood flow
pulsatility. These will now be described.

Our first studies were undertaken in open chested dogs. An electromagnetic flowmeter cuff was placed around the main pulmonary artery
and a catheter also inserted in order to measure instantaneous
pulmonary arterial pressure and flow simultaneously throughout
the cardiac cycle. At the same time, a cuff was glued around
one of the four pulmonary veins entering the left atrium to
measure vein flow continuously throughout the cardiac cycle.
The left arterial pressure and ECG were also monitered
continuously. In a number of studies the animal's chest was
then closed and capillary blood flow measured simultaneously
using the nitrous oxide plethysmograph method. Pulmonary arterial
inflow was pulsatile, lung capillary blood flow was similarly
pulsatile though attenuated compared with the main pulmonary blood
flow and slightly delayed in time due to the compliance of the
arterial system. Pulmonary venous flow was also pulsatile but
there was no arterialised pulsation to be seen.

The pulsations in the pulmonary vein were entirely different and invariably had a wave form which resembled an inverted record of the left atrial pressure. No pulsatile component of flow in the large pulmonary veins could be attributed to forward transmission of a flow pulse from the lung capillaries. Venous flow pulsatility was dominated by the changes in left atrial pressure taking place throughout the cardiac cycle (Rajagopalan et al., 1979a).

Simultaneous measurements of pulmonary vein velocity and left atrial pressure were also made in patients during routine cardiac catheterisation. These confirmed that similar relationships exist in man. In all cases the patterns of vein velocity was qualitatively similar to an inverted left atrial pressure wave. Where had the arterialised pulse from the lung capillaries disappeared to as it travelled down the pulmonary veins to the left atrium? Our next studies were designed to discover this. Again we used the dog as a model and designed experiments in which we could separate the venous outflow from the lungs to the left atrium by connecting the pulmonary vein of the left lower lobe of the lung to a constant pressure collecting reservoir to enable us to measure venous outflow independent of the left atrium. In other circumstances we could re-connect the pulmonary vein to the left atrium to measure vein flow in normal continuity with the left atrium.

When the veins were in direct continuity with the left atrium blood flow within them bore an inverse relationship to the pressure wave form in the left atrium throughout each cardiac cycle. However when vein flow was measured from the lungs with the pulmonary veins separated from the left atrium by diverting them into a constant pressure reservoir, vein flow resembled a lung capillary flow pulse, though delayed from it in time and reduced in amplitude.

The pulsatility of flow in the pulmonary veins, when separated from the left atrium, was further reduced when trans-capillary pressure was elevated by lung inflation. However in the intact state the relationship between the pattern of pulmonary vein flow and left atrial pressure remained unaffected by lung inflation and always showed an inverse relationship between pulmonary vein flow and the pressure wave form inthe left atrium. (Rajagopalan et al., 1979 b). We therefore postulated that the thin walled extra parenchymal pulmonary veins together behaved as a collapsible reservoir which could enable outflow from them into the left atrium to be determined purely by changes in left atrial pressure, in spite of variations in pulsatile inflow to the veins from the lungs.

I have already mentioned that when we compared the distensibility
of the large pulmonary veins external to the lung parenchyma with
those of the pulmonary artery we were surprised to find that at
all ages in man the pulmonary veins were virtually indistensible.
It was as if the pulmonary veins behaved as nylon tubes, while the
pulmonary arteries behaved as elastic ones. (Banks et al., 1978).
Thus we found that the pulmonary veins   acted as capacitance
vessels and damped out forward arterialised flow pulsations from
the lung capillaries in spite of being virtually indistensible.
We therefore considered that they might act by being collapsible
rather than distensible ones and this was achieved by their filling
or emptying over a very narrow transmural pressure range. This
would have the effect of damping out retrograde pressure pulses
from the left atrium to prevent them reaching the capillaries
and would also absorb any forward flow pulse coming from the
capillaries towards the left atrium. Once fully filled, the
veins could only accommodate more blood by distending. This
distension would be likely to be accompanied by a rapid
increase in pulmonary venous pressure.

The first requirement for hypothesis was that the pulmonary veins
should always assume a collapsed configuration at zero transmural
pressure. We proved this quite simply by taking pieces of main
pulmonary artery and pulmonary vein from both man and dog post
mortem and examined their shape when immersed in saline within a
glass vessel. The pulmonary artery remained almost circular
because of its more muscular walls while the pulmonary vein
collapsed flat. We called the collapsible dimension of the vein
its "minor" axis. We next compared blood flow within the pulmonary
veins with left atrial pressure and measured these changes
simultaneously with changes in the cross - sectional dimensions
of the pulmonary vein using minute ultrasonic crystals glued to
the vein walls with biological adhesive. The dimensions of both
the "major" and "minor" axes of the veins could thus be measured
(Rajagopalan et al., 1979C).

During "y" descent of left atrial pressure filling and again during
the "X" descent in left atrial pressure there was a concomitant
reduction in the dimensions of the "minor" axis of the pulmonary
vein. When pulmonary vein flow into the left atrium was reduced
during the left atrial "a" and "v" pressure waves the dimensions
of the "minor" axis of the veins increased. The changes in vein
dimensions could be corelated with changes in left atrial pressure
over a wide range. At low left atrial pressure all the changes
in dimensions took place in the "minor" axis. We used vagal
stimulation to produce alterations in left atrial contraction.
Large left atrial contractions could be produced with giant "v"
waves in the pulmonary veins. At high pulmonary venous pressure
the "minor" axis of the vein became identical to its "major" axis
so that the vein became circular. Over the normal venous

transmural pressure range of 0-12 mmHg the "minor" axis of the
pulmonary vein changed from a collapsed state to a circular one.
Above 10-12 mmHg both the minor and "major" axes of the vein
started to increase together as the vein began to distend to the
limits of it's compliance. We next measured the total capacity
of the pulmonary veins external to the parenchyma of the lung by
making silastic casts of the pulmonary venous system and left
atrium post mortem. In ten dogs we found that the average
combined volume of the extra-parenchymal pulmonary veins amounted
to 22.3 + 3.8 ml. The stroke volumes in these animals ranged
during life from 10-22 mls.

Thus the large pulmonary veins are capable of accommodating the
difference between the left atrial demands on the one hand and
the blood flow supplied to the veins from the capillary bed on
the other. We could demonstrate the importance of this by
producing pulsus alternans of the right ventricle alone by rapid
atrial pacing. Right ventricular ejection into the pulmonary
artery occurred at half the ECG heart rate while left atrial
contraction was maintained at the ECG heart rate. Pulmonary
vein flow from the lung capillaries was therefore only supplied
by every alternate beat from the right ventricle. However, when
we measured the pulmonary vein dimension we found that the episodic
dimensional changes of the "minor" axis of the pulmonary vein
distended during left atrial systole and collapsed during rapid
left atrial filling just as usual. However, the mean diameter of
the vein was larger during the cycles in which blood was supplied
from the right side of the heart and smaller during the cardiac
cycles associated with right ventricular asystole. Measurements
of blood flow rate from the pulmonary veins to left atrium
however, remain unaltered from beat to beat, indicating that the
pulmonary veins were capable of emptying into the left atrium
and maintaining left atrial filling virtually unaltered,
independant of beat to beat changes in right ventricular stroke
output.

We may thus conclude that both the arterial and venous inflow and
exit of blood flow to the lung capillary bed jealously preserve
its pulsitility and that these mechanisms are largely governed by
quite simple physical principles. On the arterial side, pulsitility
is preserved because of the reciprocal relationship between changes
in the resistance and compliance of the pulmonary arterial system
supplying the capillaries whether or not the pulmonary artery
pressure changes are as a result of physiological or pathological
causes. Within the capillaries, blood flow distribution will
depend upon the hydrostatic relationships existing between regional
alveolar capillary pressures and regional alveolar gas pressures
in mean flow terms, described by the waterfall effect (West et al.,
1964) modulated by a tidal effect due to recruitment of lung
capillaries during pulsatile ejection of blood flow by the right

ventricle. (Menkes et al., 1970).

Although we still have rather little information about how the pulmonary veins contribute to blood flow homeostasis within the lungs themselves (Smith & Butler 1975), we are reasonably confident about the role of the extra parenchymal pulmonary veins. They are collapsible structures which enable blood flow from the lungs to be accommodated and the left atrium to be supplied so that lung capillaries are effectively isolated from left atrial pressure events at physiological pressures. Only when the left atrial pressure exceeds the limits of distensibility of the large extra parenchymal pulmonary veins will retrograde conduction of pulses from the left atrium impede blood flow from the capillaries.

Why do the lungs so jealously preserve pulsatile blood flow in their capillaries? I believe the following to be a good working hypothesis; only during systole does the pressure in the lung capillaries temporarily exceed the equilibration level regulating the net inward direction of water flux between the capillaries and interstitium of the lung. During systole therefore, particularly in the dependant parts of the lung, the trans-capillary hydrostatic pressure will temporarily exceed oncotic pressure and a net flux of water outwards from capillaries to interstitium will occur. However, during diastole the intra-capillary pressure will once more fall below the oncotic pressure so that the net water flux will be back again from interstitium to capillary. During inactivity, the diastolic period of the cardiac cycle is longer than the systolic period so that the tendency will always be to maintain the alveolar capillary-interstitial system dry. However, during excercise both the heart rate and pulmonary capillary pressure will rise as a result of an increase in cardiac output. With severe exercise and diseases both tending to increase capillary hydrostatic pressure as well as heart rate, the net flux of water will tend to be outward from capillary to interstitium and the tissues will rapidly become charged with water. Breathlessnes will ensue even before clinical pulmonary oedema has occurred, because the process will reduce alveolar interstitial compliance. This will stimulate the J"receptors of Paintal (1977). These receptors are ideally placed to act as the afferent reflex sensors of breathlessnes. The result will be that the individual will stop exercising and return to his resting state with a consequent fall in heart rate so that once more the diastolic period of the cardiac cycle will become longer than the systolic period and the net flux of water from interstitium to cappillary will be reinstated once more.

The loss of intra-alveolar compliance is therefore likely to be fundamental in triggering the initial sensation of breathlessnes. An understanding of the patho-physiology of oedema therefore becomes vital knowledge. The forces governing the net fluid

movement across the capillary wall described by the Starling
relationship: -

$$Jv = Lp.A(Pc-Pi) - \sigma(\pi_c - \pi_i).$$

Where Jv = rate of interstitial fluid formation; Lp=capillary
filtration; A= filtering area of capillary wall; $(Pc=Pi)$ = transmural difference of hydrostatic pressure; $(\pi_c - \pi_i)$ = transmural difference of osmotic pressure σ = reflection coefficient.
The control of some of the hydrostatic factors affecting the
relationship between pulmonary capillary and pulmonary interstitial
fluid pressure have been aluded to above, but plainly a reduction
in capillary osmotic pressure or a rise in interstitial osmotic
pressure would also lead to an increase in fluid movement from
capillary to interstitium, with subsequent oedema. Hypoproteinemia
or over infusion with non-proteinous plasma expanders are two
obvious examples which could initiate this process in patients.
The third most important factor perturbing the Starling balance of
forces across the capillary wall, commonly overlooked by clinicians,
is an increase in capillary wall permeability by disease,particularly
hypoxia, bacterial and viral "toxins" etc.,vaso active amines,
chemicals and noxious gases.

The new challenge facing clinical investigators must surely be to
study the factors regulating lung capillary permeability in disease.
Non-invasive methods for measuring changes in capillary permeability
of the lung are now beginning to be available to us to enable these
studies to be made in patients.

REFERENCES

1. BANKS. J; BOOTH. F. V. McL; Mac Kay. E. H.;
    RAJAGOPALAN. B; & LEE. G. de J. (1978)
    The physical properties of human pulmonary arteries
    and veins. Clin.Sci. Mol..Med. 55 477.
2. BARER. G. R. (1979) Active control of the Pulmonary
    Circulation. Ex: Pulmonary Circulation in Health
    and Disease. Ed: Cumming. G. Pub;
3. GILLESPIE. W. J. ; GREENE. D. G. ;
    KARATZAS. M. B. & LEE. G. de J. (1967)
    Effect of atrial systole on right ventricular stroke
    output in complete heart block. British. Med. J. 1 75.
4. KARATZAS. N. B. & LEE. G. de J. (1969)
    Propogation of blood flow pulse in the normal human
    pulmonary arterial system: Analysis of the pulsatile
    capillary flow. Circulation. Res. 25. 11.
5. MENKES. H. A. ; SERA. K. ; ROGERS. R. M. HYDE. R. W;
    FORSTER. R. E. ; & Du BOIS. A. B. (1970) Pulsatile uptake
    of C.O. in the human lung. J. Clin. Invest. 49. 335.

6. LEE. G. de J. and Du BOIS. A. B. (1955).
   Pulmonary capillary blood flow in man.
   J. Clin. Invest. 34. 1380

7. PAINTALL. A.S. (1977). The nature and effects of
   sensory inputs into the respiratory centres. Fed.
   Proc. 36. 2428.

8. RAJAGOPALAN. B.; FRIEND. J. A. ; STALLARD. T and
   LEE G. de J. (1979a). Blood flow in pulmonary veins(1);
   Studies in dog and man. Cardiovasc. Res. in press.

9. RAJAGOPALAN. B.; FRIEND. J.A; STALLARD. T.; & LEE
   G. de J. (1979b). Blood flow in pulmonary veins (II);
   The influence of events transmitted from the right and
   left sides of the heart. Cardiovasc. Res. in press.

10. RAJAGOPALAN. B.; BERTRAM. C. D. ; STALLARD. T.; and
    LEE. G. de J. (1979c). Blood flow in pulmonary veins
    (III); Simultaneous measurements of their dimensions,
    intravascular pressure and flow. Cardiovasc. Res. in press.

11. REUBEN. S. R.; GERSH. B. J. SWADLING. J. P.; and LEE
    G. de J. (1970) Measurement of pulmonary arterial
    distensibility in the dog. Cardiovasc. Res. 4. 473.

12. REUBEN. S. R. (1971). Compliance of the human
    pulmonary arterial system. Circulation. Res. 29. 40.

13. ROUGHTON. F. J. W. and FORSTER. R. E. (1957).
    Relative importance of diffusion and chemical reaction
    rates in determining rate of exchange of gases in the
    human lung, with special reference to true diffusing
    capacity of pulmonary membrane and volume of blood in
    the lung capillaries. J. Applied. Physiol. 11. 290

14. SMITH. H. C. and BUTLER. J. (1975) Pulmonary venous
    waterfall and perivenous pressure in the living dog.
    J. Applied. Physiol. 38. 304

15. WEST. J.B. ; DOLLERY. C. T. : and NAIMARK. A. (1964)
    Distribution of blood flow in isolated lung; relation
    to vascular and alveolar pressure. J. Applied. Physiol.
    19. 713.

Discussion

CUMMING: This presentation is now open for discussion. While
people are thinking, perhaps I can ask a question to start the
discussion. In your estimates of the quantities of water in the
various compartments you showed 4.4 ml. per hundred for blood, 4.6
ml. per hundred for tissue fluid, and 2.8 ml. per hundred for
cellular contents. That adds up to 11 ml. per hundred ml. roughly
one third of the water content of lungs. Where is the remainder?

LEE: It depends very much on the volume characteristics of the
lung. That is why it is difficult to relate that curious index to
the known measurements. Because we had to have a counting volume
that we knew about. And so we had to put on very arbitrary
restrictions, and I suspect it's to do with the degree of lung
inflation.

CUMMING: It would mean that your lungs are grossly hyperinflated.
Is that the direction in which they tend to be?

LEE: No. The other thing is that we particularly used areas of
lung away from the major conducting vessels. So that is the content
of water, more or less, with least conducting vessels and most gas
exchanging vessels.

CUMMING: Yes. That would grossly change the ratios I agree.

LEE: The director of the school in his presentation talked about
history and science and referred to Aristotle. In fact Socrates
used to teach his children by asking awkward questions. And it's a
fact that Gordon's children are very intelligent. I suspect because
of the awkward father they have. First of all I have an active
prejudice which involves gravity. If you have a thin wall vessel
that is not strong enough to maintain its shape and you expose it to
gravity, it will collapse and in the open chested dog there will be
a minor and major axes in these vessels and that is what you
observe.

CUMMING: That I accept.

LEE: I cannot tell you that in the gravity less situation, that
that could occur. That is why the simple study of putting the vein
and the artery in a water bath was done. And again, the general
weight of a tissue that is not exactly identical to water produces a
collapse. This is not too important in the body, because if the
dimensions of those vessels change over a very narrow transmural
pressure, the pressure events in the left atrium will dominate the
situation and act as a pump, either sucking or preventing inflow.
And I think that's the explanation. Now, as far as the interstitial
pressure is concerned, I was very careful to say that I did not know

about the intraparenchymal pulmonary veins. I know a certain amount about the compliance of the pulmonary artery. It is an elastic structure. So throughout the lung there is a second, more dynamic reservoir working in series with the non-dynamic reservoir.

CORRIN: Grant, you just mentioned the elastic structure of the pulmonary artery. I'm sure in your studies of the pulmonary veins you have examined the structure of those and are well aware that these consist almost entirely of elastic tissue, so you must have puzzled over this apparent paradox that elastic structures are inelastic.

LEE: When we did these studies I took care to work with a professional pathologist, who preferred morbid anatomical work, undertook morphometric counts of the amount of collagen and elastin and muscle in the media or whatever. I can't remember the figures complete. They are published. In fact there is more collagen in the count than we expected, perhaps something to do with the thinness of the wall. There is some distention, but very little, you reach the limit of that distensibility. The other strange thing is that the content of the vessel changes with age. And in fact more elastic tissue, I think, if I remember rightly, occurs with age, and yet they become less distensible. This is the pulmonary artery I'm talking about now. And I believe it is all to do with the volume distention characteristics.

CUMMING: Can I confirm, Grant, that you measured volume distention and not linear extensibility, in these vessels?

LEE: I'm afraid we took circles and measured linear extensibility.

CUMMING: Did you measure the extensibility longitudinally or circularly.

BONSIGNORE: There are some discussions about the efficiency of the pulsatile flow and pulsatile volume, in comparison with constant flow and constant volume. Somebody says that constant flow and constant volume are more efficient than pulsatile ones. What is your explanation?

LEE: I'm so influenced by my teacher of the week that I have to enter semantics and ask what do you mean by efficient. The efficiency of the pump is what those people are talking about, but in terms of gas exchange another kind of requirement is necessary I believe.

BARER: Did your nitrous oxide method really tell us whether the flow in individual capillaries is pulsatile or only the whole bed.

LEE: You are absolutely right. We were only concerned with the bed, as a whole. Keith Horsfield told you a little bit about the capillaries and all sorts of different permutations take place. The dominant feature in a resting intact mammal of our size with our orientation is to recruit capillaries, until such time as all those vessels are open. Thereafter, the only way that blood can get through faster is to be pushed harder. I was interested in some of the papers earlier this week about diffusing capacity and pulmonary artery pressure. Because they differ from some of the early reading which I have worked on as a useful hypothesis. There is a very fashionable tendency in my country and, I suspect, in others for undertaking something called 'medical research'. That is doing the same experiment again, when in fact if you look at the literature there is a lot of buried information. Now, the early work on the pressure-flow characteristics in the pulmonary artery was done by Andra Cournand and he showed that pulmonary artery pressure was related to cardiac output and to oxygen consumption, in a rather special way, with an inflection point around about 12 litres or more a minute, I think 2000 cc of oxygen uptake. Another pupil of his migrated to Baltimore, named Dick Riley who did the early work on oxygen diffusing capacity. He found the situation where the diffusing capacity for oxygen went up, and then came an inflection about the same point. As a working hypothesis this tells me that recruitment is important at rest and when the vessels have been recruited the only way of increasing flow for gas exchange would be to use the membrane more efficiently by pushing the blood through it more rapidly. The diffusing capacity would tend to fall because there is not much area increase and it is at this point that the resistance of the lung becomes linear.

DENISON: Could I return to the efficiency of gas exchange in capillaries, and whether it is a good or a bad thing for blood to be moving? And I think that one of the very exciting discoveries of recent times has been that it is wiser for a blood cell to be moving than to be stationary, in order for it to pick up oxygen. And the proper image for a blood cell should be a sack full of marbles. The marbles are the haemoglobin molecules, and when the red cell moves all the marbles in the sack roll over each other, and the red cell moves along the vessel with its membrane acting as a tank track. And many elegant experiments have shown that this is a great advantage to oxygen uptake. On the other hand we can imagine that if blood is pumped into the pulmonary capillary, the longer it stays there the more oxygen it's going to pick up. And at first sight it would seem very wise to give it square wave front and then wait. I wonder if you have any information on the relative merits of these two ways of trying to transfer oxygen in the lung.

LEE: I have two reasonably firm working hypotheses that I would like to see disproved. And they will lead to Midhurst in particular. And I'm sorry to repeat them, because they know them well, but for the others it might be important. Our chairman has spent a lot of time talking about the delivery of blood molecules for gas exchange. Down the respiratory bronchioles or the main bronchi there is bulk flow, until you reach the gas exchanging areas, where the movement of those oxygen molecules becomes diffusional. By analogy you would squirt in a plug of bees, and then the bees buzz around exchanging nectar. Nectar being CO_2. So there is a random walk of molecules, so none of the alveolus is wasted, because as soon as oxygen is exchanged another molecule can take its place. If you put blood in that vessel, and it spreads over the sheet, it will exchange oxygen, and if it's done like that there will be a waste of space. But we know that with this capillary pulsation, that the exchanging systems are being recruited, generally. And when blood flow exists, plugs are delivered for gas exchange. But there's a time constant, all the path lengths to the capillaries are different, we then have to know what the state of affairs is in what Sobin and Fung called the sheet. A fenestrated sheet of capillaries with plugs in it, which are the corners of the alveoli. And Keith Horsfield is finding it very difficult to know how many supply arterioles enter and how many veins leave. In Britain it is a very common pleasure for people to ring bells in churches on Sundays. It is call change bell ringing. A good peal of bells has 8 bells, and 8 factorial combinations of tunes can be played. If there were 8 supply capillaries into a sheet, structured like a bagatelle board there will be 8 factorial ways of delivering cells through that sheet. And one would have the most enormous opportunity for a random walk of red cells. It's an absolutely diabolically exciting question, clearly difficult to get out.

ELECTRON MICROSCOPY OF PULMONARY OEDEMA

B. Corrin

St. Thomas's Hospital Medical School *

CAUSES OF PULMONARY OEDEMA

The major mechanisms responsible for pulmonary oedema traditionally come under two headings: hydrostatic and cytotoxic. Thus oedema of the lungs may be due to hydrostatic/oncotic forces acting on vessels of normal permeability, or to cytotoxic factors which enhance permeability irrespective of pressure gradients. Tracer substances normally retained within the blood stream are thought to distinguish between these two mechanisms by escaping when cytotoxic factors increase vascular permeability. It has been demonstrated however that permeability is affected by purely hydrostatic forces, so blurring the traditional distinction between hydrostatic and cytotoxic oedema (Pietra et al., 1968; Schneeberger and Karnovsky, 1971). Nevertheless it is convenient to consider the causes of pulmonary oedema as acting under one or other of these two mechanisms. Hydrostatic factors include: 1) capillary hypertension as in mitral stenosis; 2) reduction in the osmotic pressure of the blood as in overhydration; 3) self-regulatory changes in the oncotic forces of the pericapillary tissues brought about by oedema itself which diminish the further loss of fluid from the vessels; 4) lymphatic obstruction as in carcinomatosis; 5) deficiency of pulmonary surfactant, as in the respiratory distress syndromes of infancy and adult life, this substance not only preventing collapse but also keeping the lungs dry. Cytotoxic factors are primarily exogenous: 1) physical such as irradiation; 2) chemical such as paraquat, oxygen in high

* Present address: Cardiothoracic Institute, Brompton Hospital, Fulham Road, London SW3 6HP

concentrations, monocrotalline alkaloids, alloxan,α-naphthylthiourea;
3) infective; 4) allergenic. These are often augmented by the
endogenous chemicals of inflammation and shock.

DISTRIBUTION OF PULMONARY OEDEMA

        Postural effects dictate that oedema is greater in the more
dependent parts of the lung but this section is concerned more
with the distribution of the extravasated fluid between the
interstitial and alveolar spaces. Pulmonary oedema has reached a
very late stage when it can be demonstrated by wringing watery
fluid out of the excised lungs or showing microscopically that
the alveoli are completely flooded. Before this the oedema fluid
accumulates in the pulmonary interstitium which in the sheep can
absorb 500 ml before any reaches the air spaces (Staub 1974).
The pulmonary interstitium is most obvious in the centres of the
acini around the airways and arteries and in the interlobular
septa, which become evident radiologically as Kerley B lines.
Less obvious in eosin-stained sections is the connective tissue
of the interalveolar septa, but this is readily apparent in
reticulin or elastin-stained preparations. It is at this site that
oedema is first detectable with the electron microscope (Pietra
1978).

        Within the interalveolar septa the capillaries veer from
side to side, protruding first into one alveolus and then the other.
At these points gas exchange is facilitated by extreme thinning of
the alveolar epithelium and endothelium, and by the interstitial
elements being reduced to the fused basement membranes of these
lining cells (Fig.1). The total thickness of the air-blood barrier
at these points may measure as little as 0.4 nm, with the fused
basement membranes occupying as little as 0.05 nm of this.
Oedema fluid does not accumulate in this portion of the septum
until a late stage, when intra-alveolar filling has also developed.
On the opposite side of the capillary is the thick part of the air-
blood barrier where collagen, elastin, interstitial cells and nerve
fibres come between the endothelial and epithelial basement
membranes (Fig.1). The interstitial cells include alveolar macro-
phage precursors, fibroblasts and contractile myo-fibroblasts.
Associated with the scleroproteins there is abundant ground substance
consisting of hydrophilic glycosaminoglycans and these soak up the
water like a sponge. Separation of the interstitial fibres and
cells by electron-lucent oedema fluid is the first alteration
detectable in pulmonary oedema (Fig.2). Because it is situated in
the thick part of the air-blood barrier interstitial oedema fluid
does not unduly affect gas exchange, and with the rales of intra-
alveolar fluid not yet detectable, the only clinical feature of
interstitial oedema may be tachypnoea due to stretching of the
J-receptors.

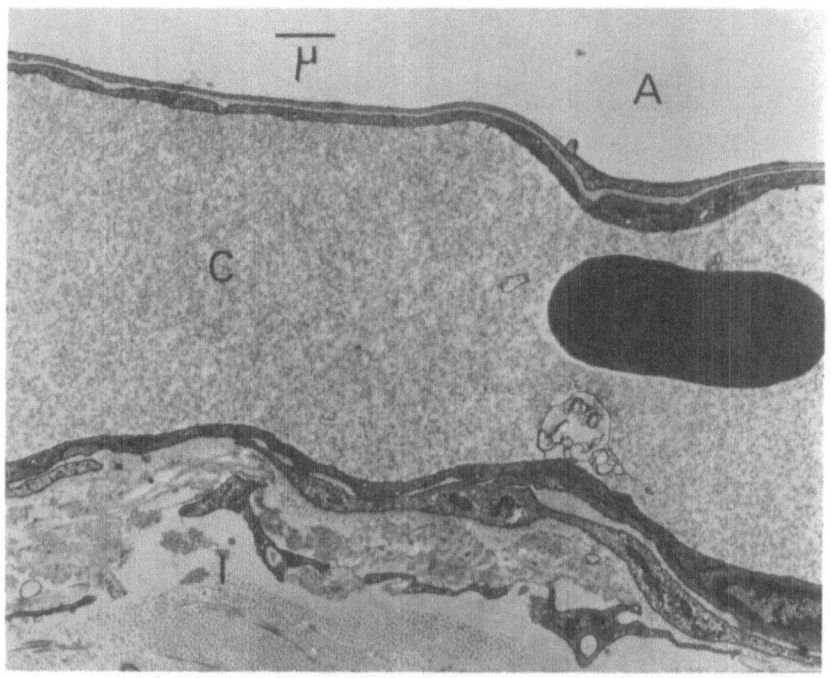

Fig. 1.   Normal interalveolar septum. Thin part of the air-blood barrier above, thick part below. A, air space; C, capillary; I, interstitium.

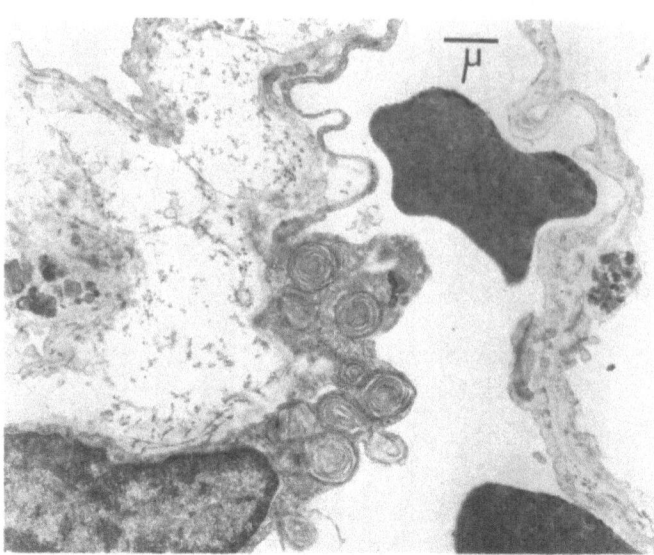

Fig. 2.   Rat subjected to heavy iprindole dosage. Lamellar
inclusions in the alveolar capillary endothelium (centre) and
epithelium (right) indicate cytotoxic damage. To the left there is
widening of the thick part of the air-blood barrier by electron-
lucent oedema fluid.

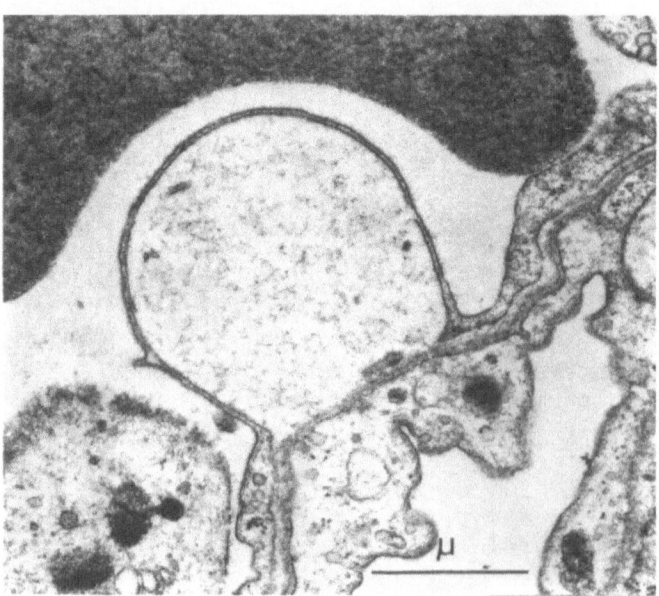

Fig. 3.   Iprindole treated rat. Interstitial oedema fluid lifts
the alveolar capillary endothelium off its basement membrane.

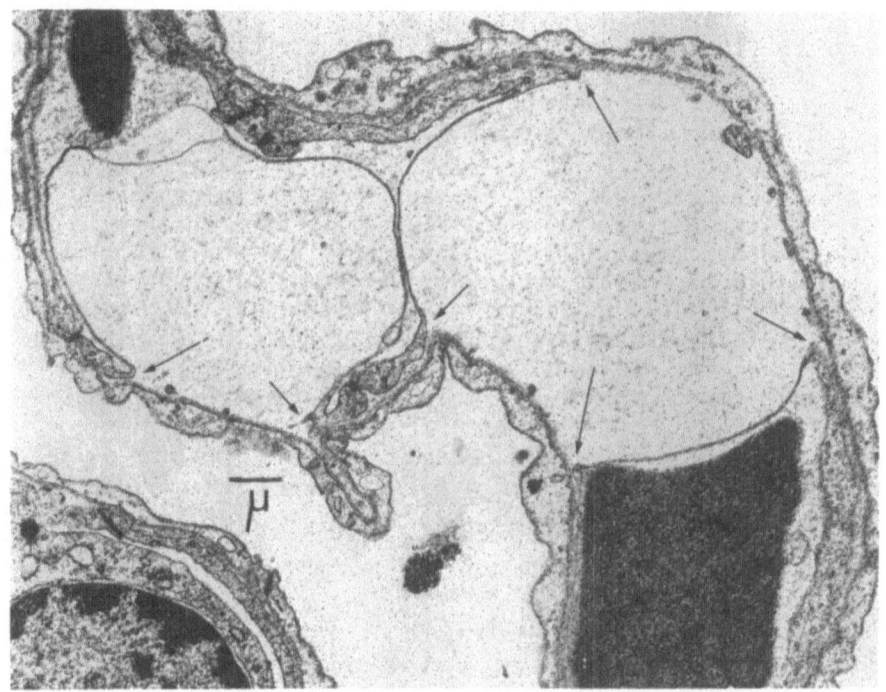

Fig. 4.   Iprindole treated rat. Extensive sub-endothelial blebbing pushes the endothelium against the opposite wall of the alveolar capillary. Arrows indicate points of reflection.

A striking feature of interstitial pulmonary oedema is a
lifting of the capillary endothelium from its basement membrane so
that it protrudes into the capillary lumen like a blister (Fig.3).
Such blebs may reach the opposite wall of the capillary and completely block the lumen (Fig.4). Obstruction of the capillary bed
in this manner may be quite widespread yet still be accommodated by
the reserve capacity of the pulmonary vasculature because it does
not appear to cause pulmonary hypertension (Vijeyaratnam and Corrin,
1974). West et al., (1965) attributed certain shifts of pulmonary
blood flow distribution to perivascular fluid permitting the
closure of small arteries, but blebbing of the capillary endothelium
could provide an alternative or additional structural basis for
these alterations in blood flow.

ROUTES OF FLUID MOVEMENT IN PULMONARY OEDEMA

Fenestrated endothelial cells may be found in the periphery
of the fibrotic lung but in the normal lung they are confined to the
bronchial capillaries (Suzuki, 1979). Although labelling experiments
indicate that it is bronchial venules which are leaky in septic
shock (Pietra et al., 1974), in most other forms of pulmonary oedema
they indicate that the fluid escapes from pulmonary capillaries and
venules (Pietra et al., 1974; Hurley, 1978), which are lined by
a continuous type of endothelium. Fluid transport across the
pulmonary endothelium is intercellular or by vesicular carriage.
Cytotoxic factors may also promote oedema by causing endothelial
fragmentation and disintegration (Fig.5).

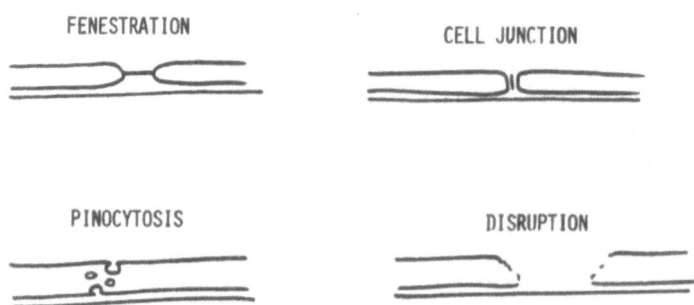

Fig. 5.   Possible routes of fluid escape across vascular
endothelia. In the lung, fenestrations are confined to the bronchial
circulation. Cell junctions have a 4 nm gap and pinocytotic vesicles
measure 50-80 nm. Gross damage results in complete disruption of
the cytoplasm.

Endothelial cell junctions in the pulmonary capillaries form belt (zonulae) rather than spot (maculae) joins but are nevertheless of adhering (adherens) rather than sealing (occludentes) type, with an intercellular gap of about 4 nm. Alveolar epithelial cell junctions on the other hand form belt seals (zonulae occludentes). Thus when Schneeberger-Keeley and Karnovsky (1968) injected horseradish peroxidase intravenously the tracer was observed between endothelial cells, within the interstitium and between epithelial cells up to their junctions, but not in the alveolar lumens. The endothelial and epithelial basement membranes appeared to present no barrier to fluid transport whatsoever. Although this work convincingly demonstrated that the epithelium formed the major barrier to fluid movements from vessels to air spaces, it appears that the ready passage of peroxidase through endothelial cell junctions was dependent on the injection of the tracer in large volumes of saline (Schneeberger and Karnovsky, 1971). At physiological pressures small molecular weight tracers such as myoglobin, horseradish peroxidase and haemoglobin are largely retained within the vessels (Table I). This blurs the distinction between hydrostatic and cytotoxic oedema by showing that purely physical forces affect permeability. More useful indicators of cytotoxic damage are large molecular weight tracers such as colloidal thorium and carbon which remain intravascular at high perfusion pressures and only escape in large amounts when there is cytotoxic damage (Table II, Fig. 6).

Table I, showing the distribution of various intravascular markers in the lung at different perfusion pressures, after Pietra (1978).

INTRAVASCULAR MARKER	MOLECULAR WEIGHT	PULMONARY ARTERY PERFUSION PRESSURE			
		5-15	30	35-50	50 mmHg
Cytochrome c	12000	I	I	I	A
Myoglobin	17000	V	I	I	A
Horseradish Peroxidase	40000	V	I	I	A
Haemoglobin	64500	V	V	I	A

V = Intravascular, I = Interstitial, A = Intra-alveolar

Table II, showing that large colloidal particles remain within
the vessels even at high perfusion pressures. Escape of these
substances indicates marked cytotoxic effects. From Cottrell
et al., 1967 and Pietra 1978.

INTRAVASCULAR MARKER	PARTICLE SIZE (nm)	DISTRIBUTION OF MARKER AT 30-40 mmHg PERFUSION PRESSURE
Horseradish Peroxidase	4	Interstitial
Colloidal thorium	7	Intravascular
Colloidal carbon	25	Intravascular

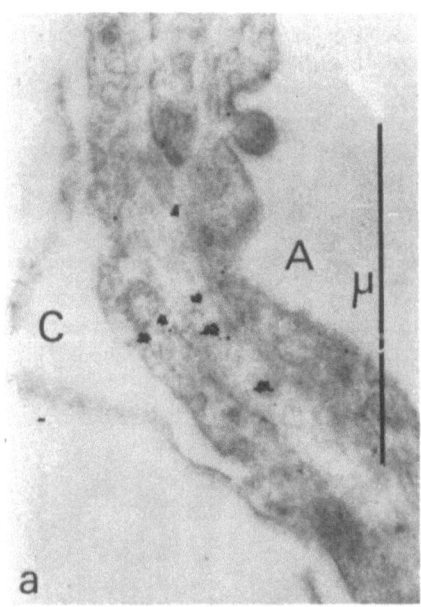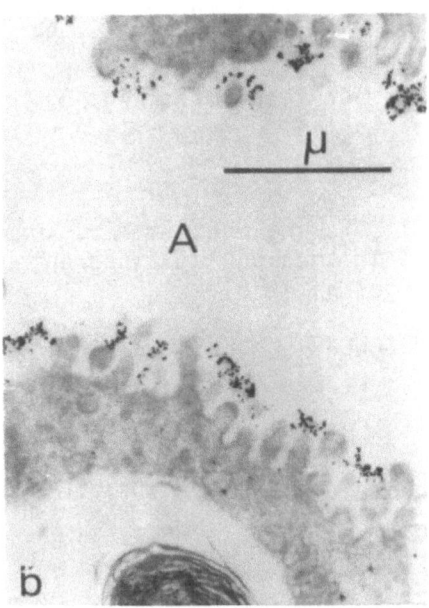

Fig. 6.   Iprindole treated rat injected intravenously with
colloidal thorium 3 minutes before being killed.
a) Thorium particles are seen within an endothelial cell junction
    and the alveolar interstitium. A, air space; C, capillary.
b) Many thorium particles are within the alveolar lumen lining
    the epithelial cell surface. A, air space

Large molecular weight colloidal tracers may escape without any obvious structural change in the endothelial cell junctions but very severe permeability alterations are accompanied by gaps in the endothelium. Such gaps may represent either foci of cytoplasmic disruption or widening of the intercellular junctions. Whilst oxygen poisoning causes extensive destruction of the endothelium (Kapanci et al., 1969) the endothelial gaps seen inα-naphthylthiourea poisoning appear to represent widening of the intercellular junctions for they are largely confined to the thick side of the air-blood barrier where the junctions are most numerous (Hurley, 1978). Widening of the intercellular clefts could be effected by contracture of the myofilaments demonstrated in pulmonary capillary endothelial cells by Bensch et al. (1964).

Small amounts of large molecular weight substances escape from normal pulmonary vessels and these are thought to pass through "pores" larger than intercellular junctions. Such "pores" are probably represented by the fusion of pinocytotic vesicles which measure 50-80 nm diameter and can be shown to take up large molecular weight substances such as ferritin (M.W. 500,000 daltons) (Schneeberger-Keeley and Karnovsky, 1968).

Extravasated fluid within the alveolar interstitium normally finds its route to the air spaces blocked by the epithelium and it drains centrally towards the more abundant connective tissue about the centriacinar arteries and bronchioles, presumably following pressure gradients. At this site are found lymphatics, vessels which do not exist at the alveolar level. Lymphatics in the lung have been extensively studied by Lauweryns (1971). They are valved and their capillaries differ from blood capillaries in the following respects: the lumen is large in relation to wall thickness; the endothelium is very thin with poorly developed junctions; adjacent endothelial cells overlap; the basal lamina is discontinuous but connected to adjacent connective tissue fibres by anchoring filaments. When the connective tissue ground substance is swollen by oedema fluid, the anchoring filaments are stretched and the lymphatics are opened up rather than compressed. Dilated lymphatics are thus a prominent feature of pulmonary oedema. It is likely that the lymphatics can increase their capacity tenfold, thereby keeping the lungs dry despite large increases in water filtration (Staub, 1970). Greater degrees of vascular fluid loss will however overload even this efficient drainage mechanism and the oedema fluid will spill over from the interstitial to the alveolar compartment. The route is unknown but it is generally assumed that there is finally an opening up of the tight junctions between epithelial cells.

SUMMARY

Intra-alveolar fluid accumulation is a relatively late feature

of pulmonary oedema which first affects the interstitial tissues.
Whereas the endothelium of the bronchial capillaries is fenestrated,
the pulmonary endothelium is normally of the continuous non-
fenestrated type with prominent pinocytotic activity involving
vesicles 50-80 nm diameter. Cell junctions in the pulmonary endothelium are zonulae adherens with a narrow (4 nm) gap. In hydrostatic oedema there are often no ultrastructural alterations in the
endothelium, but in cytotoxic oedema there may be widening of the
endothelial cell junctions and degeneration or severe disruption of
the cytoplasm. The alveolar epithelium is also continuous and shows
prominent pinocytosis, but the epithelial cell junctions are zonulae
occludentes (tight junctions) and the epithelium is the principal
barrier to fluid movement between the tissue and air spaces. The
interstitium of the inter-alveolar septim is continuous with that
around the major vessels and airways and lymphatics commence at the
level of the terminal bronchioles.

ACKNOWLEDGEMENTS

     Fig. 1 by courtesy of D. Bowes. Figs. 2,3,6b from
Vijeyaratnam and Corrin, J. Pathol. by permission. Pat Robbins,
Asit Das and Gordon Watson provided valuable secretarial and tech-
nical assistance.

REFERENCES

Bensch, K.G., Gordon, G.B. and Miller, L., 1974, Fibrillar
        structures resembling leiomyofibrils in endothelial cells of
        mammalian pulmonary blood vessels, Z. Zellforsch., 63: 759-766.
Cottrell, T.S., Levine, O.R., Senior, R.M., Wiener, J., Spiro, D.
        and Fishman, A.P., 1967, Electron microscopic alterations at the
        alveolar level in pulmonary edema, Circul. Res., 21: 783-797.
Hurley, J.V., 1978, Current views on the mechanisms of pulmonary
        oedema, J. Pathol., 125: 59-79.
Kapanci, Y., Weibel, E.R., Kapla, H.P. and Robinson, F.R., 1969,
        Pathogenesis and reversibility of the pulmonary lesions of
        oxygen toxicity in monkeys: Ultrastructural and morphometric
        studies, Lab. Invest., 20: 101-128.
Lauweryns, J.M., 1971, The blood and lymphatic microcirculation of
        the lung, in: "Pathology Annual", Vol. 6, S.C. Sommers, ed.,
        Appleton-Century-Crofts, New York.
Pietra, G.G., 1978, The basis of pulmonary edema, with emphasis on
        ultrastructure, in: "The lung", W.M. Thurlbeck and M.R. Abell,
        eds., Williams and Wilkins, Baltimore.
Pietra, G.G., Szidon, J.P., Carpenter, H.A. and Fishman, A.P., 1974,
        Bronchial venular leakage during endotoxin shock, Am. J. Pathol.,
        77: 387-406.
Pietra, G.G., Szidon, J.P., Leventhal, M.M. and Fishman, A.P., 1969,
        Hemoglobin as a tracer in hemodynamic pulmonary edema, Science,

166: 1643-1646.

Schneeberger, E.E. and Karnovsky, M.J., 1971, The influence of intravascular fluid volume on the permeability of newborn and adult mouse lungs to ultrastructural protein tracers, J. Cell Biol., 49: 319-334.

Schneeberger-Keeley, E.E. and Karnovsky, M.J., 1968, The ultrastructural basis of alveolar-capillary membrane permeability to peroxidase used as a tracer, J. Cell Biol., 37: 781-793.

Staub, N.C., 1970, The pathophysiology of pulmonary edema, Human Path., 1: 419-432.

Staub, N., 1974, Pathogenesis of pulmonary edema, Amer. Rev. Resp. Dis., 109: 358-372.

Suzuki, Y., 1969, Fenestration of alveolar capillary endothelium in experimental pulmonary fibrosis and of normal bronchial capillaries, Lab. Invest., 21: 304-308.

Vijeyaratnam, G.S. and Corrin, B., 1971, Fine structural alterations in the lungs of iprindole treated rats, J. Pathol. 114: 233-239.

West, J.B., Dollery, C.T. and Heard, B.E., 1965, Increased pulmonary vascular resistance in the dependent zone of the isolated dag lung caused by perivascular edema, Circulation Res., 17: 191-206.

Discussion

CUMMING: Thank you very much Brian. For many years there was a
battle as to which part of medicine was the most nearly akin to an
exact science, the battle raged, I think, between the physiologists
and the biochemists. There was no argument at all about who was the
bottom in the relationship to an exact science, and that was the
pathologists. It was a descriptive art. Now it seems to me, having
heard two presentations this week from pathologists, that that
branch of medicine which is now most closely akin to the exact
science has become, imperceptibly, the pathologists. Because here
we see a technique for looking at molecules of about 40,000 pieces,
4×10^4, not 4×10^{30} that Professor Zichichi was talking about;
and here we've got a method of looking at collections of cells and
finding out their precise structure, their aggregation. So, it's a
great compliment that I say to the pathologists it seems that you
now carry the banner of the approach to the exact science in
medicine.

This paper is now open for discussion.

WILLIAMS: The vesicles which you have shown as the result of toxic
substances, we have also produced.

CORRIN: Here you are referring to the subendothelial blebs?

WILLIAMS: Subendothelial vessels. We have also produced them in a
high altitude simulation chamber, with exposures as short as 12
hours. They were very prolific and totally blocked many of the
capillaries. I wonder if you'd ever quantitated these
subendothelial blebs and whether they played any part in the
deterioration of lung function seen in high altitude pulmonary
oedema in mountaineers and climbers.

CORRIN: I'm not sure whether I stressed sufficiently that these
are not a specific feature of any particular type of oedema but are
common to all forms of oedema, cytotoxic, hypoxic and hydrostatic.
My thoughts when seeing them were that the pulmonary circulation
must be arrested by them, and certainly it must be arrested in that
particular capillary. I noted the comments of West and colleagues
that interstitial oedema seems to redirect blood to other parts of
the lung, but my own suspicion was that this must surely produce
pulmonary hypertension. But, as I told you, we look for evidence
of that both microscopically and by weighing the right ventricles,
and there is none at all. So, as I said, I can only conclude that
it really demonstrates a tremendous reserve capacity of the
pulmonary vasculature. I haven't attempted to quantitate them, but
like you I have observed them, they are very easy to find and are

very numerous.

HAUGE: There is presumably a hydrostatic pressure gradient from
the interstitium to the intra-alveolar space and to the space
surrounding large vessels and bronchi. And there we have an
extra-vascular fluid pathway for oedema. This pressure gradient is
probably there also in normal situations. You mentioned that fluid
accumulation first started in the alveolar septal space and
thereafter there was a filling and a cuff formation around vascular
structures. I would have thought that if there is such a pressure
gradient removing fluid from the air spaces, that the filling up of
the alveolar walls would be a rather late event, only occurring when
these drainage pathways were in some way obstructed or if its
capacity was not great enough. In your view it was the other way
around, it was only at the later stage that the cuff was formed.
There is a group working in Copenhagen which thinks that pinocytotic
vesicles do not move at all. That they are connected by narrow
tubes to the spaces on each side of the endothelial membrane and
that materials pass through these channels. They have made serial
sections, showing that vesicles pass to and fro across the wall.

CORRIN: I've never observed any structural communications between
one pinocytotic vesicle and the next, or between a pinocytotic
vesicle and the cell membrane, until the vesicle comes in contact
with the cell membrane and then appears to fuse with it. Could you
tell me what diameter they are? Because the importance we attach to
the pinocytotic transfer is that it is capable of taking up large
molecules, such as ferritin, plasma proteins, and anything less than
the diameter of the vesicle, which is quite a substantial structure.
Anything considerably less than that could not function as a
transfer mechanism for these large molecules. It is impossible to
follow movements in fixed tissues, so I cannot be categorical about
this, but I haven't seen any evidence of any interconnecting
channels, and if there are small ones I doubt whether they would
fulfill the function that we envisage. Your other point was why is
the site at which oedema fluid congregates first in the
interstitium, in the interalveolar septum, or in the prominent
interstitial cuffs around the large blood vessels and airways. The
literature is controversial on this. Perhaps I should have
emphasised that Fishman and his co-workers believe that in septic
shock the leakage is in the peribronchiolar region. Heard has
demonstrated on the other hand that the leakage is first in the
intra-alveolar septum, but of course you are really asking where it
will rapidly move and be seen. It has also been stated that the
first site at which it becomes apparent is in the interalveolar
septum, but this perhaps does remain a controversal point.

CUMMING: If I may comment briefly on that, Anton Hauge suggests
that these are not pinocytotic vesicles, but rather microtubules.
It's a very attractive hypothesis, because if you look at transport

of molecules in the cell, the diffusion path length is far too great, by an order of magnitude, to satisfy the nutritional requirements. Thus the hypothesis that there are microtubules from which substrates can gain access to the cell is an attractive one. It is merely a theoretical concept, but it perhaps suggests that we should look with more care and see whether these are microtubules or not.

HEATH: I wonder if I might ask two questions about phospholipid, which has cropped up in your paper on two occasions. The first of these is that in Peru we noticed that the lamas, living at very high level show a pronounced degree of hyperplasia of their Clara cells in the respiratory bronchioles.

CUMMING: Would you like to say what Clara cells are?

HEATH: Yes. Clara cells are normal ciliated cells which occur in the bronchiolar tree largely and cast off the distal portion of their cytoplasm into the bronchial tree, non ciliated. They have intense activity. When you look at the Clara cells of lamas which have been born and bred in England and which have never moved into a hypoxic environment in their lives, when you look at those lamas the Clara cells are quite quiescent. I know that you believe that it is possible that Clara cells might be concerned with surfactant activity. Do you think this difference between high altitude and low altitude lamas is connected possibly with surfactant activity? The second question I would like to ask is on a related subject. You showed these pictures of pulmonary endothelial cells. Did you suggest that these represented 'indigestible remains' of some sort? I have always considered these things to be very closely related to disorders of phospholipid, especially phospholipid metabolism. We've found those structures in chlorophentermine poisoning, in which again the basic problem is disorders of phospholipid metabolism. So, are you quite certain that these structures you've shown are so non specific as you said?

CORRIN: They do have a remarkable structural similarity to the surfactant secretory bodies of the type 2 alveolar epithelial cells, which I think is quite incontrovertible evidence that that cell secretes surfactant. We did ask ourselves whether this could be excessive surfactant secretion. There is acid phosphatase in these vesicles, but then so there are in the type 2 cells, acid phosphatase being the lysosomal enzyme. We found then, as you did in the Clara cells, in the type 1 epithelium, perhaps this could represent a metaplasia towards surfactant production by these cells, but as I have shown, we found them in the endothelium. It seems beyond comprehension that the endothelial cells would be making surfactant. As far as I know the blood spaces do not require surface active agents. And in the liver and kidney, when these are subjected to chemical toxins, there is excessive lysosomal degradation of mast cell organelles by this process of autophagocytosis. The part of the chemistry of the cell which lysosomal enzymes are weakest at breaking down are the complex lipids, so these accumulate as residual bodies and because they consist of phospholipids they take up this lamellar structure which the phospholipid surfactant also takes up. So I do think this is evidence of cytotoxicity. Your other question relates to ther Clara cell, and I'm glad of this opportunity to say someting about the Clara cell. Etherton and Conning have demonstrated secretion in decapitated cells, suggesting apocrine activity. They also produced autoradiographic evidence purporting to show that this was surfactant secretion in a retrograde direction down into the alveoli. I think you and we are the only groups who report this apocrine activity of Clara cells, and I now take this opportunity in public of retracting my former views leaving you perhaps alone, Donald, because I've since observed a similar blebbing on the surface of ciliated cells. And I'm rather shifting to the view of Jeffery that this is another artefact of electron microscopy. At the moment I have no definite view of this as the function or even the means of secretion of the Clara cell but the small electron dense granules in the apical surface of the cell must be looked at with interest, and it is the secretion of these which Conning suggests is the function of the cell.

CUMMING: Thank you. May I just add a supplementary? It is a characteristic of phospholipids that they are very polar molecules, and therefore in the surface are aligned perpendicularly to it; you referred to the characteristic that they have a strong tendency to spread out in an even film, hence their name 'surfactant'. In the slide you showed, we had the surfactant heaped up, at one point it was ten times thicker than another. Do you think that can be a matter of fixation, or how do you explain this paradox of the chemical requirement for a thin film and the demonstration of a grossly different thickness?

CORRIN: The alveolus is not spherical and so in its corners we have an accumulation of lining foam which is very thick, whereas in the flatter parts it is thin.

CUMMING: I would accept that explanation, were it not for the fact that the site at which this heaping up occurred was linear. Anyway, I have raised the point, as you say, there are many complications in interpreting electron micrographs, and I thought you might consider this.

POSITIVE AIRWAY PRESSURE AND LUNG EDEMA

Anton Hauge and Gunnar Nicolaysen

Institute of Physiology
University of Oslo
Oslo, Norway

Introduction

The litterature dealing with the events which follow after induction of positive airway pressure is vast and - sometimes, bewildering. Mead and Whittenberger[1] in their chapter on "Lung inflation and hemodynamics" in Handbook of Physiology pointed out that articles on this subject commonly include the phrase "this controversial field," in the first paragraph. Since that was written our knowledge and understanding of the effect of positive airway pressure on general hemodynamics (venous return, total O_2 transport) has increased considerably. The effects on lung edema, however, still remain to be clarified.

For many years there was a commonly held opinion that positive pressure in the airways counters water accumulation in the lungs. Thus, in 1938 Barach et al.[2] wrote that this treatment will maintain a backward pressure against the pulmonary capillary wall and thereby inhibit the leakage of edema fluid. Likewise, Ashbaugh et al.[3] in 1969 stated that continuous positive pressure breathing reduces interstitial edema by increasing interstitial pressure. On the other hand Wagner et al.[4] and more recently, Alexander et al.[5] found that airway pressure per se does not influence edema formation. Demling et al.[6] even found that at comparable net intra-vascular filtration pressures, dogs ventilated at a higher end-expiratory pressure accumulated more extravascular lung water. Similar results were obtained by Thornton et al.[7].

Much of the confusion is due to the fact that observations made under special circumstances are used to formulate general relation-

ships. Methods for continuous, quantitative monitoring of pulmonary
edema formation in an intact individual do not exist. When a situation of increased transvascular fluid flux is created in an experimental animal the circulatory state at the outset and before application of positive pressure ventilation, is usually not strictly
defined. The start of positive pressure ventilation, whether it is
of the continuous or intermittent type, will cause a change in a
number of variables, all of which influence the transvascular fluid
filtration rate. The net result will therefore be difficult to
analyze.

    When we started our work in this field some years ago we
decided to avoid experimental designs which involved simultaneous
changes in a large number of variables. There was no lack of "multi-
factorial" studies. What was needed (we thought) was investigations
in which each experimental step taken should include only one
specific and defined type of change. Ultimately, results from a
number of such experiments could be pieced together, and, with luck
and perseverance, a complete and coherent picture appear. Such an
approach is common in neurobiology where investigators move from
relatively simple organisms like leeches, or from in vitro preparations to more complicated species and sub-systems in situ.
Although it is fashionable to look with disapproval on studies carried
out on isolated lung preparations, they nevertheless continue to
yield valuable information which otherwise would have been virtually
unobtainable. One unique advantage is that they allow very accurate
settings of in- and outflow pressures as well as alveolar and transpulmonary pressure.

    For the present studies we have used isolated plasma-perfused
rabbit lungs. The details concerning the preparation is published
elsewhere[8]. The perfused rabbit lungs maintain a normal vascular
resistance without spontaneous edema formation for at least 6 hr
of perfusion and ventilation. The ultrastructure of the alveolo-
capillary membrane is normal after at least 4 hr of perfusion.

    We have studied the effect of changes in airway pressure on the
net transvascular fluid filtration under conditions of constant
vascular pressures, relative to atmospheric, and, in some cases, at
constant flow. A situation of slow steady transvascular fluid flux
could be created by elevating vascular hydrostatic pressures, either
left atrial pressure only or both arterial and venous pressures.
Fluid filtration or reabsorbtion was monitored gravimetrically.
The pressure in the humidified, thermostated perfusion chambers,
outside the lungs ("pleural pressure") could be altered independently
of alveolar pressure. By this arrangement alveolar pressure could
be changed with or without a change in transpulmonary pressure and
thereby lung volume. Furthermore, a given rise in lung volume could
be obtained either by a rise in alveolar pressure or by a reduction

in pleural pressure. This was useful when the role of extra-alveolar vessels was considered. The pump and the venous reservoir were both positioned outside the perfusion chamber. Since pleural pressure in some of the experiments was used as an independent variable we chose to relate all pressures, vascular, alveolar and pleural, to atmospheric. This does not preclude the introduction of e.g. vascular transmural pressures in the analysis since pleural pressure is known, in absolute terms, throughout the study. It is important to note that the experiments were never carried to the stage of alveolar flooding. The studies on zone III lungs[9] were done in collaboration with Dr. Gunnar Bø, present address Department of Anaesthesia, Rikshospitalet, Oslo.

Simultaneous and Equal Changes in Alveolar and Transpulmonary Pressures

In these experiments the lung surfaces were exposed to atmospheric pressure and vascular pressures kept constant. A given rise in alveolar pressure would therefore increase transpulmonary pressure by the same amount, and lung volume increase. In the majority of the zone III lungs such a rise in alveolar pressure caused reversible reductions in the fluid filtration rate (FFR). A reasonable explanation is that alveolar pressure is transmitted to the perimicrovascular space in the alveolar septae. This implies that hydrostatic interstitial fluid pressure increases, thereby reducing net filtration pressure. This explanation does not, however, account for the cases in which the opposite effect, i.e. a rise in FFR, was observed. Since lung volume increased with the rise in alveolar pressure we assumed that the perivascular pressure of the extra-alveolar vessels would fall. The true extra-alveolar vessels always expand with a rise in lung volume[1], even at constant vascular pressure. Furthermore, there are observations in the litterature indicating that extra-alveolar vessels may contribute to fluid shifts in lungs[10,11,12]. What we were looking at could therefore be a combined effect of a rise in the interstitial hydrostatic pressure of the septal vessels and a fall in the perivascular pressure of extra-alveolar vessels. The balance of these two opposite effects could differ from lung to lung. One way of testing this possibility would be to exclude one of the two sets of pulmonary exchange vessels. This was done by placing the lungs in an all zone I condition, thereby excluding alveolar septal vessels from consideration[13]. The result of these experiments was again, however, that an equal rise in alveolar and transpulmonary pressure, with the concomitant rise in lung volume, caused a reduction in FFR. This was the case in 7 of 8 lungs[14]. This observation makes it unlikely that the true, expanded extra-alveolar vessels play any important role in the fluid shifts, certainly not under zone I conditions, nor in zone III.

Which vessel segments do then take part in the fluid shifts observed under zone I condition? We favour the socalled corner or junctional vessels. They appear to be mainly capillaries[15] positioned in the junctions where several alveoli come together. We have shown that they are patent in our zone I lungs[14]. Since we found that a rise in alveolar pressure caused a reduction in FFR in the zone I lungs, it follows that changes in alveolar pressure is transmitted also to the interstitial fluid around these vessels. If this is the case, corner vessels should gradually be compressed as alveolar pressure is increased. To our knowledge no information is available concerning the relation between corner vessel dimensions and lung volume, except that they are not collapsed even far into zone I[16].

It remains to explain that in a few cases, both in zone III and zone I lungs, a rise in alveolar pressure increased FFR. Since large vessels undoubtedly are radially stretched when lung volume is increased, it is reasonable to assume that the pressure just outside these vessels is reduced whenever alveolar pressure is increased at constant pleural pressure. Indirectly such an interstitial pressure reduction around larger vessels and bronchi, may well cause a pressure reduction also in the peri-microvascular space around septal and corner vessels. This would favour filtration across the exchange vessels. An additional effect of a rise in lung volume may be a reduction of the resistance in the extra-vascular fluid pathways from the peri-microvascular space to the interstitial space around larger vessels and around bronchi, where edema cuffs are formed. Such an effect would also tend to increase the net filtration pressure across the exchange vessels. Thus, what we observed, both under zone III and zone I conditions, may have been the net result of (1) the direct transmission of alveolar pressure to the peri-microvascular space and (2) the indirect effect on interstitial tissue remote from the exchange vessels. The balance of these two effects may vary from one lung to another. The volume-effects as outlined above would expectedly be most pronounced in highly compliant lungs.

Changes in Transpulmonary Pressure at Constant Alveolar Pressure

A given change in lung volume can be brought about either by a change in alveolar pressure as described above or by a reduction in pleural pressure. According to the above analysis one might have expected the same effect on transvascular fluid filtration of a lung inflation regardless of the technique employed as long as (a) the change in lung volume is the same and (b) the alveolar and vascular pressures are kept constant. Both positive and "negative" pressure inflation will decrease the interstitial hydrostatic pressure surrounding the large vessels and the airways. There is, however, an additional effect, not directly volume-related, which should also be taken into account when quantitative studies are made: When pleural pressure is reduced relative to vascular pressure the hydrostatic pressure gradient across some vessels will increase. Alveolar septal vessels are probably not influenced in this way. It is however, a distinct possibility that the interstitial hydrostatic pressure of the corner vessels is directly affected by changes in pleural pressure[17]. If this is the case these vessels are influenced both by alveolar and pleural pressure. The interstitial pressure around the true extra-alveolar vessels most likely is reduced whenever pleural pressure is lowered. This will be an effect which comes in addition to that caused solely by a rise in lung volume.

Taking these various considerations into account what type of change in FFR should one predict when pleural pressure is reduced at constant alveolar and vascular pressures in our zone III and zone I lungs? In zone III the net filtration pressure of the alveolar wall (septal) capillaries could increase slightly due to a decrease in the resistance of the extravascular fluid pathway and/or due to a decrease in the interstitial hydrostatic pressure at the end of the drainage pathway, around large vessels and bronchi, where the lymphatic network origines. The net filtration pressure of the corner vessels could increase for the same reasons and in addition, as mentioned above, due to a direct transmission of pleural pressure changes to the perivascular space of these vessels. If the true extra-alveolar vessels contribute at all to the fluid shifts it will be in the direction of an increase in FFR, since the transmural pressure will increase. The effect on corner vessels and true extra-alveolar vessels will be the same in zone I as in zone III.

Our results under both types of zone conditions are in complete agreement with these theoretical considerations: Without exception we found that a decrease in pleural pressure reversibly increased FFR.

Changes in Alveolar Pressure at Constant Transpulmonary Pressure

The above experiments suggest that a rise in alveolar pressure at constant vascular pressures cause an increase in the perivascular hydrostatic pressure in the alveolar septae (in zone III lungs) and junctions, leading to a reduction in net transvascular filtration . pressure and a reduction in FFR. This effect can be countered by a simultaneous rise in lung volume, making the net outcome as regards FFR unpredictable. If, however, lung volume is kept constant, a rise in alveolar pressure should without exception cause a reduction in FFR. This can be accomplished by elevating alveolar and pleural pressure in parallel and by the same amount. Pleural pressure elevation will reduce the transvascular pressure gradient in vessels

positioned outside the alveolar septae, and should expectedly reduce
FFR in zone I lungs. This manoeuvre is equivalent to a reduction
in vascular pressures relative to pleural pressure. It is therefore
- almost - selfevident that a smultaneous rise in alveolar and
pleural pressure will reduce the rate of transvascular fluid filtration in zone III as well as in zone I, as also pointed out by
Permutt[17].

We found without exception that this was the case, and that
the change in FFR was reversible and reproducible in each individual
lung preparation.

Concluding Remarks

Our results have been obtained under the special circumstance
that vascular pressures are kept constant relative to atmospheric.
That changes in cardiac output will influence vascular pressures
and cause transvascular fluid shifts in the lungs, is uncontrovers-
ial. Cardiac output as a variable has therefore been deleted from
our analysis.

We emphasize the following points: A rise in alveolar pressure
at constant pleural pressure cause an increase in the hydrostatic
pressure of the perimicrovascular space around alveolar septal and
corner vessels, thereby reducing net transvascular fluid filtration.
A reduction in pleural pressure at constant alveolar pressure
reduces the perimicrovascular hydrostatic pressure around the corner
vessels, thereby increasing net transvascular fluid filtration.
Both manoeuvres will cause a rise in lung volume, which has the
additional effects of decreasing the resistance in the extravascular
fluid pathway and reduce the interstitial hydrostatic pressure at
the end of the intrapulmonary drainage pathway, around large vessels
and bronchi.

A parallel and equal rise in both alveolar and pleural pressure
is equivalent to a reduction in vascular transmural pressures in all
the exchange vessels, and will always reduce the rate of fluid
filtration.

The effect of positive pressure ventilation on net transvascular fluid filtration will therefore, provided absolute vascular
pressure are kept constant, depend on whether the direct pressure-
transmission or the volume-related effects dominate. In most cases
the latter effects are, according to our findings, of minor
importance.

Our data give the alveolar corner or junctional vessels an
important role for the fluid exchange function of the lungs.

REFERENCES

1. J. Mead and J.L. Whittenberger, Lung inflation and hemodynamics,
   In: Handbook of Physiology. Sect. 3. Respiration. Vol. I.
   Washington, D.C., Amer. Physiol. Soc. (1964).
2. A.L. Barach, J. Martin, and M. Eckman, Positive pressure respiration and its application to the treatment of acute
   pulmonary edema, Ann. Internal Med., 12:754 (1938).
3. D.G. Ashbaugh, D.L. Petty, D.B. Bigelow, and T.M. Harris,
   Continuous positive-pressure breathing (CPPB) in adult
   respiratory distress syndrome, J. Thoracic Cardiovascular
   Surg. 57:31 (1969).
4. E. Wagner, P.A. Rieben, K. Katsuhara, and P.F. Salisbury,
   Influence of airway pressure on edema in the isolated dog's
   lung, Circulation Res. 9:382 (1961).
5. L.G. Alexander, W.C. DeVries, and R.W. Anderson, Airway
   pressure and pulmonary edema formation, Surg. Forum, 24:231
   (1973).
6. R.H. Demling, N.C. Staub, and L.H. Edmunds, Jr., Effect of
   end-expiratory airway pressure on accumulation of extra-
   vascular lung water, J. Appl. Physiol. 38:907 (1975).
7. D. Thornton, H. Ponhold, J. Butler, T. Morgan, and F.W. Cheney,
   Effects of pattern of ventilation on pulmonary metabolism and
   mechanics, Anesthesiology, 42:4 (1975).
8. A. Hauge, and G. Nicolaysen, Studies on transvascular fluid
   balance and capillary permeability in isolated lungs, Bull.
   Physio-Pathol. Respirat. 7:1198 (1971).
9. G. Bø, A. Hauge, and G. Nicolaysen, Alveolar pressure and lung
   volume as determinants of net transvascular fluid filtration,
   J. Appl. Physiol.: Respirat. Environ. Excercise Physiol.,
   42:476 (1977).
10. L.D. Iliff, Extra-alveolar vessels and edema development in
    excised dog lungs, Circulat. Res., 28:524 (1971).
11. H.C. Smith, V.F. Gould, F.W. Cheney, and J. Butler, Patho-
    genesis of hemodynamic pulmonary edema in excised dog lungs,
    J. Appl. Physiol. 37:904 (1974).
12. R.K. Albert, S. Lakshminaraayan, T.W. Huang, and J. Butler,
    Fluid leaks from extra-alveolar vessels in living dog lungs,
    J. Appl. Physiol.: Respirat. Environ. Excercise Physiol.,
    44:759 (1978).
13. J.B. Glazier, J.M.B. Hughes, J.E. Maloney, and J.B. West,
    Measurements of capillary dimensions and blood volume in
    rapidly frozen lungs, J. Appl. Physiol. 26:65 (1969).
14. G. Nicolaysen, and A. Hauge, Determinants of transvascular
    fluid shifts in zone I lungs, J. Appl. Physiol.: Respirat.
    Environ. Excercise Physiol., In press.

15. J. Gil, Influence of surface forces on pulmonary circulation,
       in "Pulmonary Edema," A.P. Fishman and E.M. Renkin. eds,
       American Physiological Society, Bethesda (1979).

16. D.Y. Rosenzweig, J.M.B. Hughes, and J.B. Glazier, Effects
       of transpulmonary and vascular pressures on pulmonary blood
       volume in isolated lung, J. Appl. Physiol. 28:553, 1970.

17. S. Permutt, Mechanical influences on water accumulation in the
       lungs, in: "Pulmonary Edema," A.P. Fishman and E.M. Renkin.
       eds., American Physiological Society, Bethesda (1979).

Discussion

GUNELLA: I would like to go back after these interesting logical trials on animals and come to the clinical aspect. When we have to treat patients with pulmonary oedema it has been mentioned that there is interest in ventilation by positive pressure. Now, ventilation by positive pressure is not merely a semantic matter; there are attendant technical problems concerning the positive pressure to apply. I would like to know first of all if you can give us any indication particularly as regards the type of positive pressure you use - continual, intermittent or positive pressure with possible application of a respiratory pause or a type of ventilation which today seems fashionable that is intermittent mandatory ventilation. Secondly, I would like to know if you could give us the possible repercussion of positive pressure on pulmonary arterial pressure, on the right ventricle and on cardiac output. The problem for doctors in reanimation is how to use a particular type of positive pressure without causing further damage to the haemodynamics of their patients both on the right as well as on the left heart.

CUMMING: Perhaps you could add also the benefits of breathing against a column of water.

HAUGE: Well, as you know, the experiments I was telling you about were done under very artificial circumstances, and the way we created positive pressure was to maintain a constant alveolar pressure during the periods where we measured fluid filtration rates. That is to say the lungs were not ventilated, they were just connected to a pressure source, either the airways, a lobe, or the airways and the pleural surface. This pressure source consisted of air with carbon dioxide added. So there was no ventilation in these experiments. That was the way we arranged it in order to detect a steady slope of fluid filtration and of course that is quite different from the intact situation. Concerning the effect of vascular resistance we looked specifically for effects of alveolar oedema or interstitial oedema on the pulmonary vascular resistance and we saw no systematic changes or of interstitial oedema. That was a surprise to us, we had expected that the vessels might be reduced in dimensions and that their resistance could go up. Concerning the pressure in the left atrium, another point of these experiments was that we kept atrial pressure constant. That was one of the main points. This made it easy for us, so we had time to control all the variables which the clinicians must consider. So I'm afraid I have just to escape that question.

CUMMING: That's a great pity. I think the anaesthetist would tell us that in patients with pulmonary oedema the administration of end expiratory pressure causes a more rapid resolution of the oedema, but taking Gunella's point, this often has complications for the haemodynamics, due to the raised intrapleural pressure, and its effect on the filling both of the right and left heart which I think was your problem.

HAUGE: Could I add? I think the main success of positive pressure on lung oedema is at the stage when alveolar fluid has started to accumulate because it keeps the alveoli open and presents collapse. That is an obvious benefit but I don't think it has been proved that it has a beneficial influence on interstitial filling or transvascular fluid filtration.

CUMMING: No, I agree. It is only when there is alveolar flooding - the clinical state of pulmonary oedema.

PRESSURE-FLOW-VOLUME RELATIONSHIPS IN THE NORMAL HUMAN

PULMONARY CIRCULATION AT SEA-LEVEL AND AT ALTITUDE

Alain Lockhart
Laboratoire d'explorations fonctionelles
Hôpital Antoine Béclère
92141, CLAMART, FRANCE

INTRODUCTION

Doctor Lee showed us this morning beautiful data about pulsatility of blood flow in the pulmonary circulation. That pulmonary blood flow is pulsatile in arteries, (1) and capillaries (2,3) is well documented. The distribution of blood volume in the different series components of the pulmonary circulation varies continuously throughout the heart cycle with a large fraction of right ventricular stroke volume being stored during systole in the arteries from which it runs off in to the capillaries and veins during diastole (4). Finally since ventilatory action also affects the pulmonary circulation through its effects on both intrathoracic pressure and venous return (3,5,6), it may seem naive to continue studying the relationships between mean pulmonary blood volume (PBV), mean pulmonary blood flow ($\dot{Q}$), mean pulmonary inflow (arterial) and outflow (left atrial or pulmonary wedge) pressure (Ppa and Pw respectively) whose respective values are averaged over several respiratory cycles and more cardiac cycles.

Naive though this approach may be it is the only practical one due to the anatomy of the pulmonary circulation and to the limitation of presently available techniques. Because there are four pulmonary veins which cannot be simultaneously catheterized, instantaneous flow and pressure at the outlet of the pulmonary circulation cannot be measured. This precludes two-part analysis of instantaneous pressure-flow relationships in the human pulmonary circulation. Whereas undistorted pulmonary arterial pressure waveforms are easily obtained with miniaturised transducers (7), the derivation of instantaneous blood flow from blood velocity measured with catheter mounted

electromagnetic or ultrasonic transducers is fraught with
difficulty (8). Lastly there is no technique to measure
instantaneous changes in the overall pulmonary blood volume and
in its distribution in the different parts of the pulmonary
circuit.

This presentation represents an attempt to demonstrate the
usefulness of the easily measurable time-averaged values of
PBV, $\dot{Q}$, Ppa and Pw to gain some insight on the haemodynamics of
the human pulmonary circulation.

A SIMPLIFIED MODEL OF THE PULMONARY CIRCULATION

The pulmonary circulation can be represented by a single
equivalent tube extending from the pulmonary valve to the
opening of the pulmonary veins in the left atrium. In any
given situation the "tube" contains a quantity of blood PBV and
is traversed by a steady flow $\dot{Q}$ which is associated with the
driving pressure (Ppa - Pw)

Measurement of pressure and volume

When a catheter-external manometer is used measured
pressure depends on the hydrostatic reference level the choice
of which is somewhat arbitrary since the actual location of the
hydrostatic indifferent point of the pulmonary circulation is
ill-defined (9). Therefore, whereas comparisons of pulmonary
vascular pressures in different situations may be misleading, P
can be meaningfully compared e.g. with postural changes.

PBV can only be measured in man by use of non-diffusible
indicators injected and sampled at appropriate sites in the
circulation (10). Depending on the technique used the measured
volume may include a fraction of left atrial volume, and is the
pulmonary circulating blood volume, i.e. the volume of blood in
all perfused territories. Vessels which are not perfused are
by-passed by the indicator and their volume is not included in
the measured PBV. Although attempts have been made to determine
the fraction of PBV contained in the arterial side of the
pulmonary circuit (11). PBV as usually measured yields no
information about the distribution of blood within the
pulmonary circuit. Morphometric evidence suggests that the
volume of blood in arteries, microcirculation and veins is
approximately 120, 250 and 150 ml respectively (12,13).

Pulmonary vascular resistance (PVR)

The definition of pulmonary vascular resistance is an
operational one. Pulmonary vascular resistance is the value
obtained by dividing cardiac output into the difference between

mean pulmonary arterial and mean pulmonary wedge(or left atrial pressure): $PVR = \Delta P / \dot{Q}$. It is the modulus at a frequency of zero, or in other words the D.C. component of pulmonary vascular impedance (14).

One is faced with the problem of assigning a physiological meaning to calculated PVR, this is done by applying Poiseuille s equation to the simplified model of the pulmonary circulation.
Thus,

$$PVR=(8.\eta.L)/(\pi.r4)$$

where η is the viscosity coeficient respectively of a single tube of length L and radius r, having the same energy-dissipating properties as the pulmonary vascular system. Although blood is not a Poiseuillan liquid, can be taken as constant in a given subject and comparable between subjects whose haematocrit lies within normal limits. In the geometrical factor L/r^4, L can be taken as constant. Thus r, which represents the overall cross-sectional area of the pulmonary vascular bed, is the variable factor on which Poiseuillan PVR is dependent

In such a network of parallel pathways as the pulmonary vascular bed, the cross-sectional area is a function of both number and radi of all individual units. In physiological terms r increases - and PVR falls - with recruitment and/or distension of pulmonary vessels; conversely r decreases- and resistance increases - with derecruitment and/or constriction of pulmonary vessels. Both changes in diameter and number of perfused vessels may be due to passive changes of transmural pressure of pulmonary vessels and to the tone of vascular smooth muscle (15-17). Thus, one needs to be wary before attributing changes in calculated PVR to active vasomotion.

Calculated PVR provides no insight on the longitudinal distribution of resistance along the pulmonary vascular bed. Calculations based on the morphometry of the human pulmonary arterial tree (12-13) and experimental evidence obtained with a variety of methods agree that the greater resistance lies in the most central part of the bed within a few mm of the capillaries and is almost equally partitioned between the arterial and venous side of the of the pressure drop in the capillaries (14). Therefore, a change in calculated PVR is at best circumstantial evidence of a change in tone or arterial smooth muscle.

Often calculated in the past has been the so-called total pulmonary resistance TPR which is equal to pulmonary blood flow divided into mean pulmonary arterial pressure: TPR=Ppa/Q. It should be stressed that the calculated TPR is devoid of any physical or physiological significance: i) it relies on the unacceptable assuption that under all circumstances pressure at the outlet of the pulmonary circulation is equal to the reference pressure, usually barometric pressure; ii) like Ppa, TPR changes with the chosen hydrostatic reference level. It may well be that a lot of confusion about pressure-flow relationships in the human pulmonary circulation arose from indiscriminate use of this nonsensical ratio.

SIMULTANEOUS CHANGES IN PBV IN THE PULMONARY CIRCULATION

PBV,PVR and changes in cross-sectional area of the equivalent tube.

The simplified model tells us that changes in PVR are a more sensitive index of changes in radius of the single equivalent tube than are changes in PBV. Let both length L of the pulmonary circuit and blood viscosity η be constant Then,

Since   PVR $\propto$ r^{-4}

then   PVR = Kr^{-4} and by differentiation

$$d(PVR)/dr = -4Kr^{-5}$$

and $d(PVR) = -4Kr^{-4}dr$ (1)

For small finite changes ΔPVR

$$\Delta PVR/PVR = -4 \Delta r/r \qquad (2)$$

By similar derivation for pulmonary blood volume (PBV)

$$\Delta PVB/PVB = 2 \Delta r/r \qquad (3)$$

Thus, in such a simple model of the pulmonary circulation as a unique tube a relative change in radius $\Delta r/r$ causes a relative change of PVR twice greater than the relative change in the opposite direction of PBV. This analysis relies on the assumption of even distribution of resistance and distensibility along the pulmonary vascular bed. That both are distributed parameters sets a limit to the application of this simple model to clinical data.

PVR, PBV and the actual pulmonary circulation

Changes in PVR are more sensitive than changes in PBV to
detect vasoactive changes taking place in muscular pulmonary
arteries e.g. with acute hypoxic vasoconstriction and acute
vasodilatation of previously constricted vessels. The
reasoning is as follows. The blood content of these arteries
is about one tenth of arterial blood volume and one fourtieth
of PBV, i.e. approximately 12 ml (12). Let us suppose that
resistance of these arteries is 50 per cent of PVR and
increases 66% with hypoxia corresponding to a decrease in
radius of about 16% (Eq 2). The overall PVR increases by
33%-an easily detectable change. However, the volume of blood
in the muscular arteries falls by about 32% (Eq3) or
approximately 4 ml causing no detectable change in overall PBV.
Conversely vasodilatation is likely to cause a fall in PVR and
may not cause concomitant changes in PBV. In fact,
vasodilatation of pulmonary vessels constricted by hypoxia
caused a marked fall in PVR in patients with chronic
obstructive lung disease during infusion of isoproterenol (18)
and in exercising higlanders given an enriched oxygen mixture
to breathe (19). However, PBV did not change significantly in
the highlanders. Its increase in the patients was best
explained by recruitment of previously closed pathways distal
to the small arteries since indirect evidence suggested that
distensibility of larger arteries did not change.

Vasomotor activity is usually accompanied by changes in
the pulmonary arterial pressure which may in turn modify the
degree of distension and/or recruitment of pulmonary vessels.
Passive and active changes in both PVR and PVB may be
directionally opposite and tend to cancel one another. Let me
use hypoxic vasoconstriction as an example. At normal levels
of Ppa relative arterial distensibility in man is about 45% per
k/Pa (7.5 mmHg) rise in Ppa. With 12-14% O_2 breathing in man
hypoxic vasoconstriction causes a rise in Ppa of about 0.5
k/Pa(20). Assuming no change in arterial distensibility the
computed increase in arterial blood volume is approximately
20-25% which amounts to 25-30ml This is enough to cancel out
the small reduction in PBV due to the reduced diameter of small
muscular arteries but is barely measurable with presently available techniques. In fact direct evidence for the blunting of
hypoxic pulmonary vasoconstriction by raised Ppa was provided
by experiments in dogs during both administration of serotonin
and epinephrine and alveolar hypoxia (22).

Lastly, prior to attributing changes in PVR and PBV to
vasomotor activity purely passive changes need to be
eliminated. In isolated lung preparations passive changes can
be easily produced by control of the pulmonary arterial, pulmo-

nary venous and alveolar pressure, and are responsible for the
pressure flow line being convex to the pressure axis (15, 23),
and for the relationship between PBV and Ppa being concave to
the pressure axis and plateauing once full recruitment is
achieved (24). If such passive changes do take place in the
human pulmonary circulation studied in situ, recruitment and
derecruitment may mimic vasodilation and vasoconstriction
respectively.

PRESSURE-FLOW-VOLUME RELATIONSHIP IN LOWLANDERS

PVR and PBV in supine lowlanders

The consistancy of PVR in spite of increases in both flow
and pressure in the pulmonary circulation is well documented
nowadays (Figure 1). PVR does not change significantly or
consistantly with exercise (10, 25 - 30).

Nor did PVR change in the perfused lung tissue during
unilateral occlusion of the pulmonary artery at rest and at
exercise (26,29) and during graded occlusion of up to 82% of
the pulmonery artery at rest (27).

Since these manoeuvres cause large increases in the
velocity of the blood, the comparison of PVR at different
pulmonary blood flow must take into account changes in the
kinetic energy of the blood. However, the mean kinetic energy
is about the same in the pulmonary artery and veins (14) and
will cancel out in the subtraction of mean pulmonary venous
from mean PA pressure which yields the steady component of the
pressure drop from which PVR is calculated.

PVB has been measured in a few subjects during moderate
exercise by use of radiocardiography (31) or of the dye
dilution methods (10,30). The results suggest that the rise in
PVB is minimal during exercise but this tentative conclusion
needs confirmation in a greater number of subjects exercising
at heavier workloads. Rapid infusion of up to one litre of
plasma expander in the subjects whose haemodynamics were normal
did not cause a significant rise in PVB although both left
atrial and pulmonary arterial pressure rose by an average of 6
to 10 Torr respectivly (32). It took infusions of 1000-1500ml
to cause a 15% increase in PVB (which being measured by
radiocardiography included some left atrial volume) (33).

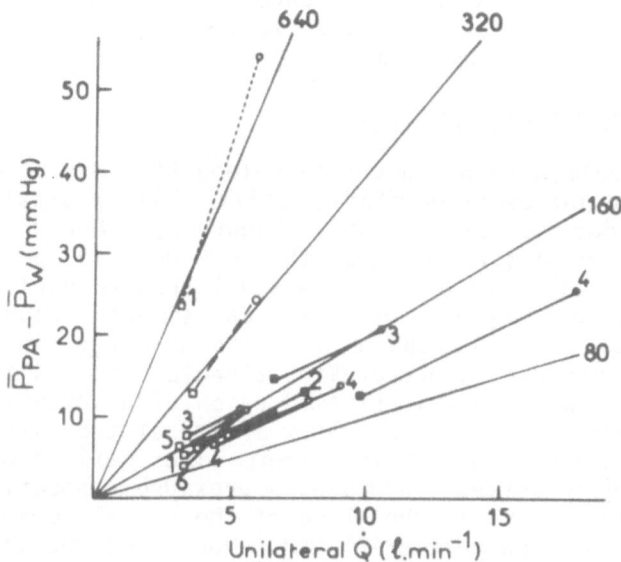

Figure 1   Effects of exercise and unilateral pulmonary arterial
           occlusion (UPAO) on driving pressure (ordinate) and blood
           flow through one lung. Control period : rest □, exercise ○
           UPAO — rest ▣, exercise ● . Solid lines = data in normal
           lowlanders at sea level : 1 = Banchero et al. (41); 2 =
           Even et al.(27); 3 = Harris et al.(26); 4 = Stanek et
           al.(29); 5 = Tartulier et al.(28); 6 = Yu(10).
           Interrupted line = normal highlanders at an altitude of
           3,750 m(19). Dotted line = normal highlanders at an
           altitude of 4,540 m(25). Four isoresistance lines have
           been drawn (cgs units). Reproduced from Lockhart et
           al.(19) by permission of the Journal of Applied
           Physiology.

"Taken together the constancy of PVR and the small and inconsistant increase in PVB suggest that in normal supine subjects no significant recruitment or distension of pulmonary vessels takes place when both blood flow and pressure increase in the lung circulation..." (30). Therefore, in normal supine lowlanders pulmonary vasiodilators are unlikely to cause significant changes in PVR or PBV. Conversely a rise in PVR is best explained by pulmonary vasconstriction, e.g. the rise in PVR during acute alveolar hypoxia.

PVR and PVB in the upright posture

Changes in pulmonary blood volume, blood flow and vascular pressures during 60 degrees head-up tilt (34) or sitting up (35) have been documented recently (Figure 2). Measured PVB fell by 29 and 30% respectively. The mean drifting pressure across the pulmonary vascular bed was not reduced pari passu with blood flow and, as a result, PVR was somewhat higher in the erect posture than supine. These results are best explained by the closure ·of derecruited alveolar vessels in the upper lung which has been demonstrated by external counting of injected radioactive isotopes. They are consistent with the existence within the lung of different zones defined by the values of pulmonary arterial and venous pressure respective to alveolar pressure. Due to the shape of the normal human lung and the level of pulmonary arterial and venous pressure at rest Zone 111 where full recruitment is present occupies most of the supine lung whereas a significant part of the erect lung corresponds to Zone 1 and 11 which are characterized by derecruitment and waterfall conditions respectively (Figure 3). It has been estimated that Zone 1 and Zone 11 occupies 11% and 34% of lung volume in the erect posture (34). Therefore, one can speculate that in the latter position increased pulmonary vascular pressures at exercise are likely to be accompanied by a progressive fall in PVR with increasing workloads until full recruitment is achieved. PBV and PVR are likely to reach supine values at this point and to remain almost constant at higher workloads. This hypothetical beaviour of PBV and PVR with increasing workloads is represented schematically in Figure 4 in which solid lines represent well documented data.

Possible Postural differences in vasomotor responses

Almost all studies in man of pulmonary vasoactive agents have been carried out in the supine posture. I know of no comparative study of the effects on PBV and PVR of such agents in the supine and upright postures. It may well be that such comparitive studies would disclose apparent difference in responses. Let me speculate about pulmonary vasoconstrictors. As disscused in a previous section agents acting on a recruited

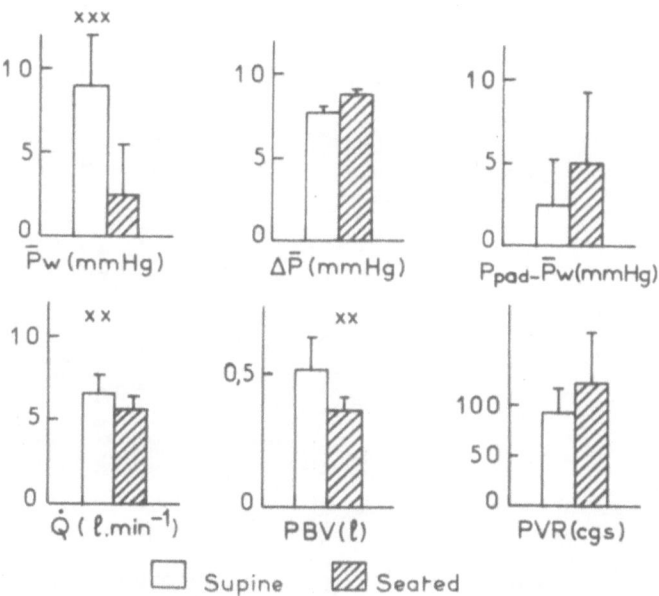

Figure 2   Effects of sitting up on pulmonary wedge pressure (Pw),
driving pressure across the pulmonary circulation (P),
pulmonary diastolic pressure difference (Ppad - Pw),
pulmonary blood flow (Q), pulmonary blood volume (PBV) and
pulmonary vascular resistance (PVR). Height of boxes =
group average values.   Vertical bar = one standard
deviation.

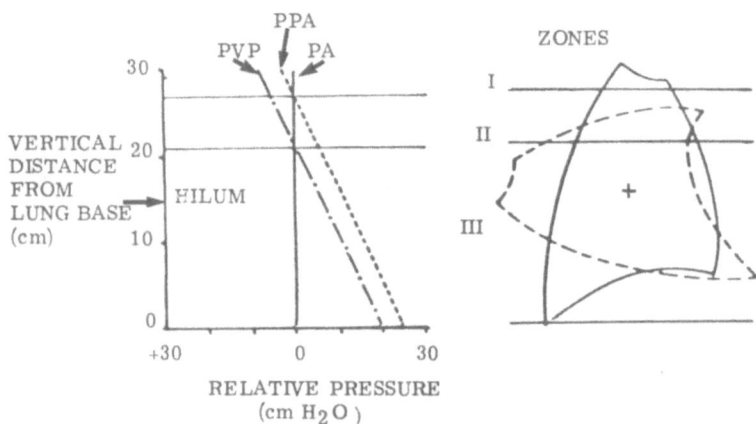

Figure 3   Left: pulmonary arterial (P_{PA}) and pulmonary venous (P_{VP})
            pressure relative to barometric pressure increase linearly
            from apex to base whereas mean alveolar pressure (PA) is
            constant and equal to barometric pressure. Zone I is
            above the upper horizontal line where $PA > P_{PA}$. Zone II is
            between the horizontal lines where $P_{PA} > PA > P_{VP}$. Zone III
            is below the lower line where $P_{PA} > P_{VP} > PA$.
            Right: Contours of upright (solid line) and supine
            (broken line) normal human adult lung. Zone III occupies
            most of the supine lung. Zones I and II occupy an
            important part of the upright lung.

vascular beds in the supine posture usually cause clear-cut rise in PVR and little change in PBV. What about the upright posture? There are two theoretical possibilities. Recruitment of vessels in the upper lung takes place under the action of a rising Ppa caused by primary vasoconstriction of perfused branches in the middle and lower parts of the lung, this would result in an immediate fall in PVR and rise in PVB and by secondary and directionally opposite changes in these variables with continuation of vasoconstrictor activiy following full recruitment of the pulmonary vascular bed. Conversely the primary increase in vascular tone may well be generalized and prevent opening of derecruited vessels in the upper lungs. This would result in an immediate increase in PVR and small changes in PVB. Whether postural differeces in pulmonary vasomotor responses do actually exist will remain purely speculative until experiments are repeated with acute alveolar hypoxia.

PRESSURE-FLOW-VOLUME RELATIONSHIPS IN HIGHLANDERS

Marked differences in the structure of pulmonary arteries of highlanders compared to lowlanders are associated with marked difference in pressure-flow-volume relationships.

Muscular pulmonary arteres and pulmonary arterioles in highlanders

There is an increased number of muscularised pulmonary arterioles in highlanders and an absolute increase in the amount of smooth muscle in distal muscular arteries and in pulmonary arterioles (36). Distal pulmonary arterioles are similar in still-born natives at altitude and at sea level (37). Therefore, it has been suggested that the normal involution of the muscularized pulmonary arterioles of the foetus to the thin-walled pulmonary arteriole of the adult at sea level does not take place in highlanders and that the hypertrophy of the media of muscular arteries is secondary to the pulmonary hypertension caused by the high resistance arterioles (38).

Pulmonary hypertension in highlanders

That pulmonary hypertension exists in adult highlanders has been repeatedly documented following pioneer observtion of Rotta et al (39). Individual data from the literature have been collected recently (40) which suggest° that a hyperbolic relationship exists between Ppa and PaO_2 of 70 Torr or more. The data from all altitudes suggest that the variation in Pa among individuals increases with increasing altitude. A large part of this variation appears to be due to variations in PaO_2, i.e. variations in the oxygen drive to breathing: however, some of the variation can be attributed to difference among individuals of reactivity to hypoxia of the pulmonary vessels.

Elevated pulmonary arterial pressure in higlanders is associated with normal cardiac output and pulmonary wedge pressure. Thus, PVR is high compared to sea level, and this high value of PVR is maintained during exercise (19, 25) (Figure 1). It has been postulated that exercise causes pulmonary vasoconstriction in highlanders (25,40). To test this hypothesis we studied the effects of unilateral pulmonary artery occlusion in 10 highlanders in La Paz (altitude 3.750 m) (19). Ppa rose less during occlusion than at exercise and unilateral PVR was less in the former. This was confirmatory evidence for pulmonary vasoconstriction at exercise in highlanders. Calculated alveolar PO_2 and Pa O_2 as well as arterial pH were comparable. Therefore aggravated alveolar hypoxia was not responsible for exercise vasoconstriction in these subjects. We postulated that the aggravated mixed venous hypoxaemia which accompanies exercise and is absent during pulmonary artery occlusion was causing pulmonary vasoconstriction. Therefore, we administered an enriched oxygen mixture (O_2 concentration 30%) to another group of highlanders at rest and at exercise and measured PBV and PVR. PVR and PBV did not change at exercise breathing ambient air. 30% O_2 breathing did not modify PVR and PBV at rest and caused a marked fall in PVR at exercise (Figure 5) which was accompanied by a small and non significant rise in PBV. The data suggest that acutely reversible hypoxic vasoconstriction is not responsible for the permanent pulmonary hypertension of highlanders and that hypoxic vasoconstriction is present during exercise.

SUMMARY

That pulmonary blood flow is highly pulstile in arteries, capillaries and veins is well documented. The distribution of blood in the different series components of the pulmonry circulation changes during the heart cycle, a large fraction of right-ventricular stroke volume being stored in the arteries during systole. Respiration also affects the pulmonary circulation through its effects on both intrathoracic pressure and venous return. It is naive to study the relationships between time-averaged pulmonary blood volume (PBV), time-averaged pulmonary blood flow ($\dot{Q}$) as well as time-averaged pulmonary arterial and pulmonary wedge pressures (Ppa and Pw) the latter being accepted as a reliable substitute to mean left atrial pressure: however, due to the anatomy of the pulmonry circulation and to the limitations of available techniques, this approach is the only one available for studies in intact

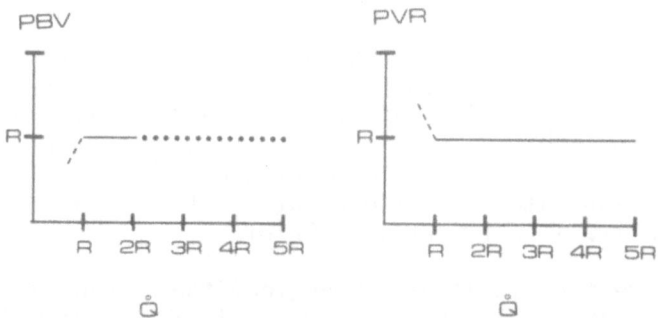

Figure 4. Schematic relationships between pulmonary blood volume
(PBV) and pulmonary vascular resistance (PVR) during
exercise and changes in posture. Cardiac output ($\overset{\bullet}{Q}$), PBV
and PVR are plotted as multiples of the control value at
rest in the supine posture (R). Solid lines represent the
well documented constancy of PVR during mild to severe
exercise and of PBV during moderate exercise in the supine
posture. The behaviour of PBV at higher workloads is
conjectural (dotted line). At rest the upright posture
PBV decreases and PVR rises (broken lines).

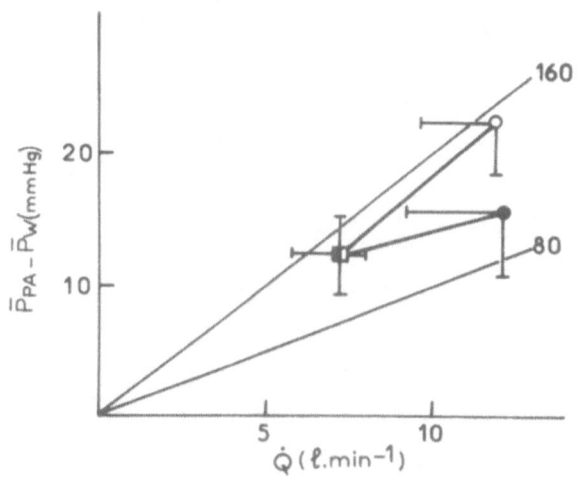

Figure 5   Effects of exercise and 30% oxygen breathing on
pressure-flow relationships in supine normal highlanders
(3,750 m). Group average values and one SD in six
subjects; control = rest □, exercise 0, hyperoxia = rest
■, exercise ● .

animals including man.

In normal supine lowlanders, the driving pressure P = Ppa - Pw is directly proportional to pulmonary blood flow when the latter is increased under the effects of physical exercise, pulmonary arterial occlusion or both. Therefore pulmonary vascular resistance PVR =ΔP/$\dot{Q}$ is constant. PBV does not increase during moderate exercise or at greatly increased Pw and Ppa caused by rapid IV infusion of fluid.

When normal resting lowlanders move from the supine to the sitting position, PBV falls by about 30%, Q falls by some 20 - 25% whereas P does not vary significantly. The resulting increase in PVR is barely significant. Some studies in the literature suggest that PVR falls at exercise to the lower supine values. There are no available studies of PBV at exercise in the erect posture.

Taken together the above data suggest:

1) that recruitment and/or distension of pulmonary vessels are almost complete in supine lowlanders in whom a useful model of the pulmonary circulation is a non-distensible tube of constant resistance traversed by Poiseuille flow.

2) that derecruitment of vessels in the apices takes place at rest in erect subjects permitting PVR to fall at exercise.

REFERENCES

1.   G. de Lee and A. B. Dubois.
       Pulmonary capillary blood flow in man.
       J. Clin. Invest, 34, 1380 (1955).

2.   B. C. Morgan, F. L. Abel, G. L. Mullins and W. G.
       Guntheroth.
       Flow patterns in cavae, pulmonary artery, pulmonary
       vein and aorta in intact dogs.
       Amer. J. Physiol., 219 : 903, (1966)

3.   E. Morkin, J. A. Collins, M. S. Goldman and A. P. Fishman.
       Pattern of blood flow in the pulmonary veins of the
       dog.
       J. Appl. Physiol., 20 : 1118, (1965).

4.   N. B. Karatzas and G. de J. Lee.
       The effect of pulsatile capillary blood flow on gas
       exchange within the lung. A consideration of some
       hydrodynamic factors which affect this pulsatility in
       man.
       Bull. Physiopath. resp., 2 : 521, (1966).

5.   G. A. Brecher and C. A. Hubay.
       Pulmonary blood flow and venous return during
       spontaneous respiration.
       Circulation Res., 3 : 210, (1955).

6.   B. C. Morgan, D. H. Dillard and W. G. Guntheroth.
       Effect of cardiac and respiratory cycle on pulmonary
       vein flow, pressure and diameter.
       J. Appl. Physiol., 21 : 1276, (1966).

7.   I. I. Gabe.
       Pressure measurement in experimental physiology.
       In: "Cardiovascular Fluid Dynamics", Vol. 1, D. H.
       Bergel, ed., Academic Press, New York and London
       (1972).

8.   C. H. Mills.
       Measurement of pulsatile flow and flow velocity.
       In: "Cardiovascular Fluid Dynamics", Vol., 1, D. H.
       Bergel, ed., Academic Press, New York and London
       (1972).

9.   D. H. Glaister.
              The effect of positive centrifugal acceleration upon
              the distribution of ventilation and perfusion within
              the human lung, and its relation to pulmonary
              arterial and intraoesophageal pressure.
              Prac. Royal Soc. Biol., 168 : 311, (1967).

10.   P. N. Yu.
              Pulmonary Blood Volume in Health and Disease.
              Lea and Febiger, Philadelphia, (1969).

11.   M. L. Lewis and C. E. Herera.
              Measurement of human pulmonary arterial volume in
              vivo,
              Bull. europ. Physiopath. respirat., 15: (1979).

12.   G. Cumming, L. K. Harding, K. Horsfield, K. Prowse, S. S.
          singhal and M. J. Woldenberg.
              Morphological aspects of the pulmonary circulation
              and of the airways.
              In: "Fluid Dynamics of Blood Circulation and
              Respiratory Flow", AGARD Conf. Proc. 65 : 23-0,
              (1970).

13.   S. Singhal, R. Henderson, K. Horsfield, K. Harding and G.
          Cumming.
              Morphometry of the human pulmonary arterial tree.
              Circulation Res., 33 : 190, (1973).

14.   W. R. Milnor.
              Pulmonary hemodynamics.
              In: "Cardiovascular Fluid Dynamics", Vol. 2, D. H.
              Bergel, ed. Academic Press, New York and London,
              (1972).

15.   J. Banister and R. W. Torrance.
              The effects of the tracheal pressure upon flow
              pressure relations in the vascular bed of isolated
              lungs.
              Quart. J. Exper. Physiol., 45 : 352, (1960).

16.   J. B. West., C. T. Dollery and A. Naimark.
              Distribution of blood flow in isolated lung; relation
              to vascular and alveolar pressures.
              J. Appl. Physiol., 19 : 713, (1964).

17.   S. Permutt and R. L. Riley,
         Hemodynamics of collapsible vessels with tone: The
         vascular waterfall.
         J. Appl. Physiol., 18 : 924, (1963).

18.   M. I. Ferrer, Y. Enson, M. M. Kilcoyne and R. M. Harvey.
         Effects of isoproterenol on the pulmonary circulation
         in patients with chronic obstructive lung disease.
         Circulation, 43 : 528, (1971).

19.   A. Lockhart, M. Zelter, J. Mensh-Dechene, G. Antezana, M.
         Paz-Zamora, E. Vargas and J. Coudert.
         Pressure-flow-volume relationships in pulmonary
         circulation of normal highlanders.
         J. App. Physiol., 41 : 449, (1976).

20.   A. P. Fishman, M. W. Fritts Jr. and A. Cournand.
         Effects of acute hypoxia and exercise on the
         pulmonary circulation.
         Circulation, 22 : 204, (1960).

21.   H. G. Borst, M. McGregor, J. L. Whittenberger and E.
         Berglund.
         Influence of pulmonary arterial and left atrial
         pressures on pulmonary vascular resistances.
         Circulation Res., 4 : 393, (1956).

22.   J. L. Benumof and E. A. Wahrenbrock.
         Blunted hypoxic pulmonary vasoconstriction by
         increased lung vascular pressures.
         J. Appl. Physiol., 38 : 846, (1975).

23.   T. C. Lloyd Jr., and G. W. Wright.
         Pulmonary vascular resistance and vascular transmural
         gradient.
         J. Appl. Physiol., 15 : 241, (1960).

24.   K. L. Zierler.
         Measurements of the volume of extravascular water in
         the lungs in intact animals and man. A review of
         tracer dilution principles, of some reported results,
         and a new hypothesis to explain the shape of
         tracer-dilution curves and certain other interesting
         relationships.
         In: "Central Hemodynamics and Gas Exchange", G.
         Giuntini, ed. Minerva Medcia, Torino, (1971).

25.   N. Banchero, F. Sime, D. Pennaloza, J. Cruz, R. Gamboa and
        E. Marticorena.
                Pulmonary pressure, cardiac output and arterial
                oxygen saturation during exercise and at sea level.
                Circulation, 33 : 249, (1966).

26.   P. Harris, N. Segel and J. M. Bishop.
                The relation between pressure and flow in the
                pulmonary circulation of normal subjects and in
                patients with chronic bronchitis and mitral stenosis.
                Cardiovascular Res., 2 : 73, (1968).

27.   P. Even, P. Duroux, F. Ruff, I. Caubarrere, P. de
        Vernejoul and G. Brouet.
                The pressure-flow relationship of the pulmonary
                circulation in normal man and in chronic obstructive
                pulmonary disease. Effects of muscular exercise.
                Scand. J. Respirat. Diseases, Suppl. 77 : 72, (1971).

28.   M. Tartulier, M. Bourret and F. Deyrieux.
                Les pressions arterielles pulmonaires chez l'homme
                normal.
                Bull. Physiopath. Respirat., 8 : 1280, (1972).

29.   V. Stanek, P. Jebavy, J. Hurych and J. Widimsky.
                Central haemodynamics during supine exercise and
                pulmonary artery occlusion in normal subjects.
                Bull. Physiopath. Respirat. 9 : 1203, (1973).

30.   A. Lockhart, P. Duhaze, J. Polianski, D. Weill and J.
        Mensch-Dechene.
                A modified double dye injection method for pulmonary
                blood volume determination. II. Results in resting
                and exercising normal subjects.
                Cardiovascular Res., 8 : 120, (1974).

31.   C. Guintini, M. L. Lewis, A. S. Luis and R. M. Harvey.
                A study of the pulmonary blood volume by quantitative
                radiocardiography.
                J. Clin. Invest., 42 : 1589, (1963).

32.   F. M. de Freitas, E. Z. Faraco, D. F. de Azevedo, J.
        Zaduchliver and J. Lewin.
                Behaviour of normal pulmonary circulation during
                changes of total blood volume in man.
                J. Clin. Invest., 44 : 366, (1965).

33.   C. Guintini, A. Maseri and R. Bianchi.
           Pulmonary vascular distensibility and lung compliance
           as modified by dextran infusion and subsequent
           atropine injection in normal subjects.
           J. Clin. Invest., 45 : 1770, (1966).

34.   M. L. Lewis and L. C. Christianson.
           Behaviour of the human pulmonary circulation during
           head-up tilt.
           J. Appl. Physiol. : Respirat. Environ. Exercise
           Physiol., 45 : 249, (1978).

35.   P. Fournier, J. Mensch-Dechene, B. Ranson-Bitker, W.
           Valladares and A. Lockhart.
           Effects of sitting up on pulmonary blood pressure,
           flow and volume in man.
           J. Appl. Physiol. : Respirat. Environ. Exercise
           Physiol., 46 : 36, (1979).

36.   J. Arias-Stella and M. Saldana.
           The terminal portion of the pulmonary arterial tree
           in people native to high altitude.
           Circulation, 28 : 915, (1963).

37.   J. Arias-Stella and Y. Castillo.
           The muscular pulmonary arterial branches in natives
           still-born at high altitude.
           Am. J. Path. Bact., 48 : 45, (1966).

38.   P. Harris and D. Heath.
           The pulmonary circulation at high altitude.
           In: "The human pulmonary circulation", 2nd edition,
           Churchill Livingstone, Edinburgh (1977).

39.   A. Rotta, A. Canepa, A. Hurtado, T. Velasquez and R.
           Chavez.
           Pulmonary circulation at sea level and at high
           altitude.
           J. Appl. Physiol., 9 : 328, (1956).

40.   J. T. Reeves and R. F. Grover.
           High altitude pulmonary hypertension and pulmonary
           edema.
           In: "Progress in Cardiology", Vol. 4, P.N.Yu., ed.,
           Lea and Febiger, Philadelphia, (1975).

Discussion

CUMMING: Thank you very much, Alan. It seems clear that the changes that take place in the pulmonary circulation in man at altitude have some survival value. Have you any idea what it is that calls for the pulmonary circulation to be at high pressure and to have a high resistance?

LOCKHART: I've not studied lamas, but there is someone in the room who has. As far as I know from Heath's paper, lamas at altitude have a normal sea level PA pressure, and they have very little muscle in their arterial walls. Therefore I submit that the response to chronic hypoxia in mammals at altitude may well not be an adaptive phenomenon since the best adapted mammal to high altitude is the lama. Now, the lama has an oxygen dissociation curve which is shifted to the left, whereas physiologists have believed for a long time that a shift to the right of the oxygen dissociation curve is the most suitable adaptive phenomenon, and again the lama is perfectly suited to high altitude living with two built-in devices, a shift to the left of the oxygen dissociation curve and a lack of responsiveness of the PA vessels to hypoxia, that are entirely different from changes that occur in other mammals and that are erroneously believed to have some adaptive value.

ZARDINI: I disagree with many things you say but one thing that I would like to tell you is that my greatest disagreement is with the pressure volume curve. I can't accept that the pressure-volume curve in the lung is linear, it is of course exponential.

LOCKHART: Are we talking of pressure volume or pressure flow?

ZARDINI: Pressure flow yes. I can't believe that the resistance can be linear because the resistance is not constant, the pulmonary circulation does not behave as undistensible tube. The reason is that recruitment and distensibility are two phenomenon that usually occur together. If you perfuse in zone II you have a straight line because with the recruitment you need much more pressure. If you make a pressure curve in the lung in zone III we have a different curve. So these are two phenomena that are occurring together in the lung. When the subject is exercised there is both distensibility in the lower zones and maybe some recruitment; in the upper part of the lung we have much more recruitment than distensibility. So, because the two phenomenon, distensibility and recruitment, they expend different pressure so they can't be linear, the pressure flow relation can't be linear.

CUMMING: Can I comment on that? It's a very common situation in science to begin a discussion with the statement: I do not believe your data. That is a perfectly proper statement to make. What I think is not proper is to say: I do not believe your data because it fails to fit my hypothesis.

LOCKHART: Well, if these were only my data I would be perfectly happy to be told you don't believe them. But they are not only mine! Peter Harris is a careful investigator, Philippe Even is a very very meticulous man as are other people in Sweden and I have taken this data to build these slides where the pressure flow plot turns out to be linear. I agree entirely with you that I can demonstrate to the students any time recruitment and distention in isolated lobes. I could demonstrate it as well, in distention in isolated lobes. I could demonstrate it as well, in sitting subjects, but I don't in supine intact lung.

CUMMING: I'm very glad to have started a controversy. I do not want the controversy to be in public, because we have a pressure on time.

ZARDINI: I didn't say that I don't believe his data. I said I am in disagreement. That's a different thing.

CUMMING: O.K. Your data and his data do not agree.

ZARDINI: You stated a different thing.

CUMMING: I accept that, I accept that. Thank you very much. I was examplifying what people say when they attack current hypotheses. I apologise if I have offended you.

OXYGEN TRANSPORT DURING EXERCISE AT ALTITUDE

Paolo Cerretelli

Dept. of Physiology
University of Geneva
Geneva (Switzerland)

INTRODUCTION

Maximal oxygen consumption ($\dot{V}_{O_2}$max) undergoes a progressive reduction in hypoxia both acute and chronic as appears from Fig. 1 where data from various authors are summarized. Such decrease, for a pressure drop of half an atmosphere (corresponding to an altitude of about 5500 meters) ranges between 30% and 45%, independent of the degree of acclimatization and of the ethnic characteristics of the subjects. Common factors known to change $\dot{V}_{O_2}$max in opposite directions in hypoxia are:

1) The decreased arterial O_2 saturation (%HbO_2) due to decreased $P_{I_{O_2}}$ and possibly to an impairment of the diffusion property of the lung. The arterial oxygen and carbon dioxide partial pressures (Pa_{O_2} and Pa_{CO_2}) of resident highlanders as well as of acclimatized lowlanders are plotted as a function of altitude in Fig. 2, along with the corresponding HbO_2 saturation values (%HbO_2). At a barometric pressure of 380 torr (5500 m) %HbO_2 drops to about 80%.

2) The increased blood hemoglobin (Hb) concentration. Hb concentration, after a prolonged exposure to 5500 m, may attain 130–140% of the sea level control value.
   Thus, the increased blood oxygen capacity reduces and may even balance the effects of low $P_{I_{O_2}}$. After 12 weeks exposure to 5500 m blood of acclimatized lowlanders was found to carry

359

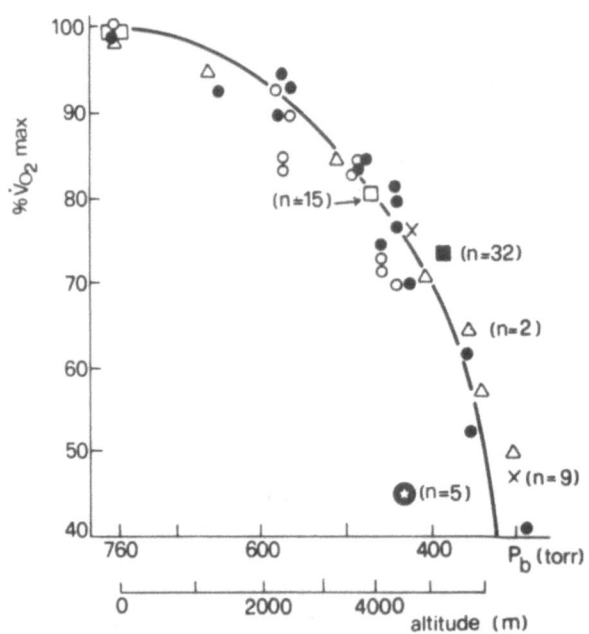

Fig. 1 : $\dot{V}_{O_2}$max (percent of the sea level values) as a function
of P_B and of altitude. Open symbols: acute hypoxia;
solid symbols: chronic hypóxia; crosses: altitude natives
(redrawn from Åstrand and Rodahl.(1970) with the addition
of data from: Cerretelli and Margaria (1961) ⊗   ;
Elsner et al. (1964) X   ; and Cerretelli (1976a):□
in a decompression chamber, Δ   breathing hypoxic mixture,
and ▉   on 32 lowlanders acclimatized to 5350 m). In
parentheses number of subjects (Cerretelli, in press).

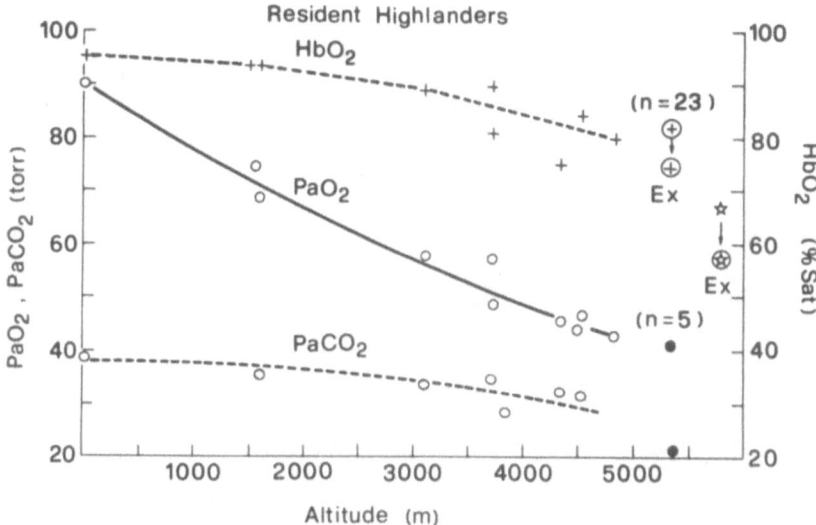

Fig. 2 : Pa_{O_2}, Pa_{CO_2} and HbO_2 (%Sat) as a function of altitude
in resident highlanders (from Biology Data Book, 1974).
Asterisks, full dots and circled crosses refer to
acclimatized lowlanders as from West et al. (1962) and
Cerretelli (1976b), respectively. Ex = exercise.

even during exercise over 20 ml of O_2 per 100 ml in spite
of an average drop of O_2 saturation to 77% (Cerretelli, 1976b).
    Additional factors involved in O_2 transport to exercising
muscles are:

3) <u>The maximal cardiac output</u> ($\dot{Q}max$). $\dot{Q}max$ may change as a
   consequence of both hypoxia and increased blood viscosity.
   Acute hypoxia corresponding to an altitude of 4000 m increases
   cardiac outptut ($\dot{Q}$) by about 15% above sea level values at
   any submaximal work load (Stenberg et al., 1966) (Fig. 3),
   the increase being mediated by higher heart rate (h.r.).
   After longer exposures, the Q response to submaximal aerobic
   work is the same as at sea level with compensatory adjustments
   of either h.r. or stroke volume (q_{st}). In acute hypoxia h.
   r. and $\dot{Q}$ seem to attain the same maximal levels as at sea
   level which would indicate that reduced Hb saturation may be
   compensated for by higher perfusion of the myocardium. By

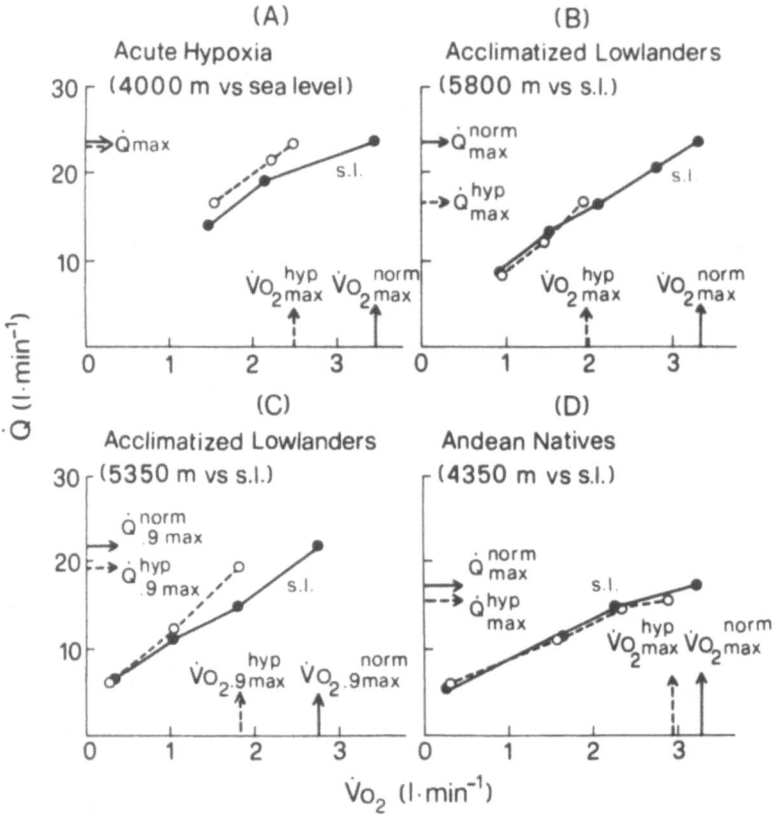

Fig. 3: Cardiac output ($\dot{Q}$) as a function of oxygen uptake ($\dot{V}_{O_2}$).
Plate A : in acute hypoxia (from Stenberg et al., 1966);
Plate B : in acclimatized lowlanders at 5800 m (from
            Pugh, 1964);
Plate C : in acclimatized lowlanders at 5350 m (from Cer
            retelli, 1976b);
Plate D : in Andean natives (4350 m) (from Vogel et al.,
            1974).

contrast, a prolonged high altitude exposure reduces maximal
cardiac output ($\dot{Q}$max) mainly through a reduction of maximal heart
rate (h.r. max). Such a decrease was found to be 20% after 2 weeks
at 4300 m (Saltin et al., 1968), 10-15% after two months at 5350 m

(Cerretelli, 1976a and b), 30% after two months at 5800 m
(Pugh, 1964) (Fig. 3). Such a decrease of $\dot{Q}max$, however,
considering the relatively high arterial blood oxygen content
would not explain the 30-45% drop in $\dot{V}_{O_2}max$ observed by all
investigators at an altitude of about 5500 m. Therefore, other
mechanisms, besides the reduction in $\dot{Q}max$, have been recently
postulated for explaining the decreased maximal aerobic power
of acclimatized lowlanders in the face of a relatively high O_2
flow to the working muscles. Among these:

4) A failure of the "power plant", i.e. a limitation of the
respiratory function of the muscles due to a) an impairment
of the respiratory function of the mitochondria induced by
chronic hypoxia or/and b) a decrease of mitochondria due to
a reduction of muscle mass. Neither of the above mechanisms,
however, seems to play a significant role in decreasing $\dot{V}_{O_2}max$
at least in animals (Gold et al., 1973; Cerretelli, 1976b).

5) Changes of muscle microcirculation, consequential to increased
central and peripheral hematocrit (Hct) and/or hypoxia, leading
to a reduced nutritional blood flow. The consequence would be
a drop of maximal aerobic power of the subject in spite of a
still relatively high blood O_2 transport potential. According
to this hypothetical mechanism, part of the peripheral blood
flow would bypass the working muscles through low-resistance
channels thus decreasing the load on the heart. The common
experimental finding that the increase of mean arterial
pressure in the course of heavy exercise is the same in
acclimatized lowlanders (Hct = 65%) as in sea level residents
is compatible with this type of circulatory adaptation.
A way of testing the validity of the latter mechanism is
to administer to acclimatized lowlanders O_2 at high (380 torr)
partial pressure and to assess their $\dot{V}_{O_2}max$. A shift from
air to oxygen breathing leads to full saturation of arterial
blood and should increase the O_2 transport to the tissues
with a substantial improvement of the performance. The absence
of a sizeable increase of maximal aerobic power could be
interpreted as the consequence of a decreased "effective" muscle
blood flow.
It has long been known, particularly to mountaineers, that
oxygen breathing during altitude climbing is not as beneficial
as expected on physiological grounds. This rather "mysterious"
finding was tentatively explained by Barcroft (1972) in the

twenties with a permanent left-shift of the oxyhemoglobin
dissociation curve. Apart from the fact that an increased
hemoglobin oxygen affinity seems to improve rather than impair
the O_2 transport in acclimatized subjects exposed to moderate
altitudes (Hebbel et al., 1978) the blood O_2 affinity of
acclimatized lowlanders appears indeed slightly decreased.
In fact, the average P_{50} value was found to be 2 to 4 torr
higher than that at sea level (Samaja et al., 1979).

The aim of this presentation is to describe the degree and
the mechanisms by which:

a) A sudden shift of $P_{I_{O_2}}$ from 80 to 390 torr,
b) A rapid increase of barometric pressure (P_B) from 390
   to 540 torr,
c) A 4 weeks sojourn at sea level following altitude
   exposure,

affect the maximal aerobic power of acclimatized lowlanders.

RESULTS

A   The effect of sudden hyperoxia on $\dot{V}_{O_2}$max.

The results of blood measurements at rest together with
the most significant exercise parameters recorded for 10
subjects in three environmental situations, i.e. at sea level
and at 5350 meters when breathing ambient air or O_2, appear
in Table I (Cerretelli, 1976b). The effects of chronic hypoxia
(6-8 weeks exposure at altitudes up to 6500 m) on blood composition
are comparable to those reported in the literature for similar
conditions, in particular, Hb concentration shows a 37% increase.
$\dot{V}_{O_2}$max determined at 5350 m by a closed circuit system dropped
to 70% of the sea level value resuming only 92% of the control
when breathing oxygen in spite of only a slight reduction of
maximal cardiac output ($\dot{Q}$max) (see Fig. 4 left and central
plates). In fact, Q determined in two among the subjects
appearing in Table I by the N_2-CO_2 rebreathing method (Cerretelli et al., 1966) during an exercise requiring 90% of $\dot{V}_{O_2}$max
at 5350 m was 19 and 20.7 $l \cdot min^{-1}$, respectively, i.e. 91% and
87% of the sea level controls. The corresponding h.r. values
were 148 and 162 beats$\cdot min^{-1}$, respectively, i.e. 83% and 91%
of the values found at sea level. $\dot{Q}$max estimated by extrapolation
of the $\dot{Q}/\dot{V}_{O_2}$ relationship to $\dot{V}_{O_2}$max was found to be 10% less
than in control conditions. Cardiac output was not measured

Table I: Age, body weight, RBC counts, hemoglobin concentration, hematocrit, arterial O_2 saturation at rest and at exercise, maximum heart rate, pulmonary ventilation (BTPS) and maximum O_2 uptake when breathing air at sea level and at 5350 m as well as O_2 at 5350 m (from Cerretelli, 1976b).

*   n = 26 subjects
**   n = 15 subjects

Subjects (n = 10)	age years	weight kg	RBC millions · l^{-1}	Hb g%	Hct %	%HbO2 rest	maximum (direct method) exercise $\dot{V}_{E\ max}$ $l \cdot min^{-1}$	h.r.$_{max}$ $b \cdot min^{-1}$	%HbO2	$\dot{V}_{O_2\ max}$ $l \cdot min^{-1}$	$\dot{V}_{O_2\ max}$ $ml \cdot kg^{-1} \cdot min^{-1}$
Sea level		72.7 ±10.6	4.73 ±0.23	15.0 ±0.9	44.7 ±1.3	98.2 ±2.1	97.4 ±13.6	185 ±9.4	97.8 ±2.8	3.21 ±0.27	45.3 ±8.6
5350 m	26.1 ±4.7 (S.D.)	67.4 ±10.3	6.57 ±0.68	20.6 ±1.4	63.8 ±4.6	82.0* ±4.2	145.1 ±21.5	161 ±15.4	77.4** ±4.0	2.26 ±0.24	34.4 ±6.7
5350 m in O_2						98.3 ±2.0	141.7 ±43.1	169 ±14.5	98.0 ±1.5	2.94 ±0.41	43.1 ±9.2

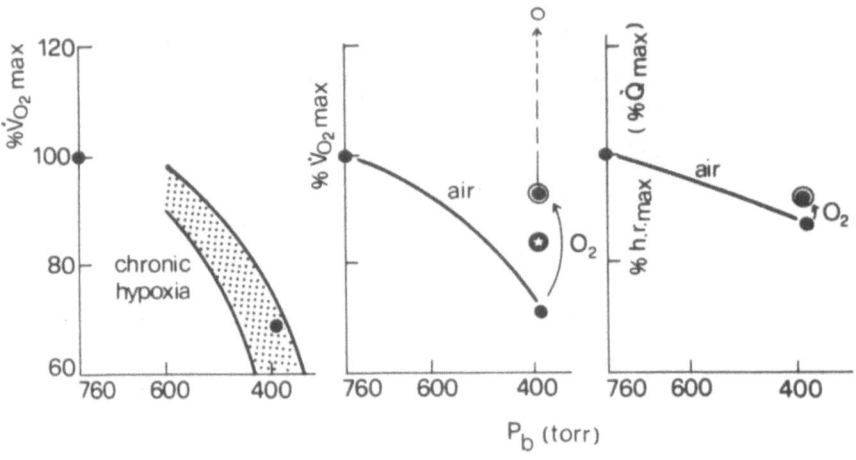

Fig. 4 : $\dot{V}_{O_2}$max and h.r.$_{max}$ (% of sea level averages) as a
            function of P_B. Left plate: the dotted area indicates
            the range of $\dot{V}_{O_2}$max as a function of altitude (see Fig.
            1). The solid dot designates the average value found
            by the author in the group under study; center plate:
            the effect of breathing oxygen is indicated by the
            arrow (see circled dots). The asterisk indicates the
            estimated $\dot{V}_{O_2}$max value in hypoxia calculated on actual
            $\dot{Q}$max and maximal potential (a - $\bar{v}$) O_2 difference. The
            latter is based on measured CaO_2 and on the $C\bar{v}_{O_2}$ value
            found at sea level during maximal exercise. The open
            circle indicates the expected $\dot{V}_{O_2}$max value when breathing
            O_2 on the assumption made in the text; right plate:
            effect of breathing oxygen on h.r.$_{max}$ (modified from
            Cerretelli, in press).

during oxygen breathing. It appears conceivable, however, that
$\dot{Q}$max be, if anything, somewhat higher than in hypoxia. This
is also compatible with the higher h.r.$_{max}$ levels attained
(169 vs. 161 beats·min^{-1}) (see Fig. 4, right plate). In
conclusion, considering the 37% increase of Hb concentration
and assuming a 10% drop of $\dot{Q}$max, the maximal aerobic power

of an acclimatized subject breathing O_2 should be 25-30% higher than at sea level. On the contrary, as previously pointed out, upon O_2 breathing $\dot{V}_{O_2}$max attains only 92% of the sea level control.

B   The effects of a rapid increase of P_B from 390 to 540 torr.

     The results of measurements of $\dot{V}_{O_2}$max, Hb concentration and h.r.$_{max}$ carried out on 13 subjects 6 to 24 hours after descent by helicopter from 5350 m to 2850 m appear in Table II (Cerretelli, 1976b). Average $\dot{V}_{O_2}$max assessed by an indirect method based on the extrapolation of the h.r./$\dot{V}_{O_2}$ relationship rose significantly (P   0.001) from 2.36 to 3.03 $1 \cdot min^{-1}$, i.e. to 97% of the sea level control. h.r.$_{max}$ rose 8 beats$\cdot min^{-1}$ to 95% of the control.

     Again, the improvement of $\dot{V}_{O_2}$max at higher P_B was less than could be expected from the increase of Hb concentration and the moderate decrease of maximal cardiac output.

C   The relationship between $\dot{V}_{O_2}$max and Hb concentration before and after altitude exposure.

     The results of the measurements of $\dot{V}_{O_2}$max and related variables carried out on 13 subjects at sea level before altitude exposure, after a 12-16 weeks sojourn at altitude and again 25-28 days after return to sea level are summarized in Table III (Cerretelli, 1976b).

     The average 5% increase of $\dot{V}_{O_2}$max ($1 \cdot min^{-1}$) found in connection to the 11.6% increase in Hb concentration when comparing return to departure values is not statistically significant (P   0.3). Thus, increased Hb concentration does not necessarily raise $\dot{V}_{O_2}$max.

DISCUSSION

     The blood O_2 partial pressure values and the systemic pressure levels in the various experimental conditions may be of some relevance for the interpretation of the results appearing in Tables I and II. In Fig. 5 (Cerretelli, 1976b) "physiological" (at actual P_{CO_2} and 2,3-DPG concentration levels) oxyhemoglobin dissociation curves are drawn for Hb concentrations of 15 and 21 g%, respectively. Measured arterial (a) and mixed venous ($\bar{v}$) points (with the exception of the venous point at exercise during

Table II: Age, body weight, RBC counts, hemoglobin concentration, maximal heart rate, and maximum O_2 uptake breathing air at sea level, at 5350 and 2850 m (from Cerretelli, 1976b).

Subjects (n= 13)	age years	weight kg	RBC millions · l^{-1}	Hb g%	h.r.max $b \cdot min^{-1}$	$\dot{V}O_2$ max (indirect method) $l \cdot min^{-1}$	$ml \cdot kg^{-1} \cdot min^{-1}$
Sea level		71.5 ± 9.7	4.70 ± 0.22	15.0 ± 0.9	187 ± 13	3.13 ± 0.29	44.3 ± 5.6
5350 m	29.1 ± 5.9 (S.D.)	66.9 ± 8.7	6.65 ± 0.7	21.6 ± 2.4	160 ± 9	2.36 ± 0.29	35.7 ± 6.2
2850 m					168 ± 15	3.03 ± 0.25	45.8 ± 5.3

Table III: Age, body weight, RBC counts, hemoglobin concentration, maximum heart rate and maximum O_2 consumption at sea level before altitude exposure, at 5350 m and at sea level four weeks after return (from Cerretelli, 1976b).

Subjects (n = 13)	age years	weight kg	RBC millions · l^{-1}	Hb g%	h.r. max $b \cdot min^{-1}$	$\dot{V}O_{2\,max}$ (direct method) $l \cdot min^{-1}$	$\dot{V}O_{2\,max}$ (direct method) $ml \cdot kg^{-1} \cdot min^{-1}$
Sea level (departure)		72.8 ±7.9	4.48 ±0.30	14.6 ±0.7	191 ±9	3.23 ±0.31	44.3 ±4.45
5350 m	25.3 ±6.1 (S.D.)	67.8 ±7.5	6.52 ±0.48	23.4 ±2.6	162 ±16	2.35 ±0.44	34.3 ±3.7
Sea level (return)		67.6 ±7.5	5.01 ±0.66	16.3 ±2.1	186 ±9	3.39 ±0.46	50.7 ±6.8

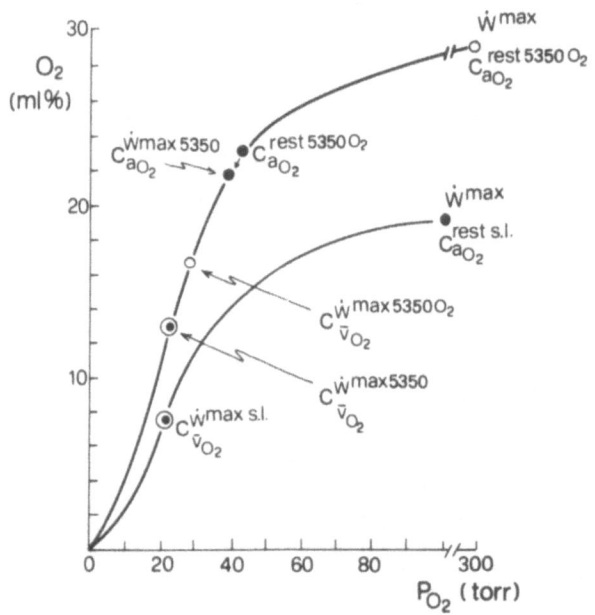

Fig. 5 :   "Physiological" O_2 dissociation curves for normal (Hb=
           15 g%) and acclimatized lowlanders (Hb = 21 g%). Arterial
           (a) and mixed venous ($\bar{v}$) points are indicated for resting
           (rest) and maximal working ($Ca_{O_2}^{\substack{\dot{W}max \\ rest\ s.l.}}$) and when
           breathing O_2 at altitude ($Ca_{O_2}^{\substack{\dot{W}max \\ rest\ 5350\ O_2}}$) are
           superimposed (from Cerretelli, in press).

maximal work (W) for both air and O_2 breathing conditions. The $P\bar{v}_{O_2}$ values during maximal exercise at altitude (both in air and O_2 breathing) appear relatively high when compared to sea level controls and to conditions of acute hypoxia. The product between measured or estimated maximal cardiac output ($\dot{Q}max$) and maximal "potential" arterio-venous O_2 difference values, i.e. calculated on actual Pa_{O_2} and on $P\bar{v}_{O_2}$ values measured during maximal exercise at sea level, yield $\dot{V}_{O_2}max$ figures much higher than those actually found at altitude both when breathing air and oxygen. In these conditions, $\dot{V}_{O_2}max$ should attain levels of 85% and 125%, respectively of the sea level controls (see Fig. 2, center plate, asterisk and open dot) as compared to the actual values of 70% and 92%, respectively).

The systemic pressure does not increase during heavy exercise in acclimatized lowlanders more than it does at sea level. This finding, considering the relatively high cardiac output and blood viscosity, necessarily implies reduced peripheral resistance to flow. This could be prompted by a dilatation of the metarterioles coupled with a contraction of the precapillary sphincteres. Such changes would cause a reduction of the O_2 flow to the muscles and would also justify: 1) the relatively low $\dot{V}_{O_2}max$ values observed in acclimatized lowlanders both when breathing ambient air or O_2 in spite of an adequate O_2 transport to the periphery and   2) the high $P\bar{v}_{O_2}$ values found during maximal exercise in both conditions.

The conclusion that may be drawn from the experiments described in (A) and (B) is that the limit to $\dot{V}_{O_2}max$ in acclimatized lowlanders is mostly peripheral and is probably attributable to a lower "effective" perfusion of the muscles. Whether this change is the consequence of a primitive increase of the central vasomotor tone due to hypoxia or of more complex adaptive mechanisms aimed at decreasing the load on the heart deriving from increased blood viscosity is still matter for investigation.

As appears from Table III, an 11.6% increase in Hb concentration a month after return to sea level is not paralleled by a significant increase of $\dot{V}_{O_2}max$. Training conditions of the subjects were the same before and after altitude exposure. The 7% reduction in body weight probably reflects more a loss of body fat than a decrease of muscle mass and should therefore not influence $\dot{V}_{O_2}max$. The latter, moreover, does not seem to depend, within broad limits, on muscle mass.

On the other hand, the effects of blood infusion on maximal aerobic power appear rather controversial. Ekblom et al. (1972) found a 9% increase in $\dot{V}_{O_2}max$ following a 13% increase of Hb

concentration by reinfusion of homologous blood. By contrast,
Williams et al. (1973) did not find differential effects of whole
blood (500 ml), RBC (275 ml) or plasma (225 ml) infusion on
endurance capacity, resting, submaximal and maximal heart rate.
In the present experimental conditions the increased Hb
concentration is a consequence of altitude exposure, thus involving
different mechanisms of adjustment of blood composition as well as
systemic and peripheral circulation. The failure of higher Hb
to increase the maximal aerobic performance of the subject by no
means implies that in ordinary normoxic conditions the factors
limiting aerobic work are peripheral. It is well known in fact
that $\dot{V}_{O_2}$max increases significantly when increasing O_2 partial
pressure in inspired air (Fagraeus et al., 1973; Margaria et al.,
1961) which indicates that the oxidative potential of the muscles
exceeds the capacity for O_2 transport by the circulation. Rather,
a change of red cell concentration in circulating blood could be
counterbalanced at the muscle level by a reduction of "effective"
blood flow. This drop, in conditions of very high hematocrit
could be more than compensatory, thus causing a reduction of the
O_2 available at the muscle level.

CONCLUSIONS

    The failure of sudden hyperoxia to raise $\dot{V}_{O_2}$max of acclimatized
lowlanders to sea level or even higher values in the absence of a
drastic reduction of maximal cardiac output could be explained with
a reduction of "effective" blood flow to the working muscles. A
similar limitation even though mediated by different mechanisms
could also explain the negative or controversial effects of blood
infusion on the maximal aerobic power of subjects at sea level.
The recently described (Zink, personal communication, 1979)
beneficial effects of hemodilution on the maximal performance of
acclimatized lowlanders could originate from an increase of
"effective" blood flow to working muscles that would more than
compensate for the decreased hematocrit.

REFERENCES

1. P.O. Åstrand, and K. Rodahl, in: "Textbook of Work Physiology",
    New York, McGraw Hill, p. 405, 573 (1970).
2. I. Barcroft, Features in the Architeture of Physiological

Function, Hafner Publ., Co., New York, p. 222 (1972).

3. "Biology Data Book", II Edition, Vol. III, pp. 1832, 1877-
    -78, 1895-96, Am. Soc. Exp. Biol., Bethesda, Maryland (1974).

4. P. Cerretelli, and R. Margaria, Maximum oxygen consumption
    at altitude, Intern. Z. angew. Physiol. 18: 460-464 (1961).

5. P. Cerretelli, J.C. Cruz, L.E. Farhi, and H. Rahn, Determination
    of mixed venous O_2 and CO_2 tensions and cardiac output by a
    rebreathing method, Respir. Physiol. 1: 258-264 (1966).

6. P. Cerretelli, Metabolismo ossidativo e anaerobico nel sogget
    to acclimatato all'altitudine, Minerva Med. 67: 11-26 (1976a).

7. P. Cerretelli, Limiting factors to oxygen transport on Mount
    Everest. J. Appl. Physiol. 40: 658-667 (1976b).

8. P. Cerretelli, Gas exchange at high altitude, in: "Pulmonary
    Gas Exchange", J.B. West ed., Academic Press (in press).

9. B. Ekblom, A.N. Goldbarg, and B. Gullbring, Response to exercise
    after blood loss and reinfusion, J. Appl. Physiol. 33: 175-
    -180 (1972).

10. R.W. Elsner, A. Bolstad, and C. Forno, Maximum oxygen
    consumption of Peruvian Indians native to high altitude, in:
    "The Physiological Effects of High Altitude", W.H. Weihe ed.,
    Oxford, Pergamon, p. 217-223 (1964).

11. L. Fagraeus, J. Karlsson, D. Linnarson, and B. Saltin, Oxygen
    uptake during maximal work at lowered and raised ambient air
    pressures, Acta Physiol. Scand. 87: 411-412 (1973).

12. A.J. Gold, T.F. Johnson, and C. Costello, Effects of altitude
    stress on mitochondrial function, Am. J. Physiol. 224: 946-
    -949 (1973).

13. R.P. Hebbel, J.W. Eaton, R.S. Kroenenberg, E.D. Zanjani,
    L.G. Moore, and E.M. Berger, Human Llamas. Adaptation to
    altitude in subjects with high hemoglobin oxygen affinity,
    J. Clin. Invest. 62: 593-600 (1978).

14. R. Margaria, P. Cerretelli, S. Marchi, and L. Rossi-Bernardi,
    Maximum exercise in oxygen, Intern. Z. angew. Physiol. 18:
    465-467 (1961).

15. R. Margaria, E. Camporesi, P. Aghemo, and G. Sassi, The
    effect of O_2 breathing on maximal aerobic power, Pflügers
    Arch. 336: 225-235 (1972).

16. G. Morpurgo, B. Battaglia, N.D. Carter, G. Modiano, and
    S. Passi, The Bohr effect and the red cell 2,3-DPG and Hb
    content in Sherpas and Europeans at low and high altitude,
    Experientia 28: 1280-1283 (1972).

17. L.G.C.E. Pugh, Cardiac output in muscular exercise at
    5800 m (19,000 ft), J. Appl. Physiol. 19: 441-447 (1964).

18. B. Saltin, R.F. Grower, C.G. Blomqvist, L.H. Hartley, and R. L. Johnson, Jr., Maximal oxygen uptake and cardiac output after two weeks at 4300 m, J. Appl. Physiol. 25: 400-409 (1968).

19. M. Samaja, A. Veicsteinas, and P. Cerretelli, Oxygen affinity of blood in altitude Sherpas, J. Appl. Physiol.: Respirat. Environ. Exercise Physiol. 47: 337-341 (1979).

20. J. Stenberg, B. Ekblom, and R. Messin, Hemodynamic response to work at simulated altitude, 4000 m, J. Appl. Physiol. 21: 1589-1594 (1966).

21. J.A. Vogel, L.H. Hartley, and J.C. Cruz, Cardiac output during exercise in altitude natives at sea level and high altitude, J. Appl. Physiol. 36: 173-176 (1974).

22. J.B. West, S. Lahiri, M.B. Gill, J.S. Milledge, L.G.C.E. Pugh, and M.P. Ward, Arterial oxygen saturation during exercise at high altitude, J. Appl. Physiol. 17: 617-621 (1962).

23. M.H. Williams, A.R. Godwin, R. Perkins, and J. Bocrie, Effect of blood reinjection upon endurance capacity and heart rate, Med. Sci. Sports 5: 181-186 (1973).

Discussion

CUMMING: Thank you very much. Would it be your wish that we discuss your paper now and then discuss again after the paper tomorrow or would it be better to have the discussion tomorrow, when you have presented the full paper?

CERRETELLI: I think probably it is better to discuss it tomorrow. Unless somebody wants to put a very specific question.

CUMMING: Right, perhaps if you can think about the questions, it would help a lot if we could have the discussion tomorrow, because we have run rather short of time and we would like the opportunity to show the film. While they are preparing to show the film, which will take a couple of moments, perhaps I could say that we have unearthed an area of great controversy and I wondered whether it would be your wish, tomorrow at 11.30 to have a round table discussion solely devoted to the problem of what is the relationship between pulmonary blood flow and pulmonary arterial pressure? The settling of this, which is a cornerstone of many hypotheses, would be a very valuable contribution that this meeting could make. I see people nodding their heads. We will begin our discussion at 11.30 which could then go on until 12.30 or until such time as we exhaust ourselves, or solve the problem. The problem may be resolvable, if we see the different evidences which we have before us and can make critical judgements upon them.

DENISON: It's a very attractive hypothesis that of a maldistribution of peripheral blood flow, and a very credible one. One could easily imagine that perhaps it would occur due to plasma skimming in the peripheral circulation, with a high haematocrit. The thing that worries me about it is that if it was going to occur in the peripheral circulation, why doesn't it also occur in the pulmonary circulation? I wonder whether you could tell us a bit more about your analysis of the passage of viscous blood through the lungs.

CERRETELLI: The problem is that little is known about the pulmonary circulation during conditions of very high viscosity, even in patients that have polycythaemia. One might even hypothesize that subjects with this plasma skimming the lungs may have an impaired gas transfer, which is not too apparent here since there is no change in arterial saturation. The saturation in the pulmonary tree is completely different from that in the muscles. It's an attractive point, and should be investigated, in the muscles first, and then in the lungs.

LOCKHART: I'm sorry but I think I missed the point you made with the slide just before the last. If we could have the slide I would like to ask you a question.

CERRETELLI: The slide before the last, please. That one.

LOCKHART: May I just make very briefly two points that support the hypothesis we've just heard about the importance of peripheral factors? Durand has conducted studies measuring kidney blood flow, ejection fraction and so forth, in highlanders. And there is some suggestion that the higher the haematocrit the more impaired are the kidney haemodynamics. Which points again to something happening in the peripheral circulation. Now, second, at sea level, in chronic bronchitis, most will stop exercising when you push them to the symptom limited oxygen uptake. When you push 'them as hard as feasible, most of them will stop with a mixed venous PO_2 which is far higher than the lowest PvO_2 that can be obtained in athletes, at a mixed venous PO_2 around 28 to 30 Torr, which is fairly high. This again suggests that with chronic hypoxia at sea level the problem does not lie with the transportation of oxygen by the blood, but with the usage of blood at the periphery, and this fits very well with what we've heard today.

CERRETELLI: That's a very interesting observation, I think it should be explored by the clinicians.

MORPURGO: I would like to ask two questions. Yesterday you mentioned that in a particular climate we can see exceptional performances such as allowed Mesner to reach the top of Everest without using oxygen. Now, undoubtedly temperature plays a part and I would like to know if there are observations either of yourself or other authors where you have been able to disassociate the influence of ambient temperature from that of altitude. Secondly, are there observations in the literature of the behaviour of systemic and pulmonary circulation times under these conditions?

CERRETELLI: In the experiments of Jacques Durand who studied the effects of temperature on the skin circulation of high altitude residents and on pulmonary circulation, I think that cold has a considerable effect. For example, exposure to cold gives an increase in pulmonary hypertension which has already been observed in acute and chronic hypoxia, and also changes cutaneous circulation. Therefore it appears that in freezing conditions, especially an altered pulmonary circulation can have repercussions on the muscles and their performance since in practice this is the same circuit. As regards the second question, considerable work has been carried out, particularly in the Andes at Morococcia. However, they were sufferers from Monge's disease and not healthy individuals. I do not have any data nor have I ever come across any on standard, healthy subjects who have been willing to undergo this sort of test, but undoubtedly this would be a very interesting study to conduct as part of a study into pulmonary haemodynamics of polycythaemic individuals. I would propose when talking of studies at sea level that we separate, for example, polycythaemia from hypoxia as a start. This can also be done in animals and that's what I am doing; trying to increase the haematocrit values in the normal dog and to see the consequences produced by polycythaemia on muscle performance in normal oxygen situations.

TRICOMI: We all noticed from the film that pulmonary oedema was prevalently apical. This leads me to formulate a hypothesis. I do not have experience with x-ray of normal subjects at high altitude, but I do have experience with highly trained sportsmen who come for check ups. One thing that immediately strikes one, especially in those who undergo prolonged muscular exertion, weight lifters and the like, is that the standard chest x-ray shows a base-apical balance of perfusion or indeed a base-apical inversion of perfusion. I think this should be gone into further and that the protocols studying these high altitude dwellers should include simple chest x-rays as a first approach. What is your interpretation of this type of chest x-ray as seen in the case of sportsmen who are trained in this way? Obviously, there is a recruitment of the apical areas. However, if these subjects undergo perfusional scintigraphy at rest we see a completely normal picture. Perfusional scintigraphy after a small amount of exertion also shows a normal picture. The conclusion being that the normal x-ray represents the completed recruitment of the apical areas which are naturally already prepared to accept the majority of the blood flow during exercise.

CERRETELLI: I am no radiological expert but I think I have understood. The picture of pulmonary oedema at high altitudes, upper zone oedema of patchy type is characteristic and well known though the pathogenesis is not. We do know that this oedema has this distribution. We have the hypotheses of Normal Staub for example who thinks that it is caused by microembolisms of lymphocytes. As regards the problem of pulmonary circulation in high altitude dwellers we must accept a well known fact that there is pulmonary hypertension in acute hypoxia and particularly in chronic hypoxia, not just in those born at high altitudes but also those exposed to high altitudes for a certain period. This would explain why there is an increase in flow, recruitment, let us call it, of the upper zones at rest and particularly during exercise. Thus, athletes under strain show recruitment of the whole lung even for fairly light exercise but probably this would also be the case even for fairly light exercise but probably this would also be the case even for non-athletes. I don't know. Perfusional scintigraphy shows a total recruitment even of the apical areas, even for non-athletes, does it not?

BONSIGNORE: What happens to cardiac output in the case of haemodilution?

CERRETELLI: I would have expected that at most the cardiac output would have a maximum increase; and it may increase greatly and this may be the reason for the benefit derived from haemodilution. It could also be an improvement in the peripheral circulation, however this is still the subject of study.

EXTERNAL IMAGING OF PULMONARY PERFUSION AND VENTILATION

Ferruccio Fazio

M.R.C. Cyclotron Unit and Department of Medicine
Hammersmith Hospital
London, W12 OHS, U.K.

INTRODUCTION

The routine chest X-ray is a standard radiographic procedure
which provides a great deal of anatomic information to the physi-
cian. Indeed, the chest X-ray will detect increased or reduced
density of lung structures, thus providing information on lung
anatomy, rather than function.

Among the various functions of the lung, the most important
is gas exchange, which depends to a great extent on the distribution of perfusion and ventilation. The most common cause of
impairment of gas exchange is ventilation/perfusion mismatching;
this can occur both at the intrazonal (or microscopical) and the
interzonal (or macroscopical) level in the lungs.

Attempts to detect macroscopic changes in regional perfusion
(and ventilation) from the chest X-ray have been made in the past,
mainly from consideration of the size and distribution of pulmonary
vessels and changes in the lung parenchyma.

In the last decade, specific techniques making use of radioactive isotopes for imaging lung perfusion and ventilation have
been developed. These techniques are based on the use of radioactive isotopes.

Techniques for Assessing Regional Perfusion and Ventilation

Lung scanning following the intravenous injection of labelled
particles is the procedure for obtaining functional images of
regional pulmonary perfusion. This technique, developed in 1964

(Taplin et al, 1964; Wagner et al, 1964; Quinn et al, 1964), is now
routinely used in virtually every department of nuclear medicine.

Human serum albumin particles of 10 to 30 μ in the poly-
dispersed (macroaggregates) or the monodispersed (microspheres)
form are now commercially available from a number of manu-
facturers and can be labelled with a variety of isotopes
(Technetium-99m is commonly used). These particles can be
injected in a peripheral vein, mix uniformly with the blood
during their passage through the right heart, and then reach
the pulmonary capillary bed where they are trapped in a way
proportional to the regional blood flow through the capillary
network. External recording of their distribution with a rectilinear scanner or a gamma camera will, therefore, yield a
functional image of pulmonary perfusion. Six views (anterior,
posterior, right and left laterals, right and left posterior
obliques) are always recommended. Right and left anterior
obliques can also be performed in the suspicion of lesions to
the middle lobe and the lingula respectively. Lateral and
oblique views are important because of the front-to-back
stratification of segments within the lung, segmental differences
being more obvious from the lateral than from the anterior or
posterior views.

Perfusion scanning using the technique described above is
now an established diagnostic procedure routinely used in the
clinical context, as it is simple, safe, does not require co-
operation of the patient and it provides functional images of
the pulmonary perfusion of high statistical accuracy and in
multiple views.

In order to produce comparable images for ventilation,
different techniques are now being used in different centres.
Indeed, none of these techniques can yet be regarded as satisfactory as the lung perfusion scan, which therefore in many
centres is still used alone, not supplemented by ventilation
measurements.

Techniques for ventilation scanning include the use of
either radioactive gases or aerosols.

a)   Radioactive Gas Methods

a.i Single Breath/Washout of Radioactive Xenon (Loken and
     Westgate, 1968; Newhouse et al, 1968).

Xenon-133 is a chemically inert gas with a half-life of
5.3 days. The patient is asked to take a deep breath of ^{133}Xe
(10-15 mCi) and then to breath-hold for 30 seconds. During
this time up to 100,000 counts can be collected on a gamma

camera (this method cannot be used with a rectilinear scanner).
The image recorded on the gamma camera will be proportional to
the regional arrival of the radioactive gas, which in turn is
proportional to regional ventilation. Re-breathing of ^{133}Xe
can then be carried out in a closed circuit for 3-5 minutes until
equilibrium is reached and another image can be obtained, which
is representative of lung volume rather than ventilation. The
patient is then switched to room air and serial pictures (every
60") are taken while ^{133}Xe is washed out. In a normal subject,
the lung empties in a uniform manner, and all the activity
should have washed out within one minute. Areas of reduced
ventilation will be seen during the wash-out phase as areas of
abnormal ^{133}Xe retention. Washout images are useful in detecting
localized areas of reduced or absent ventilation but are not
directly comparable to the perfusion images obtained with
^{99m}Tc-HAMM. On the other hand, the images obtained in the first
part of the procedure (single breath - breath-holding) require
manoeuvres which are not physiologic and are impracticable in
dyspnoeic patients. These images are usually obtained in only
one projection (due to dosimetric problems and to the build-up of
^{133}Xe background in the chest wall). They are generally of poor
quality, owing to the low counting statistics achievable during
the breath-holding. Another problem is the unfavourable physical
characteristics of ^{133}Xe. Its significant solubility ($\sim$15%) may
introduce errors in the washout phase due to uptake of tracer in
the blood and in the chest wall. Its low gamma ray energy (80 keV)
is not optimal for imaging and cannot be compared directly with
lung perfusion images obtained with ^{99m}Tc-HAMM (140 keV). The low
energy of ^{133}Xe also prevents inhalation scans from being done
after the perfusion study, which is regarded as a limitation in the
diagnostic strategy of pulmonary embolism, one of the most important clinical applications of lung scanning. Some of these problems could be avoided by using, instead of ^{133}Xe, Xenon-127 (half-
life 36.4 days) (Goddard and Ackery, 1975). This isotope has more
favourable physical characteristics, having an emission energy
of 200 keV, which is good for imaging with the gamma camera and
can easily be separated from the 140 keV of ^{99m}Tc, thus making it
possible for the ventilation study to be performed after the
perfusion study. However, ^{127}Xe is expensive and difficult to
get, as it can only be produced on high energy physics research
facilities such as linear accelerators.

a.ii Continuous Inhalation of ^{81m}Kr (Fazio and Jones, 1975;
Goris et al, 1977; Fazio et al, 1978a).

Krypton-81m is a 190 keV gamma emitting radioactive gas with
a very short half-life (13 seconds). This gas can be continuously
produced by passing air through a generator made of its parent ^{81}Rb
(Clark et al, 1976). ^{81}Rb has a half-life of 4.6 hours and can be
efficiently produced on a medium-energy medical cyclotron. The

half-life of the parent enables ^{81m}Kr to be continuously available all day after a morning (or late evening) production of ^{81}Rb. When ^{81m}Kr is continuously added to the inspired air during normal breathing, equilibrium of the isotope with alveolar gas is never reached because of the short half-life; thus the distribution becomes representative of ventilation rather than volume, unlike longer-lived radioactive gases such as ^{133}Xe or ^{127}Xe. Thus, continuous recording with a gamma camera of the activity over the chest when ^{81m}Kr is simply added to the inspired air yields a functional image of ventilation. The technique can be combined to an injection of ^{99m}Tc-labelled macroaggregates in order to perform ventilation/perfusion studies in multiple views: ventilation and perfusion can be sequentially obtained for each view by adding ^{81m}Kr to the inspired air for recording of ventilation only. Thus, ^{81m}Kr will no longer be present while recording ^{99m}Tc; when recording ventilation the 190 keV of ^{81m}Kr can easily be separated from the 140 keV of ^{99m}Tc. Both perfusion and ventilation images can be obtained in 2-4 min for each view, the patient being unaware of the switching from perfusion to ventilation. No waste disposal is required for ^{81m}Kr, due to the short half-life of the isotope and its low concentration in the expired air. ^{81m}Kr yields functional images of pulmonary ventilation under physiological conditions, that is, during quiet tidal breathing. These images can be directly compared to the standard lung perfusion scan with ^{99m}Tc-HAMM; perfusion and ventilation scans can be recorded in rapid succession without moving the patient, contain the same number of counts, and have almost identical resolution. ^{81m}Kr scans can also be used for recording a rapid sequence of physiologic events, such as the response of regional ventilation distribution to bronchodilator treatment. The major practical disadvantage of the method is the relatively short half-life of the parent, ^{81}Rb (4.6 hours), which requires considerable planning and interest on the part of the user (^{81m}Kr can only be used within 16-18 hours from the shipment of the ^{81m}Kr generator).

b)   Aerosol Methods (Taplin et al, 1966; Taplin and Chopra, 1978)

Following the inhalation, during normal tidal breathing, of aerosolized radioactive solutions, deposition of the aerosol within the lungs will take place by (a) sedimentation to the lower respiratory tract according to regional ventilation, and (b) impaction in the large airways. If all particles would sediment to the lung periphery, the images obtained following their nebulization would be representative of regional ventilation. Therefore the potential advantage of this method is to obtain images of regional ventilation of good statistical quality in multiple views and without requiring a great deal of co-operation from the patient. In fact, if the particles are sufficiently small (mass median diameter less than 2-3 μ), deposition occurs mainly for sedimentation in the small airways and, at least in subjects free from airways disease, little

is retained in the throat, trachea or large bronchi. However,
bronchial stenosis due to excessive mucus or bronchial inflammation can induce local turbulence of airflow which in turn increases deposition of particles for impaction and leads therefore
to a preferential distribution of the inhaled aerosol in the large
airways. Indeed, in patients with chronic airflow obstruction the
distribution of inhaled particles is more central than that of
inhaled gases, although by and large areas of lack of peripheral
penetration of aerosol particles correspond to areas of decreased
ventilation assessed by radioactive gas methods (Fazio et al, 1978b;
Greening et al, 1979). Thus, aerosol techniques may not be adequate
for assessing regional ventilation in patients with severe chronic
airflow obstruction. On the other hand, deposition of particles by
impaction in the large airways can be minimized by reducing the mass
median diameter of the inhaled particles (Muir, 1972). An ideal
aerosol method for the clinical assessment of regional ventilation
should have the following requirements: (a) be simple and quick to
prepare and to administer; (b) be labelled with a short-lived
isotope with energy over 180 keV. This would allow a perfusion scan
with ^{99m}Tc to be obtained first, the 140 keV of ^{99m}Tc not interfering
in higher windows. Ideally, the energy should be not more than
250 keV, because energies above this threshold are suboptimal for
the gamma camera; (c) the mass median diameter of the particles inhaled should be between 0.5 and 1.0 µ. Larger particles tend to
deposit in central airways of patients with airflow obstruction.
Smaller particles tend to be re-exhaled, therefore minimizing the
fraction of particle deposited. For an aerosol with a mass median
diameter of 1.0 µ less than 10% of the particles inhaled are retained in the lungs, more than 90% being recovered in the expired
air. This results in a considerable waste of radioactivity and in
increased radioactive risk to the operator: with the breathing
circuitry commonly used (nebulizer connected to the inspiratory
line and a filter for trapping the particles to the expiratory line),
in order to get 1-2 millicuries of a tracer into the lungs of a
patient, the operator has to start off with 20-30 millicuries.

In order to optimize the particle size, different aerosols
have been proposed by different laboratories. Simple nebulization
of a radioactive solution (even with ultrasonic nebulizers) yields
particles of relatively large size (3-5 µ) and therefore suboptimal
for ventilation scanning. Better results are achieved by nebulizing
pre-sized radioactive particles (human albumin microspheres). These
can be labelled with ^{99m}Tc and nebulized with a Venturi nebulizer,
yielding, at the outflow of the nebulizer, particles with a mass
median diameter of 1.0 - 1.5 µ. By comparing the images obtained
with those particles with ^{81m}Kr ventilation scans, it has been
found that this aerosol provides satisfactory ventilation images in
patients with chronic airflow obstruction provided that their $FEV_{1.0}$
is not less than 50% of the predicted value (Greening et al, 1979).

Excellent results are obtained using a simple and ingenious approach proposed by George Taplin (Taplin and Chopra, 1978). A solution of ^{99m}Tc-labelled DTPA is nebulized via a disposable low volume nebulizer (operated by compressed air at a flow rate of 8-10 litre/min) in a reservoir settling bag placed in the delivery line between the nebulizer and the patient's mouthpiece. This bag removes most particles and/or droplets larger than 2 μ in size by sedimentation or impaction. By using, instead of ^{99m}Tc-DTPA, ^{113m}In labelled human serum albumin, the aerosol ventilation scan can be performed following the ^{99m}Tc perfusion scan. This is preferable for the diagnostic strategy of pulmonary embolism. (The perfusion scan should be obtained first as a normal perfusion would rule out the presence of thromboembolic disease). Although systematic comparisons with other aerosols or with ^{81m}Kr are, as yet, not available, this method seems to provide, in patients with chronic airflow obstruction, less central deposition than other particle methods, including pre-sized aerosols. The technique, which is currently being evaluated in our laboratory, is to perform first the perfusion scan with ^{99m}Tc (140 keV) and to subsequently obtain a ventilation scan with ^{113m}In (390 keV), using a high energy collimator. It should be kept in mind that the two images (perfusion and ventilation) are not strictly comparable, as the coefficient of attenuation within the body for the two isotopes is different. There are also differences in resolution (even using a high-energy collimator), the energy of ^{113m}In being not optimal for the γ camera. When using ^{113m}In only the anterior, posterior and oblique views should be obtained, lateral views being meaningless due to the high penetration coefficient (and therefore the significant shine-through) of the highly energetic γ rays of ^{113m}In.

Clinical Applications of Lung Scanning

In this section the patterns of ventilation/perfusion scanning in various disease states will be described, as obtained on a large field gamma camera using the ^{99m}Tc-labelled microspheres technique for perfusion and continuous inhalation of ^{81m}Kr for ventilation. This latter technique, despite its limited clinical availability, is unique in providing images of pulmonary ventilation in multiple views which are directly comparable to the ^{99m}Tc-HAMM lung perfusion scan. Knowledge of ventilation/perfusion relationships in disease states will serve as a guideline to interpret ventilation/perfusion scans also when ventilation scanning is performed with more available but less accurate or specific techniques (such as single breath - washout of ^{133}Xe or inhalation of radioactive aerosols).

a)   The Normal Ventilation/Perfusion Scan

It has been shown, using the wash-out of radioactive gases, that in normal individuals in the upright posture (sitting or standing) there is a gradient of both blood flow and ventilation down

the lung, with greater perfusion and ventilation per unit volume
in the lower zones (West, 1977). This gradient is mainly due to
the effect of gravity on the hydrostatic blood pressure (for
perfusion) and the pleural pressure (for ventilation). The distribution of air and blood flow from the bottom to the top of the
lungs is more even when the patient is supine. A quantitative
evaluation (in terms of ventilation or perfusion per unit of
volume) of these gradients is difficult to obtain from routine lung
scanning: a lung scan is not an absolute measurement of perfusion
or ventilation per unit lung volume, but rather a map of the
regional distribution of these parameters within the lungs.

Thus, a normal lung perfusion scan obtained in the upright
position shows a gradient of perfusion toward the bases which
might be exaggerated by a geometrical problem, that is, the base
of the lung is thicker than the apices: more activity would be
recorded from the bases even if perfusion per unit of volume was
uniform. A similar (but less obvious) gradient is present in the
ventilation scan. These gradients should always be found on a
normal lung scan.

In normal erect subjects, lateral views show that ventilation
and perfusion are not only following a gravity gradient, but are
preferentially distributed to the lower lobes.

b)   Pulmonary Embolism

The diagnosis of pulmonary embolism is generally considered
the most important application of lung scanning. Pulmonary
embolism is a relatively common condition, estimated to affect as
many as 500,000 patients per year only in the United States, where
it causes some 50,000 deaths per year (Moser, 1977). Prognosis of
pulmonary embolic disease is excellent following diagnosis and early
and appropriate therapy. Nevertheless, pulmonary embolism is very
difficult to diagnose clinically. Common diagnostic procedures
(chest X-ray, blood tests, electrocardiography) are non-specific for
the diagnosis of this disease. The most definitive procedure for the
diagnosis of pulmonary embolism is pulmonary angiography. However,
this is a complex and expensive procedure, which is associated with
some morbidity and is difficult to carry out in emergencies even in
specialized centres. In addition, it is also subject to interpretive
limitations, such as the inability to demonstrate obstruction in
small pulmonary arterial branches (Dalen et al, 1966). The perfusion
lung scan is an ideal technique for this purpose, as it provides a
map of pulmonary blood flow. A negative lung perfusion scan (if
properly performed in multiple views) excludes the presence of a
significant embolus (Poulose et al, 1970; Greenspan, 1974). However,
its specificity is rather low, perfusion defects being also present
in other pathological conditions such as airways disease. The typical lung scan of a patient with pulmonary embolism shows multiple,

segmental or subsegmental defects of perfusion throughout both lungs, in presence of a normal chest X-ray and normal ventilation. Unfortunately the lesions are not always segmental, particularly if the scan is not performed immediately after the embolization and the embolus has partially resolved. The specificity of the perfusion scan is improved by combining it with a ventilation scan. This will show a normal ventilation with impaired perfusion in pulmonary embolism but a combined perfusion/ventilation defect in parenchymal lung disease. Ventilation scanning with ^{133}Xe is now extensively being used for that purpose. The specificity of this combined technique is nearly 100% for patients with multiple large defects and normal ventilation, but considerably less for patients with smaller defects and with defects corresponding to known radiographic abnormalities (McNeil, 1976).

The reason for this is probably that ^{133}Xe ventilation scanning, as discussed previously, requires co-operation from the patient, cannot be performed in multiple views, and does not yield images of good statistical quality which would be required for detecting small ventilation defects. These problems are overcome by the use of ^{81m}Kr; although a systematical comparison with angiography has yet to be made, it is possible that using the combined ^{81m}Kr/^{99m}Tc technique the specificity of lung scanning for the diagnosis of pulmonary embolism would approach 100%, even in patients with small defects and abnormal chest X-ray.

Patients with embolism without infarction typically show defects in lung perfusion with normal ventilation and clear lung fields on the chest X-ray. In patients with radiological evidence of infarction, perfusion is always absent or reduced in correspondence to the infarcted area seen on the chest film, whereas the ^{81m}Kr ventilation scan can be only minimally impaired, ventilation being in any case less impaired than perfusion.

Once the diagnosis of pulmonary embolism is made, the patient should be followed up with ventilation/perfusion scans in order to monitor the effect of treatment. Blood flow is (at least in part) restored to the affected region in about one-third of the patients (Secker-Walker et al, 1970). However, follow-up perfusion scans often show a marked redistribution of blood flow within the lungs, with restoration of perfusion to previously non-perfused or badly perfused areas and new perfusion defects in areas previously well perfused. This can be due (a) to the breaking up of large emboli into smaller fragments, or (b) to new emboli: sometimes it can be difficult to distinguish between these two possible causes of redistribution, as the lung perfusion scan is no more than a qualitative map of pulmonary blood flow. Follow-up studies are essential in that pulmonary thromboembolism does rarely present as an isolated episode; rather, it should be regarded as a recurrent disease, usually associated with the presence of deep vein thrombosis. Thus, it is also important to identify the site of origin of thrombi. Ninety-five per cent of pulmonary emboli originate from deep vein thrombosis of the legs. This can be diagnosed, apart from the clinical signs, using a number of instrumental tools (contrast venography, positive thrombi imaging with radiolabelled fibrinogen, radionuclide venography).

Radionuclide venography can be performed at the time of the perfusion scan without additional injections or administration of radioactivity or contrast medium to the patient: the labelled macroaggregates are injected in a calf vein and their arrival is recorded by collimating the γ camera over the pelvis. When deep thrombosis of the leg or of the pelvic veins are present, the arrival of the radioactive tracer is delayed; sometimes the patterns of collateral venous flow are shown. On occasions, "hot" spots can be seen, resulting from labelled particles stuck to thrombotic areas. When ventilation scanning is not available, routine radionuclide venography is recommended, as it has been shown to add specificity to the lung perfusion scan (Ahmad et al, 1979).

c)   Airways Disease

Regional ventilation and perfusion can be severely impaired in both acute and chronic airways disease, even in the presence of clear lung fields on the chest X-ray.

c.i Asthma

Lung scans can be grossly abnormal in asthma. During acute exacerbations, while the chest X-ray is normal or only shows large volume lungs, ^{81m}Kr ventilation scans reveal large, segmental or even lobar areas of reduced ventilation, with a distribution similar to that observed for perfusion in pulmonary embolism (Fazio et al, 1979a). Bronchodilators induce immediate improvement of ventilation defects and reduction of lung size but full restoration of normal ventilation can usually be achieved only following prolonged treatment (Fazio et al, 1979a).

The relationships between regional ventilation and perfusion (on a macroscopic basis) in asthma have, as yet, been poorly studied. The ventilation abnormalities can be accompanied by parallel changes of perfusion to the same areas. This perfusion impairment to poorly ventilated areas could be explained either by hypoxic vasoconstriction (von Euler and Liljestrand, 1946) or by mechanical factors (blood flow squeezed out of the hyperinflated areas). On other occasions, however, ventilation and perfusion can be mis-matched, showing preferential perfusion distribution to badly ventilated areas and vice-versa. The mechanisms responsible for these changes are, as yet, unclear.

c.ii Acute Bronchitis

Patients with acute bronchitis, either isolated or superimposed to chronic bronchitis, often show large, sometimes segmental,
defects of both ventilation and perfusion with clear lung fields at
the chest X-ray. In these patients, ventilation is usually more
impaired than perfusion. Normal patterns can be restored following
treatment with antibiotics and physiotherapy. The alteration of
ventilation seen in asthmatics and bronchitics can be explained on
the basis of functional and morphological alteration of the bronchial wall (bronchospasm, bronchial oedema, inflammation) or of the
bronchial lumen (mucus plugging), resulting in a reduced air flow
to part of the bronchial tree. This is confirmed by the fact that
these alterations can sometimes be partially reversed by coughs.
The alteration of perfusion can be attributed to functional
mechanisms induced by the ventilation impairment (hypoxic vasoconstriction, lobar shrinkage, etc.) or to direct involvement of
blood vessels by inflammatory processes (Giuntini, 1979).

c.iii Consolidation, Atelectasis

Patients with acute chest problems and presence of consolidation on the chest X-ray usually show an impairment of perfusion and
ventilation corresponding to the opacity seen on the chest X-ray.
These alterations can follow different patterns according to the
pathology underlying the consolidation. In the case of pulmonary
infarct, perfusion appears to be <u>more</u> impaired than ventilation.
On the other hand, in the presence of consolidation due to
pneumonia or bronchopulmonary infection, ventilation appears to be
more impaired than perfusion. Knowledge of these typical appearances can be useful for the differential diagnosis of acute chest
problems with and without the presence of consolidation on the
chest X-ray. Lung ventilation/perfusion scanning can also be of
great value in assessing combined pathologies, such as the association, in the same patient, of thromboembolic and infective processes (Lavender et al, 1979).

In the presence of the radiological appearance of collapse or
atelectasis of a lobe or a portion of lung, the characteristic
appearances on the lung scan are those of an absent or reduced
ventilation to the collapsed area with normal or only slightly
reduced perfusion (Lavender et al, 1979).

Why, in cases of pneumonia and collapse/atelectasis, ventilation can be almost absent while perfusion is only slightly
reduced, is not clear. Atelectasis may occur as a result of
bronchial plugging and subsequent disappearance of air from the
distal portions of the lung. Apparently, in these cases, hypoxic
vasoconstriction is not highly effective (Lavender et al, 1979).

c.iv Chronic Airways Disease

In patients with chronic airways disease predominantly of the emphysematous type (diffuse emphysema) both perfusion and ventilation show multiple, patchy areas of reduced or absent activity, the ventilation scans showing a pattern similar to that of perfusion down to the finest structural level resolved by the gamma camera. In contrast to the lung scan, only diffuse abnormalities rather than regional alterations are usually seen in these patients on the chest radiograph, the typical picture being that of large volume lungs with low diaphragms and overall reduction of the vascular markings. In bullous emphysema, the areas of reduced activity on the scans usually correspond to the bullae seen on the chest radiograph, but additional defects, presumably due to focal emphysema, can be present.

Ventilation/perfusion scans can be particularly useful when pulmonary embolism is suspected in patients with chronic airways disease: it is often difficult from the perfusion scan alone to distinguish areas of reduced or absent perfusion due to parenchymal lung disease from perfusion defects due to pulmonary emboli. A correct diagnosis can usually be obtained with an $81mKr/99mTc$ ventilation/perfusion scan while alternative methods for ventilation scanning may be inadequate. These patients can be rather ill being therefore unable to hold their breath long enough to perform the $133Xe$-single breath inhalation procedure. Only one view can routinely be obtained with this method, which reduces the chances of detecting ventilation/perfusion mismatching.

Aerosol techniques can provide a satisfactory measurement of regional ventilation in patients free from airways disease. In the presence of airways obstruction, however, there is a significant deposition of the inhaled particles in central airways, probably due to impaction of particles in stenotic airway with turbulent air flow regimen. When particles with a mass median diameter between 1.00 and 1.5 μ are used, a reasonably good peripheral distribution of the tracer can be obtained in patients with $FEV_{1.0}$ more than 50% of the predicted value (Greening et al, 1979). Using smaller particles a better peripheral penetration of the aerosol might be achieved even in patients with severe airways obstruction. This might be the alternative solution for ventilation scanning when $81mKr$ is not available.

d) Bronchogenic Carcinoma

In peripheral tumours, ventilation and perfusion are usually absent in correspondence with the mass seen on the chest film. Similar findings are observed in the case of pulmonary metastases.

In central tumours, however, both perfusion and ventilation

are often grossly reduced to the side affected by the tumour, to
an extent unpredictable from the chest X-ray. The finding of
absent ventilation and perfusion to the affected side is not uncommon. Ventilation is often less impaired than perfusion,
probably because the impairment of perfusion is at least in part
due to involvement of pulmonary vessels, particularly low pressure
pulmonary veins. These alterations of regional ventilation and
perfusion can in part be relieved by radiotherapy, unlike tests of
overall lung function like $FEV_{1.0}$ and VC (Fazio et al, 1979b).

e)   Heart Disease

       Patients with long-standing left heart disease show a variable
degree of redistribution of regional pulmonary blood flow toward
the apices (West, 1977). The lateral views of the lung scan show
that blood flow appears in these patients to be shifted not only
toward the apices, but also toward the anterior regions of the lung.
In particular, whereas in normal sitting subjects the main bulk of
perfusion is in the lower lobes, in patients with heart disease it
can be predominant in the anterior segments of the upper lobes.
These changes of the regional distribution of pulmonary perfusion
are due to several mechanisms. Blood flow redistribution can be
induced by mechanical compression from an enlarged heart. Patients
with cardiomegaly show markedly reduced perfusion to the lung bases
on the anterior (and sometimes on the posterior) view, although, in
the lateral views, perfusion to the costophrenic angles is usually
preserved. In fact, redistribution of blood flow per unit of lung
volume is largely due to factors other than heart compression, such
as the increase in left atrial pressure and the increase in pulmonary vascular resistances. Together with a redistribution of perfusion, some redistribution toward the apices of regional ventilation has also been observed in patients with left heart valvular
disease (Fazio et al, 1979c).

The Value of Lung Ventilation/Perfusion Scanning

       In a radiology department, the chest radiograph constitutes
about one-third of the work load. This is in part due to prevalence of pulmonary and cardiac disease and also to the large amount
of information present in the standard chest film. However, this
information is primarily anatomic rather than functional, as the
chest X-ray essentially detects increased or reduced density of
lung structures. Lung scanning provides now an accurate means to
assess regional lung function, in particular regional perfusion and
ventilation; despite the claim that inferences concerning regional
lung perfusion and ventilation can be derived from consideration of
the size and distribution of pulmonary vessels and changes in lung
parenchyma, there is now experimental evidence that the degree to
which regional perfusion and ventilation are impaired is difficult
to predict from the chest radiograph (Fazio et al, 1978a).

Regional function can be impaired with and without the presence of structural abnormalities seen on the chest X-ray. Therefore, a lung scan should never be interpreted without the corresponding chest radiograph, which should be taken at the time of the scan. The combination of these two techniques provides a powerful diagnostic tool for the differential diagnosis of acute chest problems. By adding a lung ventilation/perfusion scan to the routine chest X-ray it is possible to separate acute vascular (pulmonary embolism) from bronchial (acute bronchitis, asthma) disease, to assess whether the radiological finding of a consolidated lung is due to pneumonia or to infarction, and to accurately describe the pathological processes going on in patients with mixed pathologies.

However, diagnosing disease is not the only aim of lung ventilation/perfusion scanning. On occasions, lung scans can be useful to attract the attention on a particular lesion on the chest X-ray or to exactly localize a lesion: it should be remembered that lung scanning allows one to separately study the right and the left lung in multiple views, which cannot be obtained with standard radiology. Another important application of lung scanning is the staging and follow-up of lung disease. A functional evaluation of the patient's condition is nowadays as important as knowing the nature of the disease affecting the patient. The functional evaluation of patients with chest disease now rests on tests of overall and regional lung function. Spirometric measurements (for the assessment of overall function) and lung scanning techniques (for assessing regional function) are not in competition but complementary. Spirometry can be impaired in the presence of normal perfusion/ventilation scans, as these provide a qualitative assessment of relative differences of ventilation and perfusion between lung regions, rather than absolute quantitative measurements of ventilation and perfusion. On the other hand, tests of overall lung function may be relatively insensitive to detect small changes in function and are by definition incapable of detecting regional differences. With lung perfusion and ventilation scanning one can have a visual insight into the lungs, which can uncover alterations not predictable from radiological or spirometric measurements. Follow-up lung scans can be very useful in lung disease, to assess if a treatment is effective, or whether a patient is steady, improving or deteriorating.

To this aim, it is important to obtain both perfusion and ventilation scans, although a great deal of information can also be provided by the perfusion scan alone. Perfusion scanning with ^{99m}Tc-macroaggregates or microspheres is now routinely available in any hospital with nuclear medicine facilities. As far as ventilation scanning is concerned, ^{133}Xe is still widely used in the United States, although this tracer is admittedly inadequate. ^{81m}Kr would probably be the agent of choice but its availability is, as yet, limited. Aerosol ventilation scanning with ^{113m}In is very promising and warrants further consideration.

REFERENCES

Ahmad, M., Fletcher, J.W., Pur-Shahriari, A.A., George, E.A., and Donati, R.M., 1979, Radionuclide venography and lung scanning, J.Nucl.Med., 20: 291.

Clark, J.C., Horlock, P.L., and Watson, I.A., 1976, Krypton-81m generators, Radiochem.Radioanalyt.Lett., 25: 245.

Dalen, J.E., Mathur, V.S., Evans, H., Haynes, F.W., Pur-Shahriari, A.A., Stein, P.D., and Dexter, L., 1966, Pulmonary angiography in experimental pulmonary embolism, Am.Heart J., 72: 509.

Fazio, F., and Jones, T., 1975, Assessment of regional ventilation by continuous inhalation of radioactive Krypton-81m, Brit.med.J., 3: 673.

Fazio, F., Lavender, J.P., and Steiner, R.E., 1978a, ^{81m}Kr ventilation and ^{99m}Tc perfusion scans in chest disease: Comparison with standard radiographs. Am.J.Roentgenol., 130: 421.

Fazio, F., Santolicandro, A., Solfanelli, S., Palla, A., Fornai, E., and Giuntini, C., 1978b, Lung imaging following inhalation of ^{99m}Tc-labelled microspheres: A comparison with the ^{81m}Kr ventilation technique, in: "Clinical and Experimental Applications of Krypton-81m," J.P. Lavender, ed., British Journal of Radiology, Special Report No. 15, pp. 130-140.

Fazio, F., Palla, A., Santolicandro, A., Solfanelli, S., Fornai, E., and Giuntini, C., 1979a, Studies of regional ventilation in asthma using ^{81m}Kr, Lung, 156: 185.

Fazio, F., Pratt, T.A., McKenzie, C.G., and Steiner, R.E., 1979b, Improvement in regional ventilation and perfusion after radiotherapy for unresectable carcinoma of the bronchus, Am.J. Roentgenol., 133: 191.

Fazio, F., Solfanelli, S., di Ricco, G., Balbarini, A., Mariani, M., and Giuntini, C., 1979c, Regional lung ventilation and perfusion in patients with left heart valvular disease, in: "Cardiac Lung," C. Giuntini and P. Panuccio, eds., Piccin, Padova, pp. 85-96.

Giuntini, C., 1979, Personal Communication.

Goddard, B.A., and Ackery, D.M., 1975, Xenon-133, ^{127}Xe and ^{125}Xe for lung function investigations: a dosimetric comparison, J.Nucl.Med., 16: 780.

Goris, M.L., Daspit, S.G., Walter, J.P., McRae, J., and Lamb, J., 1977, Applications of ventilation lung imaging with ^{81m}Krypton, Radiology, 122: 399.

Greening, A.P., Miniati, M., Clay, M., and Fazio, F., 1979, Regional deposition of aerosols in health and in airways obstruction: A comparison with krypton-81m ventilation scanning, in: Proceedings of Sixieme Congres International de Pneumologie, Montpellier, France, 17-18 May 1979.

Greenspan, R.H., 1974, Does a normal isotope perfusion scan exclude pulmonary embolism? Invest.Radiol., 9: 44.

Lavender, J.P., Irving, H., Fazio, F., and Jones, T., 1979, Radio-
    isotope lung scanning using Krypton-81m in acute respiratory
    disease, Am.J.Roentgenol., submitted for publication.
Loken, M.K., and Westgate, H.D., 1968, Using Xenon-133 and a
    scintillation camera to evaluate pulmonary function, J.Nucl.
    Med., 9: 45.
McNeil, B.J., 1976, A diagnostic strategy using ventilation-
    perfusion studies in patients suspect for pulmonary embolism,
    J.Nucl.Med., 17: 613.
Moser, K.M., 1977, Pulmonary embolism, Am.Rev.Resp.Dis., 115: 829.
Muir, D.C.F., 1972, Deposition and clearance of inhaled particles,
    in: "Clinical Aspects of Inhaled Particles," D.C.F. Muir, ed.,
    William Heinemann Medical Books Limited, London.
Newhouse, M.T., Wright, F.J., and Ingham, G.K., 1968, Use of
    scintillation camera and 133Xenon for study of topographic
    pulmonary function, Resp.Physiol., 4: 141.
Poulose, K.P., Reba, R.C., Gilday, D.L., Deland, F.H., and Wagner,
    H.N.Jr., 1970, Diagnosis of pulmonary embolism. A correlative
    study of the clinical, scan, and angiographic findings, Brit.
    med.J., 3: 67.
Quinn, J.L.III, Whitley, J.E., Hudspeth, A.S., and Prichard, R.W.,
    1964, Early clinical applications of lung scintiscanning,
    Radiology, 82: 315.
Secker-Walker, R.H., Jackson, J.A., and Goodwin, J., 1970,
    Resolution of pulmonary embolism, Brit.med.J., 4: 135.
Taplin, G.V., and Chopra, S.K., 1978, Lung perfusion-inhalation
    scintigraphy in obstructive airway disease and pulmonary
    embolism, Radiol.Clin.N.Am., 16: 491.
Taplin, G.V., Johnson, D.E., Dore, E.K., and Kaplan, H.S., 1964,
    Lung photoscans with macroaggregates of human serum radio-
    albumin. Health Physics, 10: 1219.
Taplin, G.V., Poe, N.D., and Greenberg, A., 1966, Lung scanning
    following radioaerosol inhalation, J.Nucl.Med., 7: 77.
Von Euler, U.S., and Liljestrand, G., 1946, Observations on the
    pulmonary arterial blood pressure in the cat, Acta Physiol.
    Scand., 12: 301.
Wagner, H.N.Jr., Sabiston, D.C.Jr., Iio, M., McAfee, J.G., Mayer,
    J.K., and Langan, J.K., 1964, Regional pulmonary blood flow in
    man by radioisotope scanning, J.Am.Med.Assoc., 187: 601.
West, J.B., 1977, "Regional Differences in the Lung," J.B. West,
    ed., Academic Press, New York, San Francisco, London.

Discussion

RIEDEL: I can understand the advantages of the krypton ventilation
studies over the older xenon ones, but this krypton technique won't
be available in the majority of hospitals for years to come, so we
shall still have to rely on the xenon method. On the basis of your
experience with the better krypton technique, could you indicate
what are the main drawbacks of the xenon ventilation study, when to
use it and how to interpret it?

FAZIO: As you know we do the xenon study in the following way:
you take a single breath, and then take an image. Then you
rebreathe and look at the washout. This manoeuvre is not
physiological, since there is forced inspiration. The second
problem is that you look at only a thin layer of the lung, because
the energy of xenon, which is 80 kV does not allow you to look at
the whole depth of the lung, as you can with the high energy
krypton. During this procedure you can spot early impairment of
lung ventilation although this is not a ventilation image. Besides,
you can't obtain lateral views or perhaps only one view. These are
the major drawbacks. My feeling is that the future of clinical
ventilation scanning lies with aerosols. If we can achieve
particles small enough to truly label peripheral airways, which can
be compared with krypton ventilation studies, and which can produce
good quality functional images in multiple views, that is the
solution from my point of view.

RIEDEL: O.K. Does it mean that we should not do xenon studies?
If you say that we should abandon it completely and therefore won't
use xenon perfusion studies for diagnosing pulmonary embolism and
rely on angiography only.

FAZIO: I think it is widely recognised if one has a technique
which is more available and less invasive than angiography then that
would probably be an advantage, particularly for the follow-up of
patients with pulmonary embolic disease. I want to make the point
that I would rather not discuss techniques, because the major point
was to see the condition of the pulmonary circulation and
ventilation in different pathologies.

MORPURGO: In the last slide that you showed there seemed to be a
group of patients suffering from aortic as well as mitral valve
disease. Is there different behaviour in the two parameters shown
on the abscissa and on the ordinate for the group of mitral and
aorta patients? The question has a chemical basis since it is well
known that mitral patients behave differently to aorta patients in
respect of their ventilation.

FAZIO: There aren't really any significant differences because the number of aorta patients is limited, as we have seen. Mitral cases tend to have a more readily increased resistance compared to aorta cases, and pulmonary blood volume can be reduced in mitral disease, whereas this is not so much the case in the aorta group.

CORRIN: I'd like to recommend further correlative studies rather than old fashioned investigations. There has been no mention of post mortem confirmatory studies in any of your patients who have potentially fatal diseases, such as bronchogenic carcinoma and pulmonary emboli. When you were suggesting venous invasion by the tumour, prior consultation with the pathologist before the post mortem could lead to a definite confirmation or otherwise of this. And a lesion I would be particularly interested in looking at is the supposed pulmonary infarct. We have a radiological shadow, no perfusion, yet ventilation is shown. The conventional infarct at autopsy is completely devoid of gas. Yesterday we were discussing early interstitial oedema and the possibility that this might lead to redirection of blood flow. Have you any evidence in your perfusion scintigrams that in early oedema there might be a redirection of blood flow?

FAZIO: All the patients I showed had either a clinical diagnosis made by follow-up or by post mortem, and all patients with carcinoma of the bronchis had a histological classification. This work will appear in the literature with all these data. As far as your question is concerned, we do have indeed some data, and the data are as follows: in chronic interstitial oedema, there is a redistribution of blood flow towards the apices when this is associated with increased vascular resistances which is not frequent. If that is not the case, and in acute pulmonary oedema of the interstitial type, as in myocardial infarction, there is a slight redistribution, which is at the most a balance flow, but never a reverse flow. I have seen a couple of patients with very marked oedema localised at the lung bases and normal pulmonary blood flow.

THE ROLE OF PROSTAGLANDINS IN THE RESPIRATORY SYSTEM

Rodolfo Paoletti, Andrea Poli and Elena Tremoli

Institute of Pharmacology and Pharmacognosy, University

of Milan, Via A. Del Sarto 21, 20129 Milan, Italy

INTRODUCTION

The platelets survival time, as measured with isotopic and metabolic methods, is often shortened in patients with chronic respiratory diseases. Platelets overconsumption may be due to alterations of the intimal membranes of the pulmonary arteries, or to variations in the response of platelets themselves[1,2]. This situation is likely to contribute to the pulmonary damage, by causing the continuous formation of microthrombi reducing the arterial blood supply to the lungs: it is, then, obviously responsible of the dramatic episodes of massive thrombosis of the large pulmonary arteries[3,4].

Drugs affecting platelet aggregation are therefore potentially useful in the management of at least some of the most common chronic pulmonary diseases[5]. In this report, the theoretical basis of such therapeutic use will be discussed.

PROSTAGLANDINS IN PLATELETS AND VESSEL WALLS.

It is known that the interactions between the vessel walls and platelets are regulated, in part, by components of the prostaglandin group. All these compounds originate from a common precursor, the free fatty acid arachidonic acid, which is a normal constituent of plasma membranes in animal cells including platelets. Arachidonic acid is released from membrane phospholipids, by phospholipase A_2 [6] and then metabolized by the prostaglandin synthetase complex, which includes cicloxygenase and prostaglandin isomerase[7]. The intermediate compounds produced (endoperoxides, or PGG_2 and PGH_2) follow different pathways in the various tissues:

in platelets they are mainly transformed into Thromboxane A_2, a non-prostaglandin compound which is extremely active in reducing cAMP levels and in aggregating platelets themselves, and which exerts a marked vasoconstricting action[8] (Fig.1).

In the vessel wall, and particularly in the intimal layer, the endoperoxides are metabolized to Prostacyclin (PGI_2), a double cycled prostaglandin with pronounced antiaggregating and vasodilating properties, mediated by a stimulating effect on the adenylate cyclase[9]. The imbalance between the synthesis or release of these two antagonistic compounds may induce a thrombogenic or an hemorragic diathesis.

Arachidonic acid may follow another metabolic route: just after its release from membrane phospholipids it may be metabolized

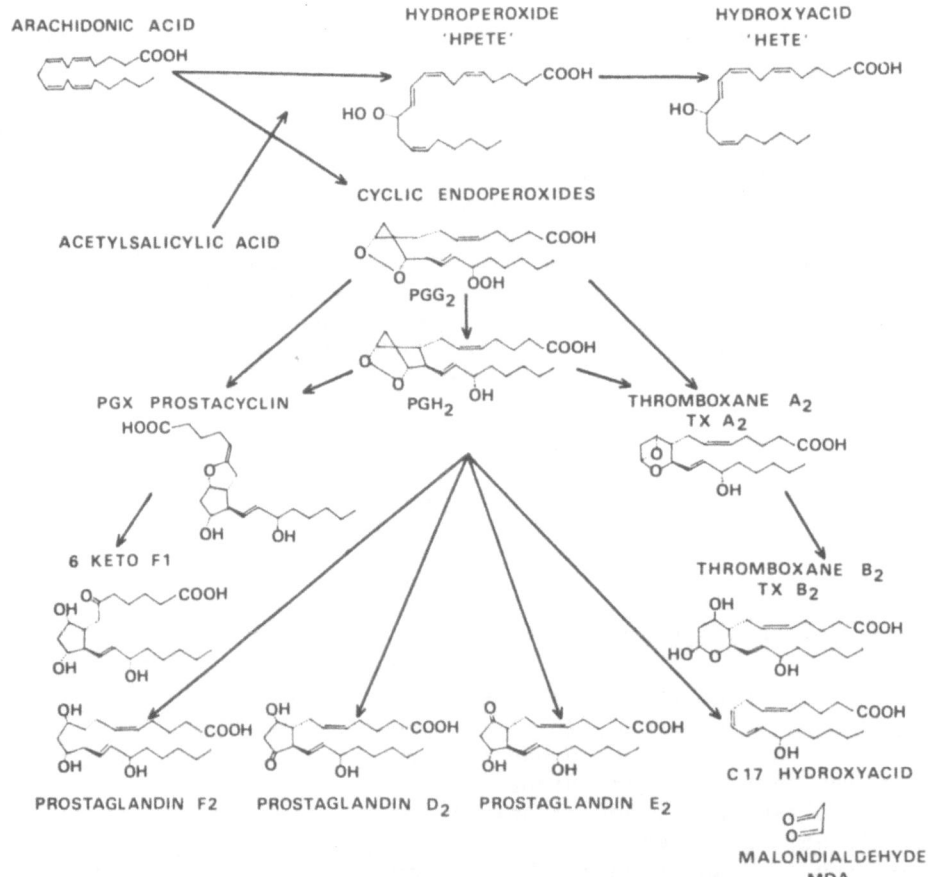

Fig. 1. Metabolic pathway of arachidonic acid.

by lipoxygenases, enzymes giving origin to not cyclized oxygenated
compounds, such as HPETE and HETE[10] (Fig. 1). The physiological
properties of these substances, much less known than those of the
prostaglandins, have recently been partially cleared by the disco-
very that SRS-A, a mediator of inflammation, originates from HPETE,
after a rearrangement of the position of the hydroxy group and its
binding to a cysteine molecule[11]. Even an imbalance between lipoxygenase and cycloxygenase activity may then be of physiopathological
interest, and expecially in lungs, where inflammatory processes may
show sometimes dramatic effects.

The metabolism of arachidonic acid may be modified for therapeutic purposes at various steps. The non-steroidal antiinflammatory
drugs exert their action by inhibiting, sometimes irreversibly (as
in the case of acetylsalicylic acid), the activity of the cycloxygenase enzyme. This action abolishes the synthesis of all the most
active compounds, such as Thromboxane and Prostacyclin[12]. On the
other hand, it may enhance the production of HETE like substances.
In psoriasic patients, for instance, this may represent a deleterious effect. The dermic lesions may become aggravated after application of salicylates, owing to the overproduction of these
compounds. A more complete antiinflammatory effect is displayed
by steroidal drugs. These substances are unable to affect the
metabolism of free arachidonate, but seem to prevent, in as yet
largely unknown manner, its release from membranes. In this way,
they reduce the synthesis of both cycloxygenase and lipoxygenase
derived metabolites. The action might be due to the membrane stabilizing effect exerted by the steroidal drugs[13], to the synthesis of
an inhibitor of phospholipase A_2 [14], or to an ipermeabilization of
the membrane to the prostaglandins and other compounds produced at
microsomal level[13].

Drugs able to affect selectively the rate of synthesis of
Thromboxane or of Prostacyclin are not yet available. Compounds of
the imidazole group are effective, in vitro, in inhibiting the
Thromboxane synthetase system without affecting Prostacyclin[15]:
they are, however, too toxic to be used in vivo.

ANTIAGGREGATING AGENTS: PHARMACOLOGICAL CONSIDERATIONS.

Even if a large group of drugs may affect platelets aggregation,
only a small number has undergone clinical evaluation.

Acetylsalicylic acid is the prototype of these drugs. It is
well characterized in its ability to suppress prostaglandin synthesis, by acetylating the active site of the enzyme cycloxygenase[12].
It is also known that all its pharmacological properties are related
to this basic mechanism of action. Enzyme inactivation following
acetylsalicylic acid exposure cannot be reversed. The direct effect
of acetylsalicylate uptake is a sharp decrease of the production of

all kinds of prostaglandin, and a correlated increase in lipoxygenase derivatives.

Sulfinpyrazone, a drug first developed as an uricosuric agent,
and later shown to reduce platelets overconsumption, normalizes
platelets shortened life[16]. Sulfinpyrazone too is able to inhibit
platelet prostaglandin synthesis. Unlike acetylsalicylic acid, its
action is competitive with respect to arachidonic acid, and fully
reversible; thus, Sulfinpyrazone must be present in the medium to
exert its action[17]. Both Sulfinpyrazone and acetylsalicylic acid
are active in the same dose-range: 500-1000 mg/day.

The third compound of the type is Dipyridamole. Its ability
to prolong platelets survival in patients has been correlated to
the inhibition induced on platelet phosphodiesterase[18]. The raised
levels of intracellular cAMP may explain its action, since this
molecule has antiaggregating properties. Recently, it has been
suggested that Dipyridamole increases Prostacyclin release from
the vessel walls[19], but this extremely interesting observation still
need confirmations. Dipyridamole is not antiaggregating in vitro:
it is thus likely that its mechanism of action is different from
that of cycloxygenase inhibitors. This consideration raises the
possibility that these two groups of drugs might act sinergistically,
as suggested also by clinical observations. Controlled clinical
studies on the clinical effects of Dipyridamole and acetylsalicylic
acid combined are presently under way[20].

ANTIAGGREGATING AGENTS: CLINICAL RESULTS.

A number of controlled or retrospective trials have been performed to assess the value of antiaggregating agents in various
fields of vascular pathology. The antiplatelet therapy seems, generally, able to produce valuable results. Both miocardial reinfarction and cerebrovascular accidents have been reduced by the use of
Sulfinpyrazone[21,22], a drug able to prolong, in vivo, the platelets
half-life. Surprisingly, the results of the trial concerning cerebrovascular accidents has shown that the benefit is confined to
male subjects. Similar results have been obtained in other trials:
it might thus be of little value to give to female subjects antiaggregating drugs, except for clear immediate indication (deep vein
pathology, etc.). These data are probably explained by the physiological difference between aggregating and antiaggregating prostaglandins in men and women.

Platelets from female subjects are generally less responsive
to aggregating agents then those of males[23]; whereas in males the
synthesis of Thromboxane seems to be prevalent. The suppression of
cycloxygenase activity induced by acetylsalicylic acid or related
compounds, would then abolish differences between the two sexes by

eliminating, in man, a potentially hazardous metabolic pathway, and thus, provinding a benefit, and on the contrary, in women a protecting one, with the consequence of negative clinical results. It must be remembered that platelet and the arterial wall cycloxygenases show different sensitivity to acetylsalicylic acid, being perhaps the latter more resistant to the action of this drug. In addition, the intimal cells, which are provided of nucleus, in contrast to platelets, may synthesize new enzymes after the exposition to the drug[24]. For these two reasons, low doses of acetylsalicylic acid (up to 400 mg) widely distributed in time (thrice a week, for example) are partially selective inhibitors of platelets prostaglandins. These doses should be theoretically more effective than the large doses used up to day (800 mg b.i.d. - 1.5 g t.i.d.) in most of the trials which have been published[23]. Evidence is increasing that prostaglandins are not only local hormones, but that at least, some of them may play a significant role even at a distance from the site of synthesis. The lung, for example, behaves as an endocrine system producing prostacyclin, but not able to inactivate it[25]. This compound enters therefore in the systemic circulation. A damage of the lung can thus affect platelet aggregation in the whole organism, and explain the epidemiological data suggesting a higher frequency of thromboembolic episodes in patients affected by chronic obstructive pulmonary disease, pulmonary hypertension, or other forms of pulmonary pathology[26].

EXPERIMENTAL DATA AND CONCLUSIONS.

The demonstration of the shortened platelet survival time in patients with chronic obstructive lung disease (COLD), and the possible role of the lung as an endocrine organ releasing prostacyclin suggests - in chronic pulmonary pathology - an imbalance among types of prostaglandins produced, favouring thrombosis. For this reason, drug affecting platelet survival could be useful in such clinical situations. Recent data obtained in our laboratory, indicate that Dipyridamole prolongs the mean survival time of human platelets, when administered at the dose of 375 mg/day to patients, even if it is unable to completely normalize this value[2] (Fig. 2). Platelet half-life has been studied, in this experiment, using a non isotopic method which seems very promising in human investigations. The ability of platelets to produce prostaglandins (which are measured in this case as one of their main metabolites, malonyldialdehyde) after a total inactivation of Prostaglandin synthesis in circulating platelets by aspirin is followed in a time sequence (Fig. 3).

The observation carried out in our laboratory and the data available from the most recent literature indicate the important role of arachidonate metabolites, notably Prostacyclin in the survival time of circulating platelets, particularly during chronic diseases of the lung.

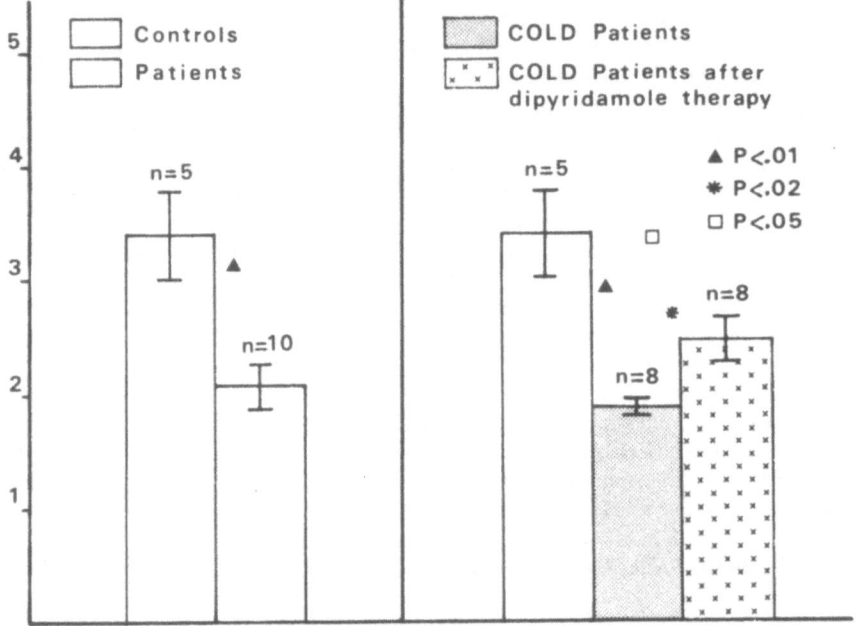

Fig. 2. Half platelet regeneration time in COLD patients before and
after dipyridamole therapy in comparison with controls.
Dipyridamole administered orally at the daily dose of
375 mg for 21 days (Tremoli et al., 1979, in press).

Direct measurements of the rate of synthesis and of the
circulatory levels of Prostacyclin and Thromboxane shall greatly
increase our knowledge of the general implications following acute
and chronic pulmonary affections.

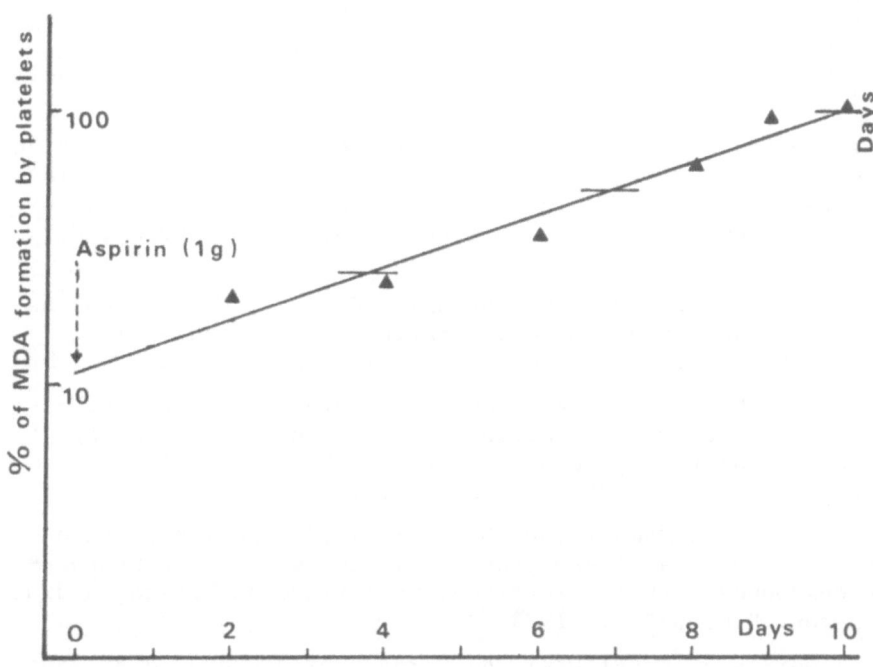

Fig. 3. Platelet survival time after aspirin administration: an
example (Tremoli et al., 1979, in press).

REFERENCES

1. M.D. Steele, J.H. Ellis, Jr., H.S. Weily, E. Genton, Platelet
   survival time in patients with hypoxiemia and pulmonary hypertension, Circulation, 55, 660-662, 1977.

2. E. Tremoli, L. Bertoli, F. Conti, R. Merlini, O. Mantero,
   Platelet antiaggregating therapy in chronic obstructive lung
   disease, in press, 1979.

3. N.O. Fowler, B. Black Schaffer, R.C. Scott, M. Gueron, Idiopathic
   and thromboembolic pulmonary hypertension, Am. J. Med. 40,
   331-333, 1966.

4. C.A. Wagenvoort, D. Heath, J.E. Edwards, "The pathology of the
   pulmonary vasculature", Springfield, Charles C. Thomas, Publ.,
   1964.

5. L.A. Harken, S.J. Slichter, Platelet and fibrinogen consumption
   in man, N. Engl. J. Med., 287, 999, 1972.

6. J.R. Vane, Inhibitors of prostaglandin, prostacyclin and thromboxane synthesis, in "Adv. Prostaglandin and Thromboxane Research", vol. IV, pp. 27-44, 1978, Raven Press, N.Y.

7. D. Nutgeren, E. Hazelhof, Isolation and properties of inter-mediates in prostaglandins biosynthesis, Biochim. Biophys. Acta 326, 448-481, 1973.

8. M. Hamberg, J. Svensson and B. Samuelsson, Novel transformation of prostaglandin endoperoxides: formation of thromboxanes, in "Adv. Prostaglandins and Thromboxane Research", vol. 1, pp. 19-27 (B. Samuelsson and R. Paoletti, eds.), Raven Press, N.Y. 1976.

9. S. Moncada, P. Needleman, S.Bunting, J.R. Vane, Prostaglandins endoperoxide and thromboxane generating systems and their selective inhibition, Prostaglandins, 12, 323-329, 1976.

10. J. Svensson, M. Hamberg, B. Samuelsson, Prostaglandins endo-peroxides. IX. Characterization of rabbit aorta contracting substance (RCS) from guinea pig lung and human platelets, Acta Physiol. Scand., 94, 222-228, 1975.

11. P. Borgeat and B. Samuelsson, Metabolism of arachidonic acid in polimorphonuclear leukocytes. Isolation of novel hydroxy-lated compounds, 4th International Conference on Prostaglandins, Washington, D.C.,U.S.A., 1979.

12. R.J. Flower, R.J. Gryglewski, K. Herdaczynska-Cedro, J.R. Vane, Effects of antiinflammatory drugs on prostaglandins biosynthe-sis, Nature, New Biol., 238, 104-106, 1972.

13. R.J. Gryglewski, Steroid hormones, antiinflammatory steroids and prostaglandins, Pharmac. Res. Comm., 8, 337-347, 1976.

14. R.J. Flower, G.J. Blackwell, Antiinflammatory steroids induce biosynthesis of a phospholipase A_2 inhibitor which prevents prostaglandin generation, Nature, 278, 456-459, 1979.

15. S. Moncada, S. Bunting, J.R. Vane, P. Thorogood, A. Raz, P. Needleman, Imidazole, a selective potent antagonist of thrombo-xane synthetase, Prostaglandins, 13, 611-618, 1977.

16. H.A. Smythe, M.A. Ogryzlo, E.A. Murphy, The effect of sulfin-pyrazone (Anturane) on platelet economy and blood coagulation in man, Can. Med. Assoc. J., 92, 818-821, 1965.

17. M. All, J.W.D. McDonald, Steroid hormones, antiinflammatory steroids and prostaglandins, J. Lab. Clin. Med., 89, 868-875, 1977.

18. D.C.B. Mills, J.B. Smith, The influence on platelets aggrega-tion of drugs that affect the accumulation of 3',5'-cyclic monophosphate in platelets, Biochem. J., 121, 185-196, 1971.

19. G. Masotti, L. Poggesi, G. Galanti, G.G. Neri Serneri, Stimulation of prostacyclin by dipyridamole, Lancet, $\underline{i}$, 1412, 1979.

20. W.F. Krol, Three large scale clinical trials of aspirin in USA, Proc. Roy. Soc. Med. $\underline{70}$, suppl. 7, 24-27, 1977.

21. Sulfinpyrazone in the prevention of cardiac death after myocardial infarction. Anturane reinfarction trial research group, N. Engl. J. Med., $\underline{298}$, 289-295, 1977.

22. The Canadian Cooperative Study Group, A randomized trial of aspirin and sulfinpyrazone in threatened stroke, N. Engl. J. Med., $\underline{299}$, 53-59, 1978.

23. P. Ramwell, Washington University, personal communication.

24. E.A. Jaffe, B.B. Weksler, Recovery of endothelial cell prostacyclin production after inhibition by low doses of Aspirin, J. Clin. Invest., $\underline{63}$, 532-535, 1979.

25. J.M. Armstrong, N. Lattimer, S. Moncada, J.R. Vane, Comparison of the vasodepressor effects of prostacyclin and 6-oxo-prostaglandin $F_{1\alpha}$ with those of prostaglandin E_2 in rats and rabbits, Brit. J. Pharmacol., $\underline{62}$, 125-130, 1978.

26. R.S. Mitchell, G.W. Silvers, G.A. Dart, T.L. Petty, T.N. Vincent, S.F. Ryan and G.F. Filley, Clinical and morphological correlations in chronic airway obstruction, Am. Rev. Resp. Dis., $\underline{97}$, 54-60, 1968.

Discussion

BONSIGNORE: This paper has very aptly crowned this symposium on the pulmonary circulation. The paper is now open for discussion.

SPINA: I would like to clarify two points. The first concerns aspirin dosage. If I have understood correctly 300 mgm per day should not be exceeded for if it is we have the contrary effect. Is this correct? Secondly, how long does treatment continue? Then, are there alternative substances to aspirin, especially given the damage aspirin can cause to some subjects if administered over the long term? Also, a further clarification: aspirin and similar substances have anti-aggregating behaviour in that they diminish platelet activity. I would like to know if the mechanism is direct in the production of healthy thrombus or if it is indirect through a diminished vitality of the platelets?

PAOLETTI: As to the first question, this is of practical interest. We calculate that at least in healthy individuals the production of prostacyclin which has also been directly measured, does not diminish following a dose of 250 - 300 mls of aspirin but it is very considerably reduced at higher doses. We do not know how it reacts in arteriosclerotic patients for example who are treated with this and who have pulmonary complications. We saw earlier that the lung is a very strong producer of prostacyclin. There remain many unanswered questions. The problem is that the usage of low doses of aspirin is not a solution to the problem; it is only a temporary solution until more selective agents are available. As regards the duration of aspirin treatment, this is less critical. It can be continued indefinitely. Aspirin can be given every 48 - 72 hours following the suggested dose of 300 mgm. Obviously the side effects will always be present because these are linked to its mechanism of action. Our laboratory has published an article in the British Journal of Oncology in February where we showed that thrombosin has importance at the bronchial level and we saw that the histamine receptors, H1 not H2, are very powerful stimualators of the formation of thrombosin at both pulmonary and bronchial levels; the inhibition of the H1 receptor prevents the formation of thrombosin. You can see how these phenomena are closely linked.

EXTRA SESSION

CUMMING: Let us make a beginning. The purpose of this meeting
this afternoon, which is not scheduled in the program, is an attempt
on the part of the organisers to let the discussions which took
place earlier today carry on to completion, because many of these
discussions had unfortunately to be terminated prematurely. Perhaps
you have had a chance to think about those papers about which you'd
like further discussion. David Denison would like to begin, and you
can all join in, either on what he talks about or what you
yourselves wish to talk about.

DENISON: My question is to Philippe Even, and I want to begin by
drawing what I believe is one of the most useful single tests of the
respiratory function, which is the flow/volume loop, and I will
remind you about it. I will draw it firstly for a normal person;
on the abscissa there is a plot of lung volume, from total lung
capacity to residual volume; on the ordinate is expiratory flow, in
this direction, and inspiratory flow in this direction. If I draw
the normal first it is a triangle, resting on a semicircle. The
semicircle is slightly bigger in area than the triabgle. And the
apex of the triangle is between 1/8 and 1/16 of the volume of the
lung. In a normal person it is immensely reproducible. When we see
something that is very reproducible in medicine and in biology it is
giving information, even if you don't know what this is. If you
look at patients with emphysema, their flow-volume loops are similar
except that they have difficulty in breathing out. They can breathe
in very easily, because on inspiration we believe that their airways
are wide open, and Philippe Even showed us a pressure curve of a
normal person breathing in, and then out, and an emphysematous
person breathing in and then out. I could not understand the
contradiction between his information and mine. And so I'm going to
ask him why it exists.

EVEN: In normal subjects the pleural pressure is like that and in
emphysematous patients there is a greater negative pleural pressure
at inspiration, and at expiration, either a slightly negative
pressure, a zero pressure, or a positive pressure depending on the
severity of the obstructive disease. Where is the contradiction?

DENISON: Your graph suggested that they have more difficulty
breathing in than breathing out, while the flow-volume loop suggests
the contrary, as does a large amount of physiology about the
construction of the airways. It's very difficult to understand why
they should have more difficulty breathing in than out.

EVEN: The driving pressure is alveolar pressure, and my graph
concerned pleural pressure, which is quite different to alveolar
pressure.

407

CUMMING: I think this is the resolution of the problem.   The measurement of intrapleural pressure does not reflect, in disease, the alveolar pressure and if the pressure during expiration rises above atmospheric, then this would itself produce difficulty in expiration.

EVEN: It would squash the airways.

CUMMING: Yes, squashing the airways. Whilst these graphs may be directly comparable, you must go through alveolar pressure in order to understand them.

EVEN: I was a little put out by your question, because I have not thought about this approach, but that is perhaps the answer.

CUMMING: Would anyone else like to give an opinion on this? Is there a contradiction in this, or not? No, you are all pretty content or bemused. Would any other member like to make a contribution or raise a question on any of the papers that we've heard today?

HORVATH: I would like to give you some of our experience in patients with mitral stenosis. We have found te average pulmonary circulation time as determined by Donato. This is interesting for the classification of the various stages of mitral stenosis. We have also worked with the distribution and redistribution of the blood circulating in the lesser circulation in the left and right heart and in the lung. There was an alteration in blood distribution in the different stages of mitral stenosis. We have evaluated volume per minute and as you have demonstrated, there are volume-flow diagrams to evaluate the work of the right heart. In this case volume was measured with radiocardiography and pressure with microcatheter according to the Grandchamps method.

LOCKART: I'd like to ask a question to Philippe Even. He has added, I think, a very significant piece of information to our understanding of type A versus type B chronic obstructive lung diseases. This information is that the A have problems in maintaining a normal cardiac output and to increase it when needed. Type A have also normal arterial blood gases at rest, whereas type B have hypoxemia, maybe also hypercapnia. Would Philippe be willing to speculate about the possible differences in the adjustment to exercise in these two groups of patients? Whether what he has found may suggest that type A patients will have more problems with exercise than type B patients, which would be my guess from his data.

EVEN: It's difficult to answer your question.   In fact, what was the question? It was a comment, not a question!

CUMMING: If I may attempt to put the question as I understand it,
is there any difference in the way that type A emphysema, without
disturbances in blood gases, and that of type B, manifested by
hypoxemia and perhaps hypercapnia, respond to exercise? Using the
principles as you have enumerated them.

EVEN: The literature suggests that the limitation to exercise in
type B patients results in bad conditions for gas exchange, as
pulmonary blood flow increases. In type B many patients have an
increaseing PaO_2 and an unchanging $PaCO_2$. In type A patients the
limitation to exercise is classically attributed to a difficulty for
gas transfer due to a limitation of gas exchange area. In fact, the
few papers where the adaptation to exercise in type A patients is
studied demonstrate that there was no significant decrease in PaO_2.
For example, in the most important paper, for exercise of 40 watts
during 5 minutes the PaO_2 changed from 73 to 61. It is significant,
but in terms of oxygen transport it is insignificant, it is equal to
perhaps 3% decrease in oxygen saturation. But I repeat I am
disappointed to find in the medical literature not a single paper
studying the respiratory response to exercise of patients with very
large distention with panlobular emphysema, type A.

CUMMING: Thank you for the brave attempt, Philippe, to answer a
very difficult question.

TRICOMI: I would like to show you some x-rays which go back to the
matter dealt with this morning and which concerns vascular
distribution in lung diseases. Unfortunately, the slides do not
particularly refer to COLD but some of these are particularly
significant. If we look at this x-ray we see a classical
hypertransparency on the left, so that there is deviation of blood
to the right with reduced vascularisation on the left. This is a
radiological sign but does not constitute a diagnosis, but it can be
confirmed by perfusion scintigraphy. Therefore whilst not
diagnostic, it is a very important indication when there is
displacement of the mediastinum to the left and elevation of the
left side of the diaphragm there is suspicion of pathology which may
be pulmonary embolus and not unilateral emphysema or that of a
carcinoma of the upper left lobe bronchus with alterations both of a
bronchial and vascular nature. Here is another case where we see a
reduced vascularisation in the lower part on the right side with an
irregular thickening in this same area, between the diaphragm and
the hilum. The left lung is more expanded. Look at the xerography
which shows a stenosis in the right main bronchus and a
peribronchial calcification. An irregular vascularisation with
excessive flow into the upper part of the lung, reduced
vascularisation in the bottom with irregular alterations in the same
area above the diaphragm. Bronchography of this case shows
bronchial compression from lymph glands which has appeared after

many years and results from primary tuberculosis.

CUMMING: I wonder if I may take a moment to tell the clinicians a piece of interesting information which I recently picked up in Sweden, concerned with the carcinoma of the bronchus which, as in England, is a very common condition in Italy. Bjorn Nordenstom who is a radiologist in Stockholm, has devised a technique by which he introduces into the tumour, transcutaneously, under radiological control, a thin electrical needle. He puts a second needle into the far end of the tumour and then passes an electric current through it. He electrolyses the tumour, releasing locally free radicals, and he has now many successes where the tumour disappears completely. I thought you might be interested to follow this up, those of you who are interested in carcinoma of the bronchus.

        Now would anyone else like to raise any general questions concerned with the papers today? To give you time to think, I wonder if you would permit me to carry out an experiment, using you, the audience, as subjects. I would like to ask three questions, and I would like an answer from each of you to each of the questions by putting up your hand. The first thing I need to do is to identify those amongst you who have clinical control of patients and who are in the business of making diagnoses. Hands up all the people who make diagnoses. Fourteen people in the audience make diagnoses. Good. Now, in the last two years how many of your fourteen clinicians have written on your case notes the diagnosis: cor plulmonale? Two people have made this diagnosis. Now, my third question is this: and it is clearly now ridiculous - do you use the criterion of right ventricular hypertrophy in order to make the diagnosis? Tricomi?

TRICOMI: No.

CUMMING: No. So, that tells a great deal about status of the diagnoses of cor pulmonale! I was interested however, that subsequent to Denolin's remarkable review of the topic we heard another clinician making a diagnosis of acute cor pulmonale. Now, is it possible to attribute the word 'acute' to right ventricular hypertrophy? Or was Philippe Even talking about acute increase in pulmonary artery pressure?

DENOLIN: I think that acute cor pulmonale is surely something else and it should not be defined as hypertrophy of the right ventricle, which takes some time to develop. We don't know how much time, but at least some time. And I think the word acute cor pulmonale should be reconsidered.

CUMMING: Yes I am not sure at all whether the diagnosis of acute cor pulmonale is acceptable.
DENOLIN: Coming back to your question. Could you ask the audience

what they put in their notes when they see such patients.

CUMMING: A good question.

DENOLIN: Perhaps a vascular complication of chronic lung disease? What word do they use?

CUMMING: Can I put it much more specifically? If you have a patient with a chronic expiratory air flow limitation, for many years, associated with shortness of breath, and he develops an elevation of the jugular venous pressure associated with dependent oedema, what do you write upon your case notes? Would anyone like to say what they write on their case notes in such a condition? Perhaps I should tell you what I write on my case notes, in order to start the discussion? I write: oedema of lung disease, and the reason I do that is a very simple one. If you measure the weight, daily, of a person with chronic lung disease, and you plot it over three months, it hardly varies. And yet when the patient comes into hospital, they have clearly got several litres of fluid dependent in the legs with an increase in blood volume, as evidenced by an increase in the jugular venous pressure. If you then treat these patients by bed rest alone, the oedema disappears. If you treat them by bed rest and diuretics, it goes more quickly. And when they have lost their fluid, what is the change in weight? Very little. Because what happens is that the fluid is redistributed in the body compartments. So the total body water is almost the same, but where it is , is different. And I cannot conceive of that as being due to a failure of the right ventricle adequately to expel its diastolic blood volume. So I write therefore: oedema of lung disease. What do you write, Henry?

DENOLIN: I think that when the patient is coming with oedema I could probably use the term 'chronic cor pulmonale', but only then. But what I write when I think that this is a problem, I ask for the measurement of the pressure in the pulmonary artery and I put pulmonary hypertension.

CUMMING: . Indeed. But the patients I have described may have an elevation of the pulmonary artery pressure by a few per cent. But while it is perfectly true to call this pulmonary hypertension, because it is greater than normal, it puts the wrong flavour on the diagnosis. It colours the diagnosis, and it colours it in a confusing way. And therefore, I choose not to do such a colouration. It's true! But at the same time it untrue. A very difficult problem.

DENOLIN: It is, it is.

CUMMING: But words are very important in this disease. Now, having given you time to think, have you any other questions you

would like to raise? No. Then I shall give you some more time to
think! When we discussed the problem this morning with Zardini,
about the diagnosis of pulmonary embolus or pulmonary infarction we
found the difficulty that the defining characteristic of this
disease is obstruction of a pulmonary artery by a non-benign
embolus. Having decided that the embolus is benign nothing happens.
How does one diagnose this? And the diagnosis was difficult. May I
ask this question: since, as Zardini suggested, there is probably
released into the circulation, subsequent to the embolus, a series
of biological amines, which are responsible for the increase in
pulmonary artery pressure, can our biochemical colleagues tell us
what we ought to look for, in order to make the diagnosis of
pulmonary embolus or infarction by taking a sample of blood and
estimating the appropriate biological amine. And I will ask Nick
Bakhle if he would like to respond to this question. He needn't if
he doesn't want to, but would he like to?

BAKHLE: I suppose that the most obvious thing that might be
generated is serotonin, from the platelets which have formed on the
embolus either primarily or secondarily, depending on the initial
tissue. The systems downstream of the embolus are probably so
efficient in metabolising the serotonin, that you will probably not
be able to find any serotonin coming out of the lung. The next
thing would be perhaps to look for either the nucleotides, which
come out of the platelets with the serotonin. But that also is very
readily metabolised by the endothelial cells. So that's another
idea that's gone. The last hope, which is always a hope, is some
prostaglandin material. Now, again, there will almost certainly be
a metabolite of the prostaglandin, but you might get an increase in
the prostacyclin, the newest one, which is not metabolised in lungs.
There might be a reflex increase in the production of prostacyclin
in the attempt to resolve the embolus and to disaggregate platelets.

CUMMING: Could I ask then: have you in your department
investigated any of the blood from patients having this disaster
occurring to them?

BAKHLE: No. We certainly haven't done that. We have tried to
estimate prostacyclin in whole blood. And it is really quite
difficult. Technically it is quite difficult to get all the zero
baseline levels down to less than 1 mg/ml. And you know that's
nonsense.

CUMMING: Would it be feasible to offer to the Royal College of
Surgeons a series of sera and run them through your screen, to see
whether there is anything obvious that may appear in the serum of
people with infarcted lungs?

BAKHLE: Yes, I think as an idea it's fantastic, as long as one has an assay which works so that it's a matter of developing an assay which is reliable.

CUMMING: I could perhaps ask someone with considerable experience of prostaglandins to give us his view about whether this is a feasible thing or not. Philippe Even.

EVEN: I think the question is a little bit more complicated, because we have not only to find a substance which is increased in the blood after an embolus but also a substance specifically increased by emboli. I am not sure that we will not find an increase in serotonin and prostaglandin during many other pathological processes in the lung. I'm not sure that would be the good way. Perhaps, perhaps not.

CUMMING: Do I understand you correctly to say you have found a specific substance, or you would like to find a specific substance?

EVEN: I would like.

CUMMING: For a moment I thought you discovered it.

DENOLIN: It is impossible today to describe any clinical condition without the help of prostaglandins. But before you consider substances why not accept the simple mechanical explanation of hypertension in emboli?

CUMMING: I think the evidence against that is this: that if you have a patient who has a small embolus and you measure the pulmonary artery pressure at the time of the embolus and observe its evolution, then the level of increase in pulmonary artery pressure is far greater than could be accounted for by the volume of lung which is itself involved in the embolic process. And therefore one must look for a greater systemic defect.

DENOLIN: Are you sure that you know the exact extent of the embolus.

CUMMING: Well, the evidence is the radiographic evolution of the embolus. If you see the embolus in day zero and the pulmonary artery pressure rises to a mean of 50, the x-ray shows nothing. The next day the pulmonary artery pressure has fallen to 35, and the third day maybe to normal levels. At the same time the shadow appears on the x-ray and the shadow is the maximum for three or four days after the pressure has gone down. So it's difficult to conceive that that mechanical event has produced the great increase in pressure.

DENOLIN: Yes, but maybe the shadow represents the most important occluded vessel and there are some microembolisations in other parts because during the last year I saw in the literature that more and more people are in favour of a mechanical explanation.

CUMMING: Yes. The difficulty with the microembolisation, attractive though the theory is, is that it needs to resolve in 24 hours. Perhaps there is the hypothesis which says there are two kinds of emboli - microemboli which resolve in 24 hours, and macroemboli leading to infarction, which take ten days to resolve. It's possible, but it's not nature.

DENOLIN: I think it's unresolved.

EVEN: In which species have you observed a discrepancy between the size of the clots and the increase in the pulmonary arterial resistences? In man or in animals during experiments where you induced emboli?

CUMMING: I cannot answer the question as you put it, because that is not what we observe. What we observe was in man having a clinical pulmonary embolus diagnosed because of hyperventilation and not feeling very well, in whom catheterisation was carried out and the pulmonary arterial pressure measured, and the evolution of the process as I have described.

EVEN: My experience is quite different. I have now catheterised 200 patients with angiographically proved emboli. And I have never seen any discrepancy between the size of the clots and the increase in the pulmonary arterial resistences. Perhaps it is a problem of the time of the diagnosis. Probably it is true if the patient is viewed the first day.

CUMMING: That's perhaps it, because after a few hours its gone.

EVEN: Yes.

DENOLIN: What time is needed to dissolve a small clot in a small arterial branch of the pulmonary circulation?

CUMMING: I can answer that question very simply. I have no idea.

ZARDINI: Sometimes 24 hours, sometimes 36, sometimes two days, sometimes three days! It depends also on the therapy. I saw in a few cases with fibrinolytic enzymes, resolution in a day. I supported the mechanical explanation because of the experimental results that I saw this morning. I now have to admit that from the clinical point of view the mechanical explanation is inadequate. When we admit patients to the intensive care unit, we put a catheter in the pulmonary artery and measure pulmonary artery pressure, cardiac output and blood gases. When it's possible we do angiography, when it's not we perform perfusion scintigraphy since we have the nuclear medicine department close at hand. We have seen cases with a great discrepancy between the level of the pulmonary artery pressure and the amount of lung which is embolised. What one can see often is that a small embolus in one region, for instance a small segment of the left lower lobe or the right lower lobe and these gave a greater increase in the pulmonary artery pressure than for instance another regional effect in the distal artery.

CUMMING: You could answer the question very simply of course, because we often produce microemboli with radio-labelled albumin. If you count the chest in successive hours you get some broad idea of how long it takes for albumin to break down and I think there is still radioactivity after a couple of days. But there are very many problems, radioactivity is decaying at the same time and so on.

DENOLIN: But if we continue in this way the next question is: why should we use thrombolytic therapy, if it is not a mechanical probelm?

CUMMING: The embolisation therapy, as I recall, is applied to the bronchial artery and not to the pulmonary.

LOCKART: I would like to support what Philippe Even has just said. In the last year I have been associated with a very aggressive type of clinician, with respect to their behaviour in cases of suspected pulmonary emboli. Each time a case is suspected on clinical grounds heart catheterisation is carried out as rapidly as possible very often a couple of hours after the onset of the symptoms. Heart catheterisation is done with pulmonary angiography, and I cannot recall in the last year or so, one case in which the value of the PA pressure came to me as a surprise when compared with the pattern of the blocked part of the PA by the emboli. The only surprise I got was a PA pressure lower than I would suspect from the size of the emboli due to a low cardiac output in cases of shock. But I have never seen the reverse. And very often a few hours after the onset.

CUMMING: If we examine a little further the mechanical hypothesis, we find a further problem. If we put a balloon into the right main pulmonary artery and occlude it completely, I think you will all agree that 55% of the circulation is being removed. The pulmonary artery pressure rises in such a condition by 3 or 4 mm of mercury perhaps. Now, are the supporters of the mechanical theory telling me that when you have a lobular segment which is infarcted, which is one fourtieth of the lung volume, that this causes a marked increase, purely by mechanical forces, in the main pulmonary artery pressure? The numbers seem to me not to agree. What Alan said: in no case was the elevation of the pulmonary artery pressure out of line with the size of the infarct which he saw. In other words, the bigger the infarct, the larger the pressure increase. And I agree with that. But in absolute terms it doesn't work.

DENOLIN: If you occlude the pulmonary artery, how long do you maintain this? I did it many many times, but never more than thirty minutes. And you have seen from what I said yesterday that in exercise and other conditions it takes probably either one or two hours of arrested circulation.

CUMMING: Well I take that point and we can take the next piece of evidence. If you embolise a dog's pulmonary artery with microspheres of plastic, non expanded polystyrene, you can eliminate four fifths of the pulmonary circulation before there is a marked increase in the pulmonary pressure. And that's a chronic experiment, not an acute one.

DENOLIN: Yes.

MORPURGO: I suppose that you are speaking about different kinds of patients. Patients having or not having pre-existing cardiac or pulmonary disease. The discrepancy between haemodynamic data and the size of the embolus can be observed in patients having pre-existing cardiac or lung disease.

CUMMING: Yes, that's a good point.

EVEN: We have obstructed, sometimes, the pulmonary artery of the right inferior lobe, or the main branch of the pulmonary artery of the left side, or both together, in ten patients. And we have been able by this method to observe the pressure changes in the pulmonary circulation up to a very high level of flow, equivalent practically to 30l/minute through the right upper lobe. And we have obtained a perfect straight line, passing through the origin - driving pressure flow - up to 30l/minute. We have compared that line with many data in the literature, especially the data of Donald, I think the patient was Gordon Cumming but you were 32 years old at that time. You have found a slope quite similar.

CUMMING: Yes.

EVEN: So, about two mm of mercury per litre of increase of cardiac output. After that we have projected all your measurements of driving pressure, in pulmonary emboli, taking into account percentage of obstruction measured by angiography. The superposition of all points was excellent, so excellent as it can be in that kind of physiological measurements.

CUMMING: Can you tell me how you assessed the volume of lung that was infarcted?

EVEN: I have excluded a part of my cases. Particularly when there was a very important retraction of the lobe, with an elevation of the diaphragm and a large infarction with pleural involvement because it is very difficult to make any reasonments.

CUMMING: Then the remainder, how did you assess the volume of lung that was involved? You see the hypothesis is that the volume of lung enables you to determine the size of the 'infarcted' area. You measured flow through the remaining lung?

EVEN: Yes, through the remaining lung.

CUMMING: What that tells me is that the part of the lung that is not infarcted behaves as if it were not infarcted, which seems to be a trivial conclusion.

BARER: Which suggests the chemical nature of the embolus and not the mechanical.

CUMMING: The evidence is by no means clear. I have really made this discussion in order to interest the audience in the problem. I don't, myself, have a fixed view on the topic, though I am quite willing to put a fixed view if you wish me to. This is a very difficult problem which we have not yet solved, but I want to make the point that the mechanical hypothesis is by no means certain.

The chemical hypothesis is by no means certain. But if we wish to understand it we must look at both and try and find the solution to the problem.

ROUND TABLE

CUMMING: Ladies and Gentlemen, thank you very much for coming so promptly to our additional session this morning. The purpose of this session is to attempt to resolve a current controversy in physiology, and that is the two points of view about the way in which the pulmonary circulation conducts blood in relation to the pressure which is applied to this conduction. We saw yesterday that these two points of view are of considerable importance. Now, before beginning, I want to tell you a story, which concerns a famour lawyer in England, who became the Lord Chancellor of England, and his name was Smith, and later Lord Birkenhead. When he began his career in law he worked at Downing College in Cambridge and the undergraduates at both Oxford and Cambridge are noted for their rowdy behaviour when they have something to drink. One Saturday evening everybody had several drinks and there was a fierce fight as the students fought the police, and one of the policemen's helmets was knocked off. An undergraduate was arrested for having knocked off the helmet. Now, when the trial came to court, F.E. Smith was being questioned by the lawyer about what the Sergeant of police had said. The Sergeant of police had said "I saw this man knock off the policeman's helmet". And the judge said to Smith "do you agree with that statement?" "No" said Smith "I do not agree with that statement". "Are you calling the Sergeant a liar?" "No, I am not calling the Sergeant a liar". "You must be calling him a liar, if he says this and you say no". And Smith said a very important thing. He put up five fingers. He said "No there is not one choice, there are five choices: firstly, that the sergeant is telling a lie; secondly, that I am telling a lie; thirdly, that although the sergeant said what he saw, and he believes that he saw it, he is mistaken; fourthly, that although I am saying what I believe I may be mistaken and fifthly, although both of our observations are correct, there may be an explanation which we have not yet found which makes both of them perfectly acceptable". Now, that is a common situation in science. There's never one thing which is right and the other thing which is wrong. So there are five possible solutions to this controversy, and not one. Having said that, let us extend the discussion, because we now have to explain the observations made in the experiments we are talking about, measuring flow and pressure, and listen to the two sides to see if there is anything in the experimental procedure, in the way it is measured, in the species and so on, to see if we can say: "they are both right, for this reason". That's step number one. Then we have to look at other evidence, because it is agreed amongst all of us that if you look at radioactivity in the pulmonary circulation, there is more at the bottom than there is at the top. And when you exercise this distribution becomes more even. Can we take this observation and apply it to the flow measurements, so that each gives the same answer. And then we have to ask a third question; given that we have an area of the lung which has got a different behaviour in respect to flow, can we get any quantitative evidence about how much of the lung is so involved? And then add all together and come out with a hypothesis in which Zardini is right and Even is right and Fazio is right, because all adds up together. That would be a very nice outcome. So, let us address ourselves to that problem. And the first thing I will ask Zardini to tell us the technique, - we know the result - to tell us what his evidence is in support of the view that the ratio between driving pressure and flow is curvilinear.

ZARDINI: When I worked with West at Hammersmith in 1963 the pulmonary arterial pressure-flow relationships were measured in the dog lung and this gave not a linear relationship but a curvilinear one. This curve was then divided into the famour three zones. In a subsequent study the relationships between pulmonary arterial pressure, venous pressure, alveolar pressure and blood distribution were investigated and this led to the theory of the vascular waterfall in Zone 2 and Zone 3. In Zone 3 the blood flow diminishes from base to apex, due to the fact that the capillaries are more distended at the base even though they are in the same Zone.

In 1973 I was interested to investigate the fashionable controversy about recruitment and distensibility and divided the pressure-flow curve into two components and attempted to confirm this using isolated dog lungs. Experiments were done with the whole lung in Zone 2 or in Zone 3 conditions. In Zone 3 conditions the pressure-flow curve was rectilinear, but in Zone 2 the relationship is curvilinear and these results were identical in 9 experimental preparations of the isolated lung. The vascular resistance in Zone 2 is therefore non-linear since there are two types of flow at the same driving pressure, and transition between Zone 3 and Zone 2 demarcates the point at which alveolar pressure is equal to venous pressure. The existance of Zone 1 in the lung was questioned by workers from San Francisco and West and his collaborates documented the existance of pulsatile capillery flow and also questioned the existance of Zone 1 under physiological conditions. To investigate this further we carried out a further seven experiments with a negative venous pressure and an alveolar pressure of zero so that the transpulmonary pressure was -12 cm of water. This gave the control reading with the lung in Zone 2. The lung was then collapsed for a few minutes and then re-expanded with -12 cm. of water pressure. This moved the pressure flow curve to the left. Expanding then with a pressure of -25 cms of water followed by estimation of the pressure-flow curve for a third time at -12 cms of water gave the third curve.

With the lung in Zone 2 increased flow results in a recruitment of new vessels, resulting from variations in the distensibility of the pulmonary vascular bed and a rectilinear plot is obtained. The critical closing pressure in the lung is very low, West gave a value of 1.5 - 2.0 cms of water in a series of 100 experiments. In our 500 experiments we found slightly higher values of 4 - 5 cm of water. Critical closing pressure can be measured by the method of Burton in which the declining flow rate in the pulmonary circuit is measured after inflow is stopped. The pressure at which flow ceases represents the critical closing pressure. The flow curve at the point of flow cessation is curvilinear for the same reason that the curve with increasing flow is curvilinear, anyway that is my impression, I don't know. The lung in pulmonary oedema shows similar properties, with a difference in the critical closing pressure. I have found a linear flow pressure curve in the isolated atalectatic lung, in which flow did not begin until a pressure of 14 cm of water and then showed a rectilinear response to pressure. This is the only case where we have this behaviour.

Therefore when the pressure-flow relationships of the lung are discussed it is necessary to define whether it is under Zone 2 or Zone 3 conditions. The application of isolated dog lung data to the human is difficult because of the co-existance of these zones. I cannot conceive that the whole pulmonary circulation is extensible from the pulmonary artery to the periphery, and that capillaries can be collapsible but not distensible. I think that this would go against a law which regulates the pressure-flow curve.

CUMMING: Thank you very much, you have put the case very fairly for the behaviour of the isolated erect dog lung. Now, I think our problem is going to be to relate such experiments, as you rightly said, to the erect intact man. Before we see if we can make such a correlation, would anyone like to clarify any of the points that Zardini has raised in order to make sure that we are talking about the same thing. David Denison. I want us all to be quite clear about what the other is saying, and then we might understand.

DENISON: I want to be clear too that I have understood this precisely. It seems to me that both Lockart and Zardini have described linear relationships between flow and pressure. Where they differ, if they differ at all, is that Lockart finds a constant pulmonary vascular resistance and he does not. And this implies that the only difference between them is that Lockart's straight lines go through the origin and Zardini's do not. And all I want to do is to be clear about the problem. Because if it is so, we have to be very careful about the measurement of pressure.

CUMMING: Indeed. Can I extend that argument to make this point. If one plots flow against pressure, is it true to say that the slope of the line represents the resistance? It is not because, as David said, it depends critically on whether the line passes through the origin or not. The slope represents resistance only when it passes through the origin. It is important to be clear about that. We have identified that the difference hinges critically on the slope, which both agree is rectilinear, not going through the origin in one case, and going through the origin in the second case. And that is a very important distinction. We could now start looking at how the pressure is measured in the two situations. Alan, do you want five minutes to put the other point of view?

LOCKART: No. I just want to say that I don't think I fully agree about the linear relationship of the pressure-flow curve. I was very careful to state yesterday that this is a linear relationship in supine normal lowlanders, whereas in sitting or erect man, it is non-linear. I said very clearly that resistance tends to increase on sitting up, and it will decrease with exercise. Blood volume decreases with sitting up, and it will follow that it is possible for blood volume to increase with exercise. The pressure-flow plot is linear in a supine man, crossing the origin, or at least with no significant positive intercept on the pressure axis, whereas it is not linear in sitting man. If you accept the hypothesis that there is such a thing as a closing pressure in humans, studied in normal, non artificial situations, you have to reconcile the prediction of this hypothesis with the observation that there is no pressure difference at end diastole when flow ceases, between PA pressure and left atrial pressure. Flow ceases at end diastole and there is no pressure difference in normal lowland man. So again, I think this is a very strong argument against the existance of a critical closing pressure in the normal supine lowlander. Behaviour in sitting and supine subjects is entirely different and I believe that most of the confusion and controversy in the literature is due to the fact this is not clearly realised and people do not use the same words with the same meaning.

LEE: I would like to try and help resolve the controversy, because I really believe that we are all talking about different tings. If we take, and I subscribe very much to Alan Lockart's explanation, if we take a sitting or lying man and we place a cardiac catheter into any portion of the lung and wedge it, we see a transcapillary pressure which is very closely related to the left atrial pressure. And if that is measured directly, there will be a hydrostatic difference depending on whether or not the left atrial catheter tip is higher or lower than the other. If you now leave those catheters wedged in the upper part of the lung, and put the subject into the erect posture on the catheter table, the left atrial pressure at a critical moment cuts out, depending on the alveolar venous manometer relationship.   If you turn the man the other way around, you will see an augmentation of that pressure by the same hydrostatic amount, with the catheters above. I believe that is all we are arguing about.   And that under these circumstances it is absolutely essential to have very clear ideas of the position of your catheter in relation to the known facts about the isolated lung.
CUMMING: You give us the observation. Would you like to interpret

it for us?

LEE: The interpretation is that, depending on the shape of the
subject, the anteroposterior dimensions are actually less than
either the left atrial pressure, keeping the veins open at the top
of the so called waterfall or the pulmonary artery pressure. Why
did Andre Cournand not find that with Rejane Harvey in the old days?
It's a long long time ago now, and there was then a certain fear of
cardiac catheterisation, and certainly it was normal for us to have
the patient lying flat on the x-ray table. The x-ray table was in
fact tilted slightly, and there were usually pillows under the head
and chest to make the subject comfortable. That is where the
controversy lies.

CUMMING: Thank you, Grant. Looking at history often tells us
something important.

ZARDINI: I agree with that. I am in perfect agreement.

CUMMING: Could I ask you then, Zardini, to try and explain for us
the observations that are made and seem to be pretty well agreed by
everybody, of the linearity of the flow pressure difference in
supine intact man.

ZARDINI: One cannot measure the complete pressure flow curve in
the human in the supine position. So I can't say if in the human
being the flow pressure curve is linear. I think that nobody has
the experimental data, starting from very low blood pressure and
going up with blood flow and pulmonary artery pressure. So I don't
believe that you can in a human with a closed chest make a pressure
flow curve.

CUMMING: It is certainly true that using experimental animals
makes one's job a great deal easier, because so many things are
under control and one can give extreme stresses at all points, I
think if one stresses a man, with PA occlusion and exercise and
change his output from 5 litres to 30 litres, I think that's enough
to show this to be curvilinear. Wouldn't you agree?

ZARDINI: Well, I give you another answer. In 1976 there was a
meeting in Florence on the cardiac lung, and I presented data, on 25
patients, with a left to right shunt from bilateral septal defect.
We checked in these patients the distribution of blood flow, to know
where the blood flow passing through the atrial septal defect, was
going; to the lower, medial or upper lobe. The patients were in
the sitting position, and the lung was scanned from bottom to top.
What we found was that the increased blood flow through the lung was
distributed mainly to the lower zones. These were patients with
atrial septal defect, an increased pulmonary blood flow, but with
normal pulmonary artery pressure. When I talked with our

cardiovascular surgeon and he said "it is curious that the lower zones of the lung in these patients are receiving a large blood flow". After one week he called me and said "we made the operation yesterday of the atrial septal defect and found that soon after the patch was put in the arterial septal the patient became hypoxic for one or two hours, and then became normal. If I find that the distribution of the increased blood flow is to the lower zones, I believe that the branch of the pulmonry artery is distensible, I must believe that also the capillary must be distensible.

FAZIO: There was a point about the distribution of blood flow in left to right shunt which is quite important, because it's the transposition of what you are talking about to the pathological situation. Now, in our experience, we never published a full paper on that, in our experience the distribution of blood was as follows: at the beginning there is an increased flow. Suppose the pressure stays the same, then there is a low pulmonary vascular resistance, lower than normal. The distribution of blood flow is normal. When there is the same flow, with normal vascular resistances, which, for a normal flow, means a pathological condition, there is then a uniform distribution from base to apex.

CUMMING: This is after closure?

FAZIO: No, when the patient gets worse.

So there is an increase in pulmonary vascular resistances. Then the patient can get even worse. In that case you can have a reverse flow, when in addition to having increased pulmonary vascular resistances, and increased blood flow, there is an increase in pressure. A second condition is where there is a uniform distribution of blood flow from base to apex, and you operate on the patient. Then you can have a reversion to the first condition, whereby there was increased flow. We clearly have two situations in which, in the first with normal regional recruitment or distensibility; and the second when the patient gets worse, you definitely have recruitment.

EVEN: Please may I have the third slide, a historical slide with pioneer work of many people before John West. We have established the pressure flow relation in man driving pressure, equivalent flow, control measurements in normal men in supine position at rest, during the occlusion of 50% of pulmonary circulation and during the occlusion of 80% of pulmonary circulation with a balloon. We obtained a straight line passing through the origin. After that we have restudied the same patient and compared the results in the supine and erect positions. We observed a transposition of the curve towards the top suggesting that at some point the pressure flow relation becomes curvilinear and demonstrating, I think, the appearance in the erect position of zone I and II in the lung. In another experiment we studied a normal patient with the same method in the supine position, breathing air and then a hypoxic mixture containing 10% oxygen. We obtained again a transposition of this line above the control suggesting that a part of the lung was in zone Iv of West, due to the constriction of extra-alveolar vessels by the hypoxic mixture. I think this is a demonstration in man of the variability of the pressure flow line, according to the distribution of total flow in zone III or with all the zones of West represented. Now I will ask a question to Grant Lee about his presentation yesterday, because you have drawn the pressure flow relation quite differently to Zardini or Lockart. You have described a curve in the reverse direction. It is a third solution, suggested at the beginning by the work of Cournand. You have described pulmonary artery pressure flow and the curve like that. Cournand studied pneumonectomised patients and there was, I think 17 points distributed like that, and one point there, and Cournand drew that line by eye, but I think from the statistical point of view it is a little disputable.

LOCKART: I just want to remind you of a point about establishing pressure flow curves in man. We are using measurements that are crude and not sensitive to small changes. When weuse data, either from our own laboratory or from the literature, and sort them out to get a straight line relating driving pressure and flow, which crosses or almost crosses the origin, this does not say at all that more precise measurements would not achieve a curved line. But to the best of our availability, using the techniques that can routinely be used in a laboratory, the line is straight. Were it slightly curved, it would demonstrate some recruitment even in supine man. However, it cannot be established with the available techniques, and I think one should be very very conscious about the fact that pressure flow curves and pulmonary blood volume measurements in man cannot be measured to any degree of accuracy comparable to that used in isolated lobes. And that may also be part of the difference.

CUMMING: There is another problem concerning measruement, and when Cournand spent a few days with us, eighteen months ago, we looked at the problem of whether the Fick principle is applicable in the lungs. We came jointly to the conclusion that it was not so applicable. So it may be that even our measurement of flow is not precise, as well as the measurement of pressure. So, I think, ladies and gentlemen, this can end our discussion, I think we have cleared the air considerably, we each see the other point of view, and I tink now we can go back happy in the knowledge that we can look at our results, and compare them with those of others. Before you go, since this is the last meeting that we shall have, may I, as the person who had to sit in this chair and be cruel to you all for the whole week, thank you very much for your kindness, and your courtesy, and the general feeling of good will that I have the whole week, thank you very much for your kindness, and your courtesy, and the general feeling of good will that I have experienced throughout. Thank you.

INDEX